CAPSAICIN - SENSITIVE NEURAL AFFERENTATION AND THE GASTROINTESTINAL TRACT: FROM BENCH TO BEDSIDE

Edited by **Gyula Mózsik, Omar M. E. Abdel-Salam and Koji Takeuchi**

Capsaicin - Sensitive Neural Afferentation and the Gastrointestinal Tract: from Bench to Bedside
http://dx.doi.org/10.5772/57289
Edited by Gyula Mózsik, Omar M. E. Abdel-Salam and Koji Takeuchi

Contributors

Pal Perjesi, Monika Kuzma, Gyula Mozsik, Tibor Past, Koji Takeuchi, Eitaro Aihara, Kimihito Tashima, John V. Priestley, Syunji Horie, Kenjiro Matsumoto, Masaki Raimura, Takao Namiki, Katsutoshi Terasawa, Kikuko Amagase, Klara Gyires, Predrag Sikiric, Janos Szolcsanyi

Published by InTech

Janeza Trdine 9, 51000 Rijeka, Croatia

Publishing Process Manager Danijela Duric

Technical Editor InTech DTP team

Cover InTech Design team

First published July, 2014

Printed in Croatia

Additional hard copies can be obtained from orders@intechopen.com

Capsaicin - Sensitive Neural Afferentation and the Gastrointestinal Tract: from Bench to Bedside, Edited by Gyula Mózsik, Omar M. E. Abdel-Salam and Koji Takeuchi

p. cm.

ISBN 978-953-51-1631-8

For EU product safety concerns:
IN TECH d.o.o., Prolaz Marije Krucifikse Kozulić 3, 51000 Rijeka, Croatia,
info@intechopen.com or visit our website at intechopen.com.

Meet the editors

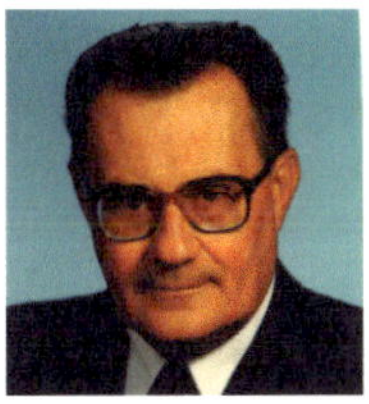

Gyula Mózsik, MD, PhD, ScD (med): professor emeritus of medicine at First Department of Medicine, Medical and Health Centre, University of Pécs, Hungary. He was the head of this Department from 1993 to 2003. His specializations: internist, gastroenterologist, clinical pharmacologist. His research fields are the biochemical pharmacological studies of gastrointestinal tract and the role capsaicin-sensitive neural afferentation in human gastrointestinal tract. He published more than 350 papers in peer-reviewed journals, 200 book chapters, 18 monographs and edited 28 books. From his students, fourteen full University Professors were appointed in Cuba, Egypt and Hungary.

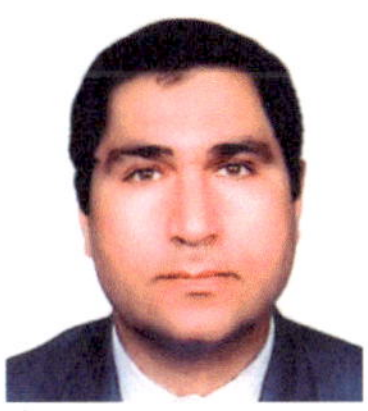

Omar M.E.Abdel-Salam, MD, PhD is a professor of Pharmacology and the head of the Department of Toxicology and Narcotics, Medical Division, National Research Centre, Cairo. He received his medical degree and M.Sc. in Internal Medicine (1991) from the Faculty of Medicine at Cairo University, and later received his Ph.D. in Medical Sciences in 1997 from the Hungarian Academy of Sciences in Budapest. His research interests include: gastric acid secretion and its regulation; gastric mucosal injury; role of sensory nerves in gastric mucosal protection; hepatic protection; bile secretion; inflammation, analgesia, modulation by different agents; the role of antidepressants and the serotonin reuptake inhibitors in inflammation and nociception; neurodegeneration and neuroprotection. He authors or co-authored 162 research papers and 7 book chapters.

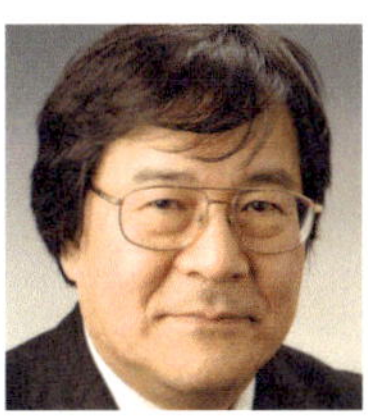

Koji Takeuchi, PhD received his Ph.D. degree from the University of Tokyo, Tokyo, Japan. He is a Professor Emeritus & Guest Professor of the Kyoto Pharmaceutical University as well as a Guest Professor of Doshisha Women's College of Liberal Arts. His research interest covers numerous areas of GI pharmacology and physiology, and his most notable contribution is to understanding of mucosal defense, focusing on the regulation of acid/bicarbonate secretion, the role of capsaicin-sensitive afferent neurons, and the influences of non-steroidal anti-inflammatory drugs and prostaglandins; their mode of action, cyclo-oxygenase isozymes, receptors that drive physiological responses, and their role in mucosal injury, protection and healing. He published more than 400 papers in the peer-reviewed journals and about 20 book chapters.

Contents

Preface

Capsaicin, the hot principle of red peppers or chilli (paprika) is a favorite spice in culinary practice.

Since the time man started gathering food, the additional of small amounts of some plan materials may have been used for the powerful impact they had on the appearance or eating quantity. Initially, these additions were valued for masking the off-flavor of stored, decomposing foods; late on, in medieval Europe, they were imported as rural spices for their capacity to slow down deterioration during storage. Gradually, when definitve ethnic cuisines developed, the individual spices came to be valued in the modern sense for their contribution, which is to flavor generally insipid meat and cereal foods and to make more acceptable and preferred. Spices have became indispensable in the modern kitchens on individual homes, institutions, and the food manufactoring industries. They provide individually to the dishes and distinquishing gourmet foods.

Among the spices, capsicums are the most colorful in appearance, and are important in terms of their history, antiquity, and influence on many cuisines of the world.

During the first expedition, Colombus (1492-1493) observed that the natives of the New World used a colorful red fred fruit calls **aji** or **axe** with most of their foods. This additive was found to be much stronger than the black pepper of Asia (Piper nigrum L.) in search of which he had undertaken this expedition. He took samples of this fruit back to Spain and named it „red pepper". De Cuneo, who accompanied Colombus on the second voyage to the New World in 1495, made the more definitive observations that „rose-like bushes have fruits as long as cinnamon, full of small grains, as biting as pepper; those Caribes and Indians eat that fruit like we eat apple".

Chanca, the physician with expedition, observed that the natives used this food additive bot has a condiment and in medicine. Other travelers, who extensively traveled in Spanish America in the 16th and 17th centruries, decribed the popular use of **Uchu** , a colorful fiery pod of a plant, in the food of Peruvian Indians. Since early Indians of northern Guatemala has been recorded. The highly irritating smoke from the burning dried fruit is reported to have used by the native Indians against Spanish invaders.

The chilli pepper (paprika) is one of the very old domesticated plants of Middle America. The Valle de Tehuacan (Puebra) which is one of the best documented examples on an early settlement in Mesoamerica, archeological evidence for the consumption of chilli pepper dates back to the seventth millennium B.C., long before the cultivation of maize and beans.

Capsicum has been known since the beginning of civilization in the Western Hemisphere. It has been a part of the human diet since about 7500 B.C. It was the ancient ancestors of the native people, who took the wild chilli piguin and selected the values types known today.

The Capsicum is a genus of the family of Solanaceae and is closely related to another genus, Solanum, which covers many economically important plants such as potato (Solanum tuberosum L.), eggplant (S. melengere L.), tomato (Lycopersieon esculentum Mill.), and tobacco (Nicotiana tobacum L.).

Some 20 to 30 species of *Capsicum* are reported in the world. The following five major species are mophologically definable: *Capsicum annuum var. Annuum L., Capsicum frutescences L., Capsaicum chinense Jacq, Capsicum baccatum var. Pendulum wild, Capsaicum pubescens Riuz and Pav).*

Seven capsaicinoids (capsaicin, dihydrocapsaicin, nordihydrocapsaicin, homodihydro-capsaicin, homocapsaicin, nonanoic acid vanillylamide and decanoid acid vanillylamide) can be extracted from the different Capsicum species. The first five compounds represent capsaicin homologues, meanwhile the last two represent capsaicin analogues.

In physiological and pharmacological basic research, the term of „capsaicin" as „one" chemical compound" is generally used, meanswhile the fine chemical trading firms (including Sigma Aldrich and all of others) obtain the capsaicin from plants (*Capsicum*). According to the chemotaxonomic key, the different species of *Capsicums* contain different amounts of capsaicin homologues and analogues. So, the commercially available natural capsaicin preparation are mixtures of capsaicin and natural capsaicinoids.

The capsaicin preparation can be used as an active pharmaceutical ingredient (Capsaicin Natural) is described by the United States Pharmacopeia (USP). The 2006 edition of USP30-NF25 described its definition, identification, melting range and the content of capsaicin, dihydrocapsaicin and other capsaicinoids. According to the USP requirements Capsaicin Natural should contain not less than 90 percent of total capsaicinoids. The content of capsaicin and dihydrocapsaicin should not less than 75 percent, and the content of other capsaicinoids should not more than 15 percent calculated on dried basis (USP30-NF25 Page 1609).

The principal requirements of the European Authorities capsaicinoid content of natural capsaicin preparations for medical therapy are the as those of USP30-NF25.

The capsaicin (capsaicinoids) modify the functions of capsaicin-sensitive afferent nerves, however, this (these) action(s) is(are) on dose-dependent manner. This (these) compound (s) stimulates (stimulate) in smaller doses and inhibits (inhibit) in higher doses of capsaicin-sensitive afferent nerves. The capsaicin-.induced actions on capsaicin-sensitive afferent nerves are associated with changes of vascular microcirculation, relaese of different neuropeptides, modifications of functions of immune cells, hormonal system, etc. Consequently the the capsaicin(oids) is (are) able to produce gastrointestinal mucosal protection and mucosal damage.

Because of capsaicin(oids), the hot principle of red peppers or chill is (are) a favorite spice in culinary practice and therefore it's (their) role in gastrointestinal tract has (have) been tested in animal experiments and in human observations. The obtained results were contradictory ones in gastrointestinal tract of animals and of humans (patiensts). The capsaicin was given in very different (from small to extremely high) doses of capsaicin int he different observations.

Szolcsányi and Barthó (1981) firstly demonstrated that the capsaicin given in 5-50 μg/mL (given intragastrically) prevents the development of gastric mucosal damage in rats, meanwhile it enhances the gastric mucosal damage given in higher doses. It was important discovery that the gastroprotection produced by small doses of capsaicin does not associated with the decrease of gastric acid secretion (volume and H^{st} output) and of pepsin secretion (details in a book chapter of this book).

Robert el al. (1979) described the phenomenon of „cytoprotection" to prostaglandins. The essetial point of this discovery was that the small doses of prostaglandins are able to protect the gastric mucosal damage produced by intragastric administration of 96% ethanol, 0.2 M NaOH, 0.6 M HCl and 25% saline sulution in rats, without presence of any decrease of gastric acid secretion.

The capsaicin-induced gastroprotection differs from the „classical cytoprotection", beacuse the mechanism of gastroprotection by capsaicin mediated by subepithelial enhanced of microcirculation, meanwhile in case of the „classic cyoptoprotection" produced by different chemicals produce in fact a destroy the superficial protective layer of the stomach (mainly mediated by prostaglandins). In many other observations indicated that the chemicals-induced mucosal damage (produced according to the method of Robert et al.,1979) can be protected by many other compounds (SH-inhibitors, retinoids, carotenoids, etc) as the prostaglandin system.

Prior to these basic observations in animal models we had previously performed studies in humans with anticholinergic agents. We employed conventional clinical pharmacological studies using methods that were then established in our group in time period of 1962 to 1970. Our attention was focussed on the changes of gastric secretory responses in patients with duodenal ulcer during a chronic atropine treatment. We were very surprised to find that the patients with duodenal ulcer healed following chronic (2 to 4 weeks) treatment with atropine. However, the gastric secretory responses of patients were not decreased (as basal acid output, BAO, and after application of superliminal (but submaximal) of dose of histamine (0.5 mg given s.c.), thus showing that the duodenal protection could be obtained independent of effects on acid secretion (Mózsik et al., 1965). In 1978, we found that the gastrointestinal anti-ulcer effects of atropine, cimetidine and carbenoxolone were superior to that of placebo in a multicentre, randomized, prospective and comparative study in duodenal ulcer patients. However, no significant difference was obtained in the beneficial effects of atropine vs. cimetidine vs. cabenoxolone (Tárnok et al., 1978). Since carbenoxolone, has no inhibitory action of gastric acid secretion in DU patients could be considered independent of any effects on acid secretion. We did not know anything about the „classical cytoprotection", and we gave a clinical pharmacological explanation (namely the development of tolerance to drug used in the treatment and together development of „pharmacological denervation") for the first our observation, and in the second case, we suggested that the increase of mucus secretion (and no the gastric acid secretion) took place in the duodenal protection in DU patients.

Discoveries of both of these two kinds of gastroprotective mechanims in rats opened new gates of research in the gastrointestinal tract. These studies run, in some meaning, in different and separated ways, meanwhile these studies have been combined together in our days.

Many new pathways were found in the field of „classical cytoprotection „in our days, and as well as in the field of capsaicin research. There are no questions that the principal regulatory functions exist in basic research of animals and in humans. However, there are some differences between the results (and explanations) of basic research and human observations in the GI tract in human beings.

Many observations with capsaicin were carried out from last decades in the animal experiments and in human observations. It's true that number of capsaicin studies much more higher in animals and than in humans.

The explanations for the small number of human observations are complex, namely. 1. the solution of the ethical problems of human observations; 2. permission from the national and international Authorities for investigating compound (presently the capsaicin) based on the internationally accepted laws; 3. of course, the grants to help the carried out of observations; 4. existence of special internationally accepted institutes (wards) for doing these types of observations.

It is also important to mention that the different extractions of Capsaicums (without exact knowledge of their chemical composions) were used (instead of pure chemical composions) in the earlier periods of the human studies.

To receive permission for human use - for orally given as a drug substance - of capsaicin preparation from the National and Inteernational Regulatory Authorities we have to present the following details: 1. specification of the Capsaicum species; 2. climatic regulations of places of Capsicum cultivation; 3. chemical treatments of Capsicum plants during their cultivation; 4. details of treatment of Capsicum plants (their collection, drying, extractions, storages, etc.); 5. analytical results supporting the chemical composition of the plant origin capsaicinoids extract; 7.the chemical stability of the natural capsaicin (capsaicinoids); 7. analytical results showing the (possible) contamination of the capsaicin product with organic phosphates, pesticides, fusariums, aflatoxin; 8. international certification (including Food and Drug Administration, FDA) on capsaicin (capsaicinoids) content of the natural preparation. Data above mentioned fact given by internationally accredited laboratories. These data are collected in Drug Master File (DMF).

In our case we found only one natural capsaicin preparation with Drug Master File (DMF) (Asian Herbex Ltd., Asdhra Pradesh, India), which is signed in the documentation of Food and Drug Administration (FDA) in USA („ 17856 A II 26.10.2004 Asian Herbex Ltd: Capsicum USP as manufactured in Andhra Pradesh, India") for orally applicable drug substance in healthy human subjects and in patients.

The fine chemical trading firms (concerning capsaicin supply) had no DMF for their capsaicin preparation. Independently., several trade firms keep the natural capsaicin(oids) preparation on the market they can not have, however , exact knowledge on the circumstances of cultivation, details of preparation extract, stability of the product. They have no exact information on the quantities of residues of organic phosphates, pesticides, fusariums, aflatoxin in the preparation of origin capsaicin (proved by certification of different internationally accredited laboratories).

We wanted to use this (these) capsaicin(oids) as the only component or one of the components for orally applicable drug or drug combinations for in human healthy beings and patients.

We compiled the documentations for the National Institute of Pharmacy to ask permission for human clinical pharmacological studies with this capsaicin preparation: 1. expert's opinion; 2. results of all toxicological studies; 3.chemical stability of the natural capsaicin preparation; 4. results of pharmaceutical formulation from the natural capsaicin; 5. different permissions from University; 6. documentation of health insurance of volunteers; 7. preclinical dossier; 8. documented valid permission on the accreditation of Clinical Pharmacological Unit for human phase I and II examinations – which accreditaion controlled by the National Insitute in Hungary – were prepared for the National Instutute of Pharmacy in Hungary; 9. exact protocols for human clinical pharmacological studies; 10. written informations on the planned examinations, for volunteers; 11. request for authorization of a clinical trial on medical product for human use the competent authorities and for of opinion of the ethical committees in the community; 12. lists of investigators (together with their CV), places institutes (departments) participating in the study.

Of course, after receiving all of the permissions from the authorities, the human observations with capsaicin were carried out respected the conditions of Good Clinical Practice (GPC).

This book gives a special collection of our update knowledges in the capsaicin research in the gastrointestinal ttract: from bench to the human bedside [including the main mechanisms of gastroprotection, available methods for measurements of capsaicin(oids) from different spices of Capsicums and their necessary regulatory chemical qualification required by the international authorities,observations with isolated gastic cells from rats, main lines on animal capsaicin research and finally approach of capsaicin action in the human gastrointestinal tract and clinical pharmacological requirements for development and pharmaceutical production of capsaicin containing and orally applicable drug or drug combinations in the human healthy subjects and in patients].

The authors of the different book chapters are internationally well known and accepted researchers (chemists, pharmaceutist, pharmacologist, internist, gastroenterologist, clinical pharmacologist, pharmaceutical industrial expert, who are working in the basic and clinical research).

The editors wishes to express their thankfulness for the excellent work of the contributing authors.

The editors are specilally thankful on the excellent support given by Ms.Danijela Duric (Head of Book Publishing) from the Intech Open Access Publisher. Without her help this book would not be possible.

Gyula Mózsik, MD, PhD, ScD
First Department of Medicine, Medical and Health Centre,
University of Pécs, Hungary

Omar M.E.Abdel-Salam, MD, PhD
Head of the Department of Toxicology and Narcotics, Medical Division,
National Research Centre, Cairo, Egypt

Koji Takeuchi, PhD
Kyoto Pharmaceutical University, Japan
Doshisha Women's College of Liberal Arts, Japan

Section 1

Historical, Physiological and Pharmacological Backgrounds of Capsaicin(oids) in Gastrointestinal Tract

Chapter 1

Discovery and Mechanism of Gastroprotective Action of Capsaicin

János Szolcsányi

Additional information is available at the end of the chapter

http://dx.doi.org/10.5772/58684

1. Introduction

Capsaicin, the hot principle of red peppers or chilli is a favorite spice in culinary practice and therefore it's role in gastric ulcerations has been tested since a long time. In early clinical practice sudies in this line using intake of pungent pepper flavoured foods resulted in contradictory conclusions and for patients having peptic ulcers intake of hot spicy foods was forbidden (Schneider et al., 1956, Lennard-Jones and Babouris, 1965, Viranuvatti et al., 1972, Solanke, 1973). Furthermore, animal experiments (Sanchez-Palomera 1951, Makara et al., 1965) were neither conclusive. In the latter study aggravation of gastric ulceration in rats was observed by capsaicin application into the stomach while pungent paprika extract in oil inhibited the reserpine-induced gastric ulcerations in the rat. The authors supposed that protective effect of carotenoids in the extract counteracted the ulcerogenic effect of capsaicin (Makara et al 1965).

Studies in our laboratories on the actions of capsaicin in the guinea-pig isolated ileum revealed that capsaicin acting in a highly selective way elicits in low concentration a new type of neural contraction which after higher doses are completely abolished (Barthó and Szolcsányi 1978, Szolcsányi and Barthó 1978). This effect was elicited by neuropeptides as substance P released from the sensory nerve terminals in response to capsaicin. The neuroselective action of capsaicin was shown by it's lack of effect on function of cholinergic, adrenergic, purinergic, enteric peptidergic neural responses (Szolcsányi 1984, 1996). These capsaicin-sensitive unorthodox sensory nerve terminals served as nerve endings mediating both afferent sensory and mediator releasing efferent functions. On "capsaicin-sensitive" neural elements the presence of a "capsaicin receptor" was predicted (Szolcsányi and Jancsó-Gábor 1975) which was later cloned (Caterina et al 1997) and is now named as Transient Receptor Potential Vanilloid Type-1 (TRPV1). TRPV1 is a nonselective cation channel gated by long list of exogenous and endogenous chemical agents including H^+as well as noxious heat (Jordt et al. 2000, Szolcsányi and Sándor 2012).

The capsaicin-sensitive cutaneous and visceral sense organs correspond to the C-and Aδ – polymodal nociceptor group of primary afferent neurons (Szolcsányi 1996, 2014).

Capsaicin elicits cutaneous enhancement of microcirculation which can be elicited also by antidromic dorsal root stimulation. Antidromic vasodilatation evoked by dorsal root stimulation was known since over a century (Bayliss 1901) but our recent laser-Doppler results revealed that it can be activated at subnoxious level of stimulation applying very low frequency of discharges (0.1Hz or less). Thus this highly efficient efferent function of these sense organs elicits maximum cutaneous vasodilatation from lower level of stimulation than it causes sensation (Szolcsányi 1996, 2004). These fibers with "sensory-efferent" functions differ from the theoretical so called "nocifensor" nerves of the posterior root system proposed by Sir Thomas Lenis (1937) since he predicted that they have only efferent but no sensory function. (Szolcsányi 2013).

On the basis of our results with the "sensory-efferent" function of TRPV1-expressing "capsaicin-sensitive" sense organs of the skin it was tempting to test whether it could operate also in the stomach mucosa where the acidity of the gastric juice, spicy foods or drugs like acetyl salicylic acid seemed a rational site where this local neuroregulatory vasodilator system might operate and play an important role in gastroprotection. On this ground we started to analyze from the late seventies the effect of blocking or stimulation these capsaicin-sensitive nerve endings on gastric ulcer formation in the rat.

2. First evidence for the gastroprotective role of capsaicin-sensitive nerves

In the first series of experiments on rats (Szolcsányi and Barthó 1981) gastric ulcers were provoked by pylorus ligation (Shay et al 1945) or by acid distension (Gáti and Guth 1976). In rats pretreated with capsaicin (50+100mg/kg s.c 6-8 days before the experiment) a systemic blockade of capsaicin-sensitive nerve endings was achieved. These rats did not react to capsaicin if it was instilled into the eye and as revealed earlier this state of loss of nociceptive function was coupled with ablation of sensory nerve-mediated neurogenic inflammation (Jancsó et al 1967) or other sensory-efferent responses (Szolcsányi 1996). Fig 1A shows the effect of this capsaicin-induced blockade of sensory nerve endings on gastric ulcer formation in the Shay ulcer model. In the pretreated group mucosal lesions appeared as early as at the 7th hour after pylorus ligation and at the 9th hour deep extensive nearly perforating lesions were observed in the forestomach. On the contrary out of the 20 control rats terminated 7-9 hours after ligation petechial and minimal mucosal lesions appeared only in two animals. At the 14th hour incidence of perforation was only 13% in the control group and 75% in the group of capsaicin-pretreated rats. Differences at 7th, 9th and 14th hours in ulcer indexes of Fig 1A were highly significant ($P< 0.01$; n=8-11 of each group).

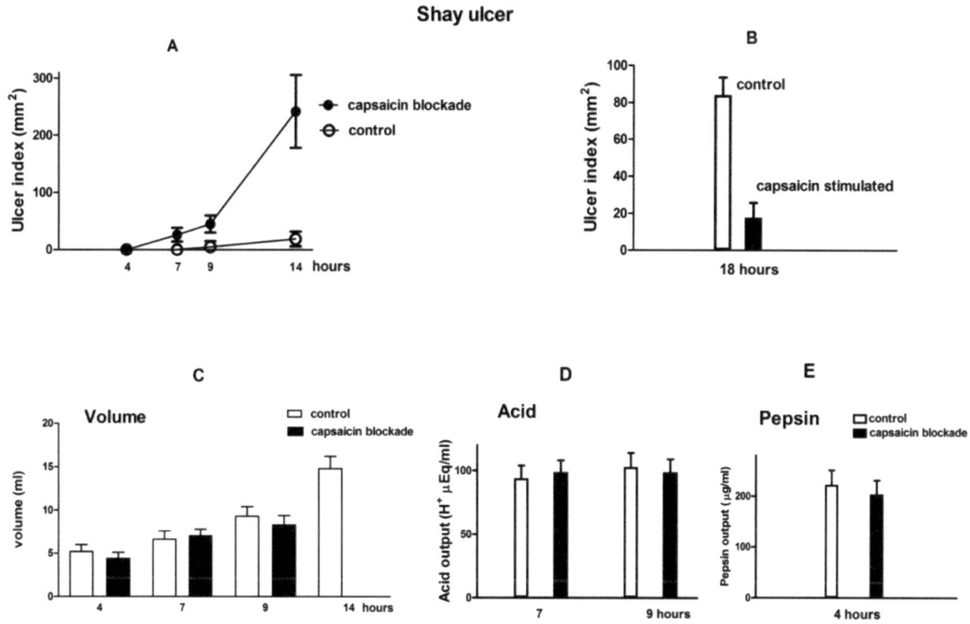

Figure 1. Effect of blockade of capsaicin-sensitive sensory neurons on gastric ulceration in rats evoked by pylorus ligation (A), on volume of gastric juice (C) as well as on gastric acid (D) and pepsin secretion (E) at different time points after pylorus ligation. Gastric ulcers of control rats and that of rats which received by oral application low dose of capsaicin (0.5 µg/0.5 ml and 4 hours later 50 µg/0.5 ml) given into pylorus ligated rats (B).

Aggravation of gastric ulcer formation was not due to enhancement of aggressive factors responsible for mucosal damage. Gastric secretion of the capsaicin pretreated group of animals did not differ from that of the controls as shown on Fig 1C, D and E. The volume, acidity and pepsin concentration of the gastric juice as measured at different time points were similar. Since at the 7th hour petechiae appeared in the capsaicin pretreated group the pepsin concentration was determined only at the 4th hour. Thus it has been concluded that in rats where the function of capsaicin-sensitive nerve endings were abolished in the stomach the gastroprotection is severely impaired against the injurious effect of secreted gastric content inducing H^+ back-diffusion and distension. This conclusion was supported also in another model when constant acid-distension was used (Gáti and Guth 1976). In these experiments the animals under pentobarbitone anaesthesia (40mg/kg ip) received 0.1M HCl in 6ml/100g volume through the duodenum and thereafter both the esophagus and the duodenum were ligated. The animals were sacrificed one hour later and mucosal lesions of the removed stomach was determined. In 17 control rats the incidence of lesions was 59% and the area of damaged mucosa (ulcer index) was 19±7mm^2. In 15 rats where the functions of capsaicin-sensitive sensory nerve ending were abolished all rats had mucosal erosions and the gastric ulcer index was 41±11mm^2 ($p<0.002$).

On the basis of these remarkable clear results it has been concluded that capsaicin-sensitive nerve endings of the stomach have a gastroprotective effect in peptic ulcer models of the rat.

In another series of experiments it was also revealed, that this gastroptective sensory-efferent mechanism is enhanced in rats where sensory stimulating low concentration of capsaicin was applied in the Shay model of gastric ulcer. Since it had been shown earlier (Szolcsányi and Jancsó-Gábor 1976) that topical application of capsaicin up to a concentration of 10 μg/ml stimulates the sensory nerve endings in the conjunctiva without causing desensitization this concentration was applied: 5μg capsaicin in 0.5ml was introduced into the stomach after pylorus ligation and 50μg four hours later when the volume of gastric juice was shown to be enhanced to 5ml (Fig 1C). 18 hours after pylorus ligation all control rats had severe forestomach lesions (ulcer index 84.1±9.5), while in the group of rats where low concentration of capsaicin was introduced into the stomach for stimulation of the nerve endings clear gastroprotective effect was observed (ulcer index 17.8±8.0 mm^2). The difference between the two groups was highly significant ($p=0.002$).

Threshold concentration of capsaicin on the human tongue which elicits recognizable slight warm sensation is about 0.2μg/ml and a concentration of 1-2μg/ml causes the well known hot spicy sensation (Szolcsányi 1977). Thus, in this range of culinary practice commonly used slightly hot foods capsaicin is gastroprotective and inhibits the development of mucosal erosions. Capsaicin content of pungent chilli pods varies between 0.2-1.4%. Thus, regular intake of very hot foods can produce 1) local desensitization of gastric TRPV1-expressing capsaicin-sensitive sensory nerve endings; 2) enhance vagal reflexes causing smooth muscle contractions and producing gastric discomfort or even pain if gastric ulcers are already present; and 3) induce focal oedema with mucosal inchaemia (Viranuvatti et al 1972) probably mediated by neurogenic inflammation (Jancsó et al 1967, Szolcsányi 1996).

On the basis of the first results and considerations the effect of capsaicin on gastroprotection had been presented in a shematic way as shown on Fig 3. Acid back-diffusion activates both the capsaicin-sensitive sensory nerve endings and release vasodilator mediators from mast cells which enhance mucosal microcirculation and protect the epithelial barrier against erosions which could produce peptic ulcer formation. This natural protective mechanism can be enhanced by low concentration of capsaicin present e.g in spicy flavoured foods. The significance of the capsaicin-sensitive neural part in this protective hyperaemic response is underlined by the fact that if these nerve endings are not functioning under experimental conditions described above severe ulcerations will develop in acid-back diffusion models of gastric ulcers. It is important to note, however, that no erosions in the stomach develop after capsaicin-induced sensory blockade under control conditions. Thus without aggressive factors TRPV1-expressing capsaicin-sensitive nerve endings are not required for gastroprotection.

It is worthy to emphasize, that the mechanism of gastroprotection mediated by subepithelial enhancement of microcirculation clearly differs from the cytoprotection of the epithelial cells described by Robert et al (1979). Cytoprotection is mediated by the release of prostaglandins mainly PGE_2 which inhibit ulcerations induced by tissue damaging necrotic agents (96% ethanol, 0.6M HCl, 0.2 M NaOH, 25% NaCl) which in fact destroy the superficial protective layer of the stomach. Using these aggressive treatments in rats where the capsaicin-sensitive nerve endings were blocked by capsaicin pretreatment no difference in number of lesions, but a significant reduction in the severity of the mucosal damage was observed (Szolcsányi and

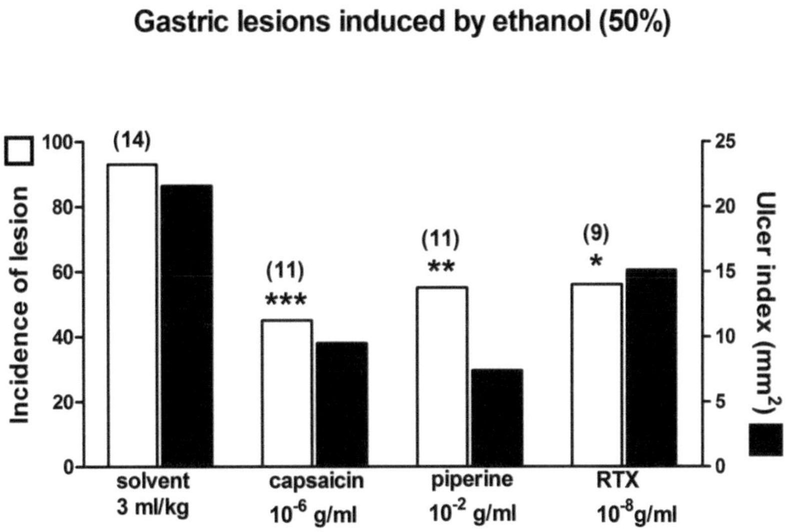

Figure 2. Gastric ulcers of rats induced by ethanol (50%) containing capsaicin, piperine or resiniferatoxin (RTX) in doses indicated. Number of rats in each groups in brackets. Significance ***: P<0.01, **<0.02, *<0.05 from the values obtained on rats which received ethanol with solvent as control.

Mózsik 1984), just in contrast to the H^+back-diffusion models discussed earlier. It has been concluded that in this case ulcerations evoked by profound tissue damaging chemical agents resulted in inflammatory reaction and part of it was mediated by the release of substance P (Sharkey et al 1984) released from the capsaicin-sensitive nerve endings (neurogenic inflammation) which are released at higher frequencies of stimulation than the release of CGRP which induces gastroprotective enhancement of microcirculation (Szolcsányi 1996, 2004).

3. Gastroprotection induced by capsaicin-sensitive nerves in animal experiments

Five years after we described the first data and a proposed mechanism for explaining the effect of capsaicin on gastric ulcer formations other groups also supported our results on the gastroprotective effect of capsaicin. Holzer and Sametz (1986) reported that in adult rats treated in the neonatal age by capsaicin which induces a permanent loss of sensory neurons including also a major group of TRPV1 –expressing neurons for ref (Szolcsányi and Pintér 2013) gastric ulcers evoked by indomethacin is aggravated although the release of prostaglandin E_2 remained unchanged. Proposal for the involvement of the adrenals in this capsaicin-sensitive gastroprotective effect in the indomethacin-induced ulceration was raised by another group (Evangelista et al 1986). One year later it has been revealed by immunohistochemistry that in the digestive tract of rats the highest concentration of the potent vasodilator neuropeptide, calcitonin gene-related peptide (CGRP) is present in the stomach (45±2.8pmol/g wet weight).

After neonatal capsaicin pretreatment the peptide content was reduced by greater than 95% (Sternini et al 1987). Subsequently our data about the gastroprotective effect of intragastric low concentration of capsaicin was supported in case of the ulcerogenic effect of 25% ethanol (Holzer and Lippe 1988). This study provided also evidence against the involvement of autonomic nervous system in the gastroprotective effect of capsaicin and subsequently this group described that intragastric capsaicin (62-640μM) had no effect on nonstimulated acid output of the rat stomach and by light and scanning electron microscopy no signs of mucosal damage was observed (Lippe et al 1989). It is worthy to mention here, that in 1988 it was also reported that in humans using videoendoscopy no visible mucosal damage was observed in individuals who have eaten hot Mexican meal with chili but in those subjects who was taken bland meal plus aspirin multiple erosions developed (Graham et al 1988).

Beyond capsaicin other TRPV1 agonists also induced gastroprotection (Szolcsányi 1990). Fig 2 shows that in these experiments 50% ethanol was given through a stomach tube to conscious rats which evoked mucosal lesions in almost all rats as detected one hour after ethanol exposure (first two columns of Fig 2). Capsaicin, piperine, the pungent principle of black pepper and resiniferatoxin (RTX), the highly potent irritant of Euphorbia resinifera as TRPV1 agonists (Szállási and Blumberg 1999, Szolcsányi 2004) were dissolved in the ethanol and given to three groups of rats (n=9-11). Fig 2 shows that the three TRPV1 agonists given in similar pungent potency ranges induced similar significant gastroprotection against ethanol-induced mucosal ulcerations (Szolcsányi 1990). RTX similarly as capsaicin induces enhanced blood flux of the stomach wall as detected by laser-Dappler flowmetry (Abdel-Salam et al 1996).

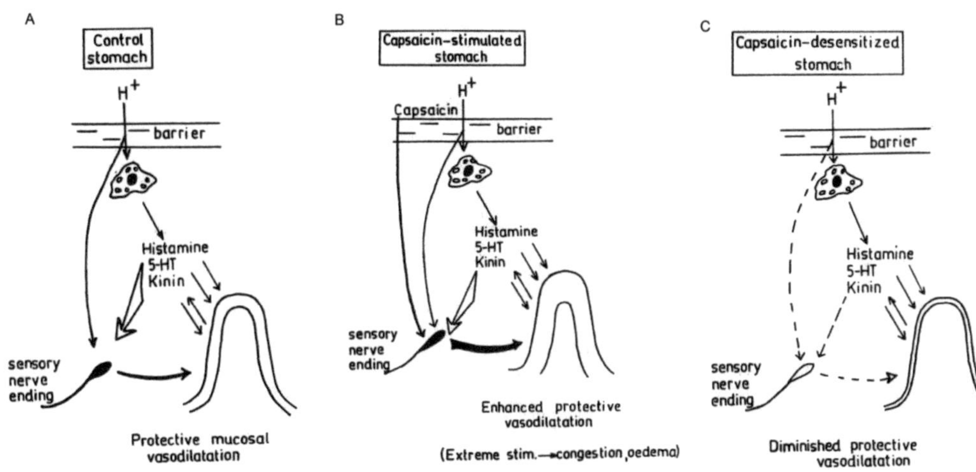

Figure 3. Schematic representation of the hypothetical role of capsaicin-sensitive sensory nerve endings in response to acid distension models which induced gastric mucosal erosions and ulcerations (reproduced from Szolcsányi and Barthó, 1981 with kind permission of the Akadémiai Kiadó, Budapest). A. H^+back-diffusion through the epithelial barrier activates both capsaicin-sensitive chemoceptive nerve endings and mast cells which release vasodilator mediators and enhance mucosal microcirculation. B. Low concentration of capsaicin in the stomach enhances the gastroprotective vasodilatation. C. Blockade of capsaicin-sensitive nerve terminals induces depletion of the sensory neuropeptides. In these rats the natural gastroprotective mucosal vasodilatation is impaired.

4. Mechanism of action of gastroprotection of capsaicin

In the defense mechanism to maintain the structural integrity of the gastric mucosa unstirred layer of mucosa-bicarbonate-phospholipid barrier (Fig 4) and the surface epithelial cell layer with tight and gap junctions form the superficial layers of gastroprotection including cyto-protection (Robert et al 1979, Whittle 1993, Abdel-Salam et al. 1999, 2001, Mózsik et al. 2007). Subendothelial enhanced microcirculation proposed to be the main site where capsaicin and TRPV1 agonists (Fig 3) induce the gastroprotective effect was supported by several lines of evidence beyond the opposite effect of capsaicin desensitization on H^{+}back-diffusion models and on ulcers provoked by epithelial necrotizing agents suitable to be inhibited by the cytoprotective prostaglandins.

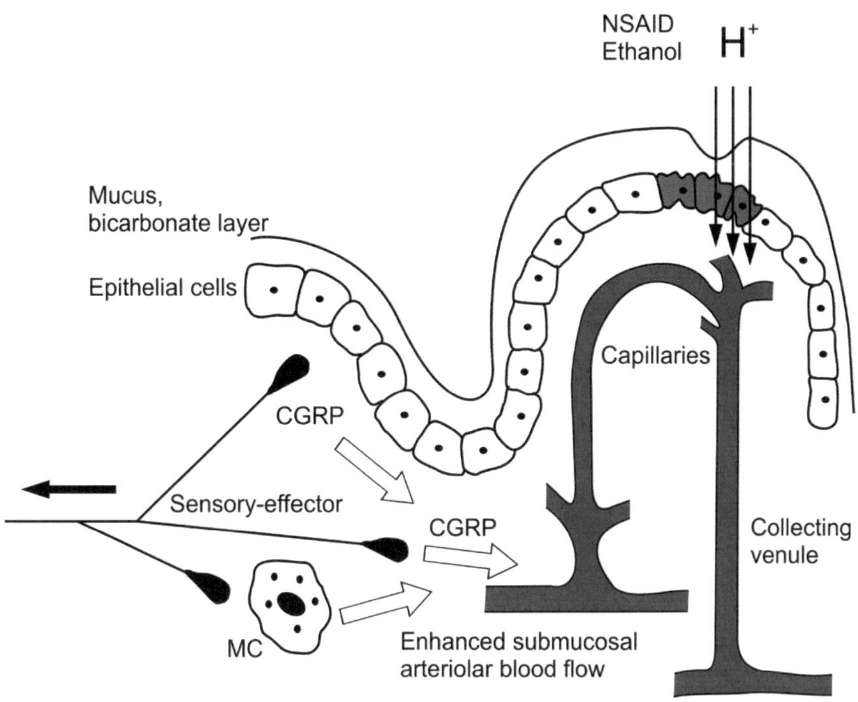

Figure 4. Mechanism of capsaicin-sensitive sensory-effector nerve terminals in gastroprotection depicted on a modified scheme of Whittle (1993). Black arrows: H^{+}backflow through the epithelial barrier damaged by nonsteroid anti-inflammatory drugs (NSAID), ethanol or other aggressive agents. White arrows release of CGRP from capsaicin-sensitive nerve endings or other vasodilator mediators released during degranulation of mast cells (MC). The released mediators induce enhancement of mucosal microcirculation. Thick black arrow: action potentials of sensory message to the central nervous system.

TRPV1 is a non-selective cation channel with preferential gating to Ca^{++}over Na^{+}(Caterina 1997, Szolcsányi and Sándor 2012) and there is firm evidence in the skin that both CGRP and TRPV1 are coexpressed in the sensory receptors terminating in the epidermis (for ref see Szolcsányiand Pintér 2013). Furthermore it has been shown that in vitro no inhibition of sensory neuropeptide release ensues in the presence of blockade of axon reflexes by tetrodo toxin or lignocaine (for ret Szolcsányi 1996, 2013).

Thus CGRP is released from the sensory nerve ending which in an unorthodox way serve in a bidirectional neuroregulatory sensory-efferent function. Nevertheless, capsaicin prevented deep but not epithelial mucosal damage and local intra-arterial infusion of tetrodotoxin prevented the capsaicin-induced gastroprotection (Holzer at el 1991).These results indicate, that if the stomach mucosa was perfursed with capsaicin in 25% ethanol nerve terminals excites the superficial layers and evoke axon reflexes (Fig 4). In this case mainly those sensory nerve endings situated deeper near to the vessels are activated through branching axon collaterals and mediators released by Ca^{++}influx through the TRPV1 channel in the subepithelial sensory nerve endings play minor role in enhancement of mucosal microcirculation. There is, however, no evidence to suppose that in axon reflex arrangement in the periphery some nerve endings of primary sensory neurons might have nerve terminals specialized for efferent, mediator releasing function in antidromic vasodilation (Szolcsányi 1996, 2013).

Recently another hypothesis for gastroprotection (Holzer and Maggi 1988), in fact a revival of Lewis's "nocifensor" fiber theory was raised according to which vasodilator mediators are released from nerve endings of capsaicin-sensitive DRG fibers which have only efferent function without mediating messages to the central nervous system. In other words these authors in this paper proposed that peripheral release of neuropeptides in the stomach mucosa takes place from effector nerve terminals of a subset of DRG neurons which have only efferent function. They showed that acid challenge of the mucosa elicited rapid c-fos mRNA activation in the nucleus tractus solitarii but not in the spinal cord, while capsaicin-induced mucosal vasodilation was abolished by splanchnic nerve denervation but remained intact after vagotomy. (Holzer and Maggi 1998). Subsequent data (Blackshaw et al 2000) indicated that most of the vagal afferents excited by low pH are capsaicin-insensitive fibers from where neuropeptides are not released (Szolcsányi 2004). Thus they could mediate the c-fos activation in the nucleus tractus solitarii. It has been shown earlier that for release of sensory neuropeptides a very low frequency of activity is already maximal (see Introduction and Szolcsányi 1996 2013). Therefore pronounced mucosal vasodilatation without c-fos activation can be evoked (Szolcsányi and Barthó 2001). More recent data of Peter Holzer's group seems to support our conclusion, since the lack of c-fos activation in the dorsal half of the spinal cord by mucosal HCl application was in contrast to the effect of capsaicin which evoked c-fos activation both in the nucleus tractus solitarii and particularly in the lamina I of dorsal horn of the spinal cord (Holzer et al 2005). Distension of the stomach enhanced c-fos expression and CGRP expression both in the spinal cord and medulla oblongata (Zhang et al 2006).

The pivotal role of CGRP in gastroprotection due to an enhancement of mucosal microcirculation (Peskar et al 1993) in response to stimulation of peptidergic capsaicin-sensitive vagal and spinal sensory neurons are supported by several further lines of evidence. Gastric hyperemia to intragastric capsaicin or acid back diffusion (0.15M HCl +15% ethanol) was blocked by the CGRP antagonist hCGRP 8-37 (Li et al 1991, 1992). Some data indicate that beyond the vascular effect of CGRP it induces also release of somatostatin (Inui et al 1991). Furthermore a subpopulation of capsaicin-sensitive vagal sensory neurons contain also somatostatin which is released by electrical nerve stimulation of the nerves both from the thoracic and abolominal parts of the nerves (Than et al 2000).

Recently it has been shown, that $TRPV_1$ and neuronal nitric oxide synthase (nNOS) are coexpressed in sensory fibers around the vessels of the gastric mucosa and the capsaicin-induced enhancement of mucosal blood flow appeared to be diminished by nNOS inhibition (Raimara et al 2013). Epidermal growth factor (EGF) reduces gastric mucosal lesions evoked by ethanol by activating capsaicin-sensitive sensory nerve terminals (Matsumoto et al 2001).

The role of prostaglandin E_2 and its receptors EP1 in cytoprotection against necrotizing agents is well established and has been discussed to be different from the effects of capsaicin. Recent data using EP1 and prostacyclin (IP) knockout mice showed that capsaicin-induced gastro-protection is present in gene-deleted mice of EP1 but disappeared in IP knockout mice (Takeuchi, 2014). The role of prostacyclin in capsaicin-induced gastroprotection seems to be interesting for further research. For further reviews see Abdel-Salam 2001, Pawlik et al 2001, Evangelista 2009, Mózsik et al 2007, 2014, Luo et al 2013).

It is important to note that stimulation of capsaicin-sensitive perivascular nerve terminals in vitro elicits slow inhibitory junction potential (IJP) and dilator response on mesenteric smooth muscle cells. IJP evoked by capsaicin or electrical stimulation was unaffected by endothelial removal or pharmacological blockade of autonomic neuroeffector mechanism by pharmaco-logical treatments with guanethidine, 6-hydroxydopamine, propranolol, atropine, α, β-methylene ATP (Meehan et al. 1991).

The role of mast cells in gastric mucosal injury evoked by H^+back-diffusion, NSAID, ethanol and other aggressive chemicals has been described since a long time (Fig 3, 4) (Szolcsányi and Barthó 1981, Takeuchi et al 1997, Rydning et al. 2004). Recently it has been reported, that mast cell deficient Sash mice are highly susceptible to piroxicam-induced gastric ulceration. Thus, it seems that beyond the potent gastroprotective effect of capsaicin-sensitive nerve endings described earlier and presented in humans (Mózsik et al.,2014 in this volume) mast cells play also role through releasing vasodilator mediators (Rydning et al., 2002), but by releasing histamine it enhances on H_2 receptors gastric acid secretion which in these mice did not interfere with the ulcer formation (Hampton and Hale, 2013).

5. Conclusions

CGRP release from the capsaicin-sensitive TRPV1-expressing sensory nerve endings induces potent enhancement of submucosal microcirculation which results in marked gastroprotective effect. CGRP, substance P and somatostatin are released from these nerve endings which by arborizations could induce effector tissue responses also by axon reflexes.

Capsaicin-sensitive sensory nerve-mediated vasodilation together with mast cell degranula-tion participate in the gastroprotective effect against mucosal injuries induced by aggressive agents as H^+back-diffusion, ethanol or nonsteroid anti-inflammatory drugs (NSAID) and provide therapeutic means for gastroprotection.

Acknowledgements

I thank Ágnes Kemény and Éva Szőke for drawing the figures and Brigitta Incze for typing the text. The work was supported by the grant SROP U.2.2.A-11/1/KONV-2012-0024.

Author details

János Szolcsányi*

Address all correspondence to: janos.szolcsanyi@aok.pte.hu

Department of Pharmacology and Pharmacotherapy, University of Pécs, Hungary

References

[1] Abdel-Salam O.M.E., Szolcsányi J, Pórszász R, Mózsik G. (1996) effect of capsaicin and resiniferatoxin on gastrointestinal blood flow in rats Eur. J. Pharmacol. 305, 127-136

[2] Abdel-Salam O.M.E., Debreceni A, Mózsik G, Szolcsányi J. (1999) Capsaicin-sensitive afferent sensory nerves in modulating gastric mucosal defense against noxious agents, J. Physiol (Paris) 93, 443-454

[3] Abdel-Salam O.M.E., Czimmer J, Debreceni A, Szolcsányi J, Mózsik G. (2001) Gastric mucosal integrity: gastric mucosal blood flow and microcirculation. An overview. Journal of Physiology 95, 105-127

[4] Barthó L, Szolcsányi J. (1978) The site of action of capsaicin on the guinea-pig isolated ileum. Naunyn-Schmiedeberg's Arch. Pharmacol. 305, 75–81

[5] Bayliss WM. (1901) On the origin from the spinal cord of vaso-dilator fibres of the hindlimb and on the nature of these fibres. J Physiol 26, 173-209

[6] Blackshaw L.A, Page A.J, Partosoedarso E.R. (2000) Acute effects of capsaicin on gastrointestinal vagal afferents, Neuroscience 96, 407–416

[7] Caterina M.J, Schumacher M.A, Tominaga M, Rosen T, A., Levine J.D., Julius D. (1997) The capsaicin receptor: a heat-activated ion channel in the pain pathway. Nature 389, 816–824

[8] Evangelista S, Maggi C.A, Meli A. (1986) Evidence for a role of adrenals in the capsaicin-sensitive "gastric defense mechanism" in rats, Proc. Soc. Exp. Biol. Med. 182, 568–569

[9] Evangelista S (2009). Role of calcitonin gene-related peptide in gastric mucosal defense and healing. Curr Pharm Des. 15, 3571-6

[10] Gáti T, Guth, P. H. (1976) Acid-distension gastricmucosal lesions in the rat. In: Mózsik, Gy, Jávor, T.(Eds.) Progress in Peptic Ulcer, pp. 597-603. Akadémiai Kiadó, Budapest.

[11] Graham DY, Smith JL, Opekun AR. (1988) Spicy food and the stomach. Evalutuion by videoendoscopy. JAMA 16, 3473-5

[12] Green T, Dockray GJ (1988) Characterization of the peptidergic afferent innervation of the stomach in the rat, mouse and guinea-pig. Neuroscience. 25, 181-93

[13] Hampton D.D., Hale P (2011) Mast cells are critical for protection against peptic ulcers induces by the NSAID Piroxicam. Plos One 6(8), e23669

[14] Holzer P and Sametz W (1986) Gastric mucosal protection against ulcerogenic factors in the rat mediated by capsaicin-senitive afferent neurons Gastroenterology 91, 975-981

[15] Holzer P, Lippe IT. (1988) Stimulation of afferent nerve endings by intragastric capsaicin protects against ethanol-induced damage of gastric mucosa. Neuroscience 27, 981-7

[16] Holzer P, Livingston E.H, Guth P.H. (1991a) Sensory neurons signal for an increase in rat gastric mucosal blood flow in the face of pending acid injury, Gastroenterology 101, 416–423

[17] Holzer P, Livingston E.H, Saria A, Guth P.H. (1991b) Sensory neurons mediate protective vasodilatation in rat gastric mucosa, Am. J. Physiol. 260, G363–G370

[18] Holzer P, Maggi C.A. (1998) Dissociation of dorsal root ganglion neurons into afferent and efferent-like neurons, Neurosci. 86, 389–398

[19] Holzer P, Painsipp E, Shuligoi R.(2005) Differential effects of intragastric acid and capsaicin on gastric emptying and afferent input to the rat spinal cord and brainstem. BMC Neurosci 6, 60-69

[20] Inui T, Kinoshita Y, Yamaguchi A, Yamatani T, Chiba T. (1991) Linkage between capsaicin-stimulated calcitonin gene-related peptide and somatostatin release in rat stomach, Am. J. Physiol. 261, G770–G774

[21] Jancsó N (the late), Jancsó-Gábor A, Szolcsányi J. (1967) Direct evidence for neurogenic inflammation and its prevention by denervation and by pretreatment with capsaicin. Br J Pharmacol 31, 138-151

[22] Jordt SE, Tominaga M, Julius D. (2000) Acid potentiation of the capsaicin receptor determined by a key extracellular site. Proc Natl Acad Sci USA. 97, 8134-9

[23] Lennard-Jones, J.E., Babouris, N. (1965) Effect of different foods ont the acidity of the-gastric contents in patients with duodenal ulcer. I. A comparison between two „therapeutic" diets and freely chosen meals. Gut 6, 113-124

[24] Lewis T. (1937) The nocifensor system of nerves and its reactions, Br. med. J. 194, 431–435

[25] Li D.S, Raybould H.E, Quintero E., Guth P.H. (1991) Role of calcitonin gene-related peptide in gastric hyperemic response to intragastric capsaicin, Am. J. Physiol. 261, G657–G661

[26] Li DS, Raybould HE, Quintero E, Guth PH. (1992) Calcitonin gene-related peptide mediates the gastric hyperemic response to acid back-diffusion. Gastroenterology 102, 1124-1128

[27] Lippe IT, Pabst MA, Holzer P. (1989) Intragastric capsaicin enhances rat gastric acid elimination and mucosal blood flow by afferent nerve stimulation. Br J Pharmacol 96, 91-100

[28] Luo Xiu-Ju, Liu Bin, Dai Zhong, Yang Zhi-Chun, Peng Jun. (2013) Stimulation of calcitonin gene-related peptide release through targeting capsaicin receptor: a potential strategy for gastric mucosal protection. Dig Dis Sci. 58: 320-325

[29] Makara, G. B., Csalay, L, Frenkl, R, Somfai, Zs, Szepesházi, K. (1965) Effect of capsaicin on experimental ulcer in the rat. Acta Med. Acad. Sci. hung. 21, 213-216

[30] Matsumoto Y, Kanamoto K, Kawakubo K, Aomi H, Matsumoto T, Setsuro I, Masatoshi F. (2001) Gastroprotective and vasodilatory effects of epidermal growth factor: The role of sensory afferent neurons. Am J PhysiolGastrointest Liver Physiol 280, G903

[31] Meehan A.G, Omar D. Hottenstein, Kreulen D.L. (1991) Capsaicin-sensitive nerves mediate inhibitory junction potentials and dilation in guinea-pig mesenteric artery. J. Physiology 443, 161-174

[32] Mózsik G, Abdel-Salam O.M.E., Szolcsányi J (1997) Capsaicin-sensitive afferent nerves in gastric mucosal damage and protection, Akadémiai Kiadó, Budapest

[33] Mózsik G, Dömötör A, Czimmer J, Szabó JL, Szolcsányi J (2014) Capsaicin-sensitive afferent nerves and the human gastrointestinal tract. In: MózsikGy, Abdel-Salam OME, Takeuchi K (Eds) Capsaicin-sensitive neural afferention and the gastrointestinal tract: from bench to bedside (in press).

[34] Pawlik M, Ptak A, Pajdo R, Konturek PC, Brzozowski T, Konturek SJ. (2001) Sensory nerves and calcition gene-related peptide in the effect of ischemic preconditioning on acute and chronic gastric lesions induced by ischemia-reperfusion. J PhysiolPharmacol 52, 569-81

[35] Peskar BM, Wong HC, Walsh JH, Holzer P. (1993) A monoclonal antibody to calcitonin gene-related peptide abolishes capsaicin-induced gastroprotection. Eur. J. Pharmacol. 30, 201-203

[36] Raimura M, Tashima K, Matsumoto K, Tobe S, Chino A, Namiki T, Terasawa K, Horie S. (2013) Neuronal nitric oxide synthase-derived nitric oxide is involved in gastric mucosal hyperemic response to capsaicin in rats. Pharmacology 92, 60-70

[37] Robert A, Nemazis JE, Lancaster C, Hanchar A. (1979) Cytoprotection by prostaglandins in rats.Prevention of gastric necrosis by alcohol, HCl, NaOH, hypertonic NaCl and thermal injury. Gastroenterology. 77, 4433-4442

[38] Rydning A, Lyng O, Falkmer S, Gronbech JE. (2002) Histamine is involved in gastric vasodilation durig acid back diffusion via activation of sensory neurons. Am J Physiol Gastrointest Liver Physiol 283, G603-G611

[39] Rydning A, Bakkelund K, Chen D, Falkmer S, Gronbech JE. (2004) Role of bradykinin in gastric vasodilation caused by hypertonic saline and acid back diffusion. Regulatory Peptides 119, 139-148

[40] Sanchez-Palomera, E. (1951) The action of spicesontheacidgastricsecretion, onappetite and onthecaloricintake. Gastroenterology 18, 254-286

[41] Schneider, M. A., de Luca, V., Gray, S. J. (1956) The effect of spiceingestionuponthestomach. Amer. J. Gastroent. 26, 722-732

[42] Sharkey KA, Williams RG, Dockray GJ. (1984) Sensory substance P innervation of the stomach and pancreas. Demonstration of capsaicin-sensitive sensory neurons in the rat by combined immunohistochemistry and retrograde tracing. Gastroenterology 87, 914-21

[43] Shay, H.,Komarov, S. A.,Fels, S. S.,Merance, D., Grunstein, M., Siplet, H. (1945) Simple method for uniform production of gastric ulceration in rat. Gastroenterology 5, 210-226

[44] Solanke, T. F. (1973) The effect of red pepper /Capsicumfrutescens/ on gastric acid secretion. J. Surgical Res. 15, 385-390

[45] Sternini C, Reeve JR Jr, Brecha N. (1987) Distribution and characterization of calcitonin gene-related peptide immunoreactivity in the digestive system of normal and capsaicin-treated rats. Gastroenterology 93,852-62

[46] Szállási Á, Blumberg P.M, (1999) Vanilloid (capsaicin) receptors and mechanisms, Pharmacol. Rev. 51, 159–211

[47] Szolcsányi J (1977) A pharmacological approach to elucidate of the role of different nerve fibres and receptor endings in mediation of pain, J. Physiol. (Paris) 73, 251–259

[48] Szolcsányi J. (1984) Capsaicin-sensitive chemoceptive neural system with dual sensory-efferent function. In: Chahl LA, Szolcsányi J, Lembeck F (end) Antidromic vasodilatation and neurogenic inflammation. AkadémiaiKiadó, Budapest, pp 27-56

[49] Szolcsányi J. (1990) Effect of capsaicin, resiniferatoxin and piperine on ethanol-induced gastric ulcer of the rat, Acta Physiol. Hung. 75, 267–268

[50] Szolcsányi J. (1996) Capsaicin-sensitive nerve terminals with local and systemic efferent functions: facts and scopes of an unorthodox neuroregulatory mechanism, Progr. Brain Res. 113, 343– 359

[51] Szolcsányi J. (2004) Forty years in capsaicin research for sensory pharmascology and physiology. Neuropeptides 38, 377-384

[52] Szolcsányi J. (2013) Neuroregulation of cutaneous microcirculation: the shadow of Sir Thomas Lewis Trends. Pharmacol. Sci. 34, 591-592

[53] Szolcsányi J. (2014) Capsaicin and sensory neurons: a historical perspective. In: Abdel-Salam OME (Ed) Capsaicin as a Therapeutic Molecule Springer, Basel pp1-38

[54] Szolcsányi J, Barthó L. (1978) New type of nerve-mediated cholinergic contractions of the guinea-pig small intestine and its selective blockade by capsaicin, Naunyn-Schmiedeberg's Arch. Pharmacol. 305, 83–90

[55] Szolcsányi J, Barthó L.(1981) Impaired defense mechanism to peptic ulcer in the capsaicin-desensitized rat, in: Mózsik G, Hänninen O, Jávor T (Eds.), Gastrointestinal Defense Mechanism. Adv. Physiol. Sci. Vol 29 pp. 39–51.Akadémiai Kiadó,Budapest-Pergamon Press, Oxford.

[56] Szolcsányi J, Barthó L.(2001) Capsaicin-sensitive afferents and their role in gastroprotection: an update. J. Physiology 95, 181-188

[57] Szolcsányi J, Jancsó-Gábor A. (1975) Sensory effects of capsaicin congeners. I. Relationship between chemical structure and pain producing potency of pungentagents. Arzneim.-Forsch. 25, 1877-1881

[58] Szolcsányi J, Jancsó-Gábor A.(1976) Sensory effects of capsaicin congeners II. Importance of chemical structure and pungency in desensitizing activity of capsaicin-type compounds. ArzneimForsch (Drug Res) 26, 33-37

[59] Szolcsányi J, Mózsik G. (1984) effects of capsaicin on the development of gastric mucosal damage by different necrotizing agents and of gastric cytoprotection by PGI_2 atropine and cimetidine in rats. Acta Physiol Hung 64, 287-91

[60] Szolcsányi J, Pintér E. (2013) Transiens receptor potential vanilloid 1 as a therapeutic target in analgesia. Expert Opin Ther Targets 17, 641-657

[61] Szolcsányi J, Sándor Z. (2012) Multisteric TRPV1 nocisensor: a target for analgesics. Trends Pharmacol Sci 33, 646-655

[62] Takeuchi K, Kato S, Yasuhiro T, Yagi K. (1997) Mechanism of acid secretory changes in rat stomach after damage by taurocholate: role of nitric oxide, histamine, and sensory neurons. Dig Dis Sci. 42, 645-53

[63] Takeuchi K. (2014) Gastric cytoprotection by prostaglandin E_2 and prostacyclin: relationship to EP1 and IP receptors. J Pharmacol. 65, 3-14

[64] Than M, Németh J, Szilvássy Z, Pintér E, Helyes Zs, Szolcsányi J. (2000) Antiinflammatory effect of somatostatin released from capsaicin-sensitive vagal and sciatic sensory fibres of the rat and guinea-pig, Eur. J. Pharmacol. 399, 251–258

[65] Viranuvatti V, Kalayasiri C, Cherani O, Plengvanit U. (1972) Effects of capsicum solution on human gastric mucosa as observed gastroscopically. Amer. J. Gastroent. 58, 225-232

[66] Whittle B.J.R. (1993) Neuronal and endothelium-derived mediators in the modulation of the gastric microcirculation: integrity in the balance, Br. J. Pharmacol. 110, 3–17

[67] Zhang FF, Mo JZ, Chen XY, Peng YS, Chen SL, Xiao SD. (2006) Gastric distention enhances c-fos and calcitonin gene-related peptide expression in the spinal cord and brain of rats. Chin J Dig Dis 7, 19-23

Section 2

Plant (natural) origin capsaicin(oids) and their necessary regulatory chemical qualifications required by the international authorities

Chapter 2

Pharmacobotanical Analysis and Regulatory Qualification of *Capsicum* Fruits and *Capsicum* Extracts — A Survey

Mónika Kuzma, Tibor Past, Gyula Mózsik and Pál Perjési

Additional information is available at the end of the chapter

http://dx.doi.org/10.5772/58812

1. Introduction

Capsicum fruits contain *coloring pigments*, *pungent principles*, resin, protein, cellulose, pentosans, mineral elements and a small amount of *volatile oil*, while seeds contain *fixed (non-volatile) oil*. Besides these organic constituents *Capsicum* fruits also contain inorganic constituents, mostly potassium and sodium, calcium, phosphorus, iron, copper and manganese.

Paprikas derive their color in the ripe state mainly from *carotenoid pigments*, which range from bright red (capsanthin, capsorubin) to yellow (cucurbitene). The *pungent principles* capsaicin and its structurally closely related homologs (so-called *capsaicinoids*) and analogues, are contained only in small amounts, as low as 0.001 to 0.005% in "mild" and 0.1% in "hot" cultivars. The characteristic aroma and flavor of the fresh fruit is imparted by the *volatile oil* containing a range of alkylmethoxypyrazines and a structurally diverse group (alcohols, aldehydes, ketones, carboxylic acids, and esters of carboxylic acids) of oxygenated hydrocarbons. Apart from capsaicinoids, the taste of paprika is mostly due to the *fixed oil* which is comprised mainly of triglycerides of which linoleic, linolic, stearinic and other unsaturated fatty acids predominate.

The first part of the chapter summarizes the chemical characterization of the three classes of *Capsicum* ingredients (*coloring pigments*, *pungent principles*, and *volatile oils*), the most important analytical methods used in pharmacobotanical studies or acknowledged by different regulatory bodies.

Capsicum extracts are frequently used as active pharmaceutical ingredients (API) in manufacturing pharmaceutical products. For such applications *Capsicum* extract should be qualified not only on the basis of the amount of API(s) but on the basis of the amounts of possible impurities/contaminants as well. Among the most important impurities/contaminants (a) *toxic metals,* (b) *pesticides,* (c) *mycotoxins,* (d) *foreign organic matters,* and (e) *radioactivity* (if there is cause for concern) should be mentioned.

The second part of the chapter describes the Pharmacopoeial and other internationally recognized methods for determination of pesticides in *Capsicum* fruits and extracts.

2. Structure and biosynthetic pathways of the most important ingredients of *capsicum* fruits

Capsicum is a versatile plant used as vegetable, pungent food additive, colorant and raw material for pharmaceutical products. The genus *Capsicum,* which is commonly known as "chili", "red chili", "tabasco", "paprika", "cayenne", etc., is a member of the family *Solanaceae,* and closely related to eggplant, potato, petunia, tomato and tobacco. After much work by taxonomists concerning the classification of the presently domesticated species, they have been considered to belong to one of five species, namely *Capsicum annuum, Capsicum frutescens, Capsicum baccatum, Capsicum chinense* and *Capsicum pubescens* (Bosland, 1994).

Capsicum types are usually classified by fruit characteristics, i.e. *pungency, color, fruit shape,* as well as by their use. *Capsicum* species are commonly divided into two groups, *pungent* and *non-pungent,* also called hot and sweet.

The word "paprika" was borrowed from Hungarian (paprika). It entered a great number of languages, in many cases probably via German. In the end, also "paprika" is derived from a name of black pepper, in this case Serbian pepper. In most languages, "paprika" denotes the dried spice only, though in some (e.g., German) it is commonly used for the vegetable bell pepper.

Capsicum fruits contain *coloring pigments, pungent principles,* resin, protein, cellulose, pentosans, mineral elements and a small amount of *volatile oil,* while seeds contain *fixed* (non-volatile) *oil.* Besides these organic constituents *Capsicum* fruits also contain inorganic constituents, mostly potassium and sodium, calcium, phosphorus, iron, copper and manganese (Thresh, 1846; Brawer and Schoen, 1962; Brash et al., 1988; Pruthi, 2003).

The pungent principles capsaicin and its structurally closely related homologs (so-called *capsaicinoids*) and analogues, are contained only in small amounts, as low as 0.001 to 0.005% in "mild" and 0.1% in "hot" cultivars. Apart from capsaicin, the taste of paprika is mostly due to the *fixed oil* which is comprised mainly of triglycerides of which linoleic, linolic, stearinic and other unsaturated fatty acids predominate. The fixed oil content of the *Capsicum* seeds also play an important role in the visual sensing of the paprika powder since it can dissolve and homogeneously distribute the colored substances during grinding of the dried fruits. The characteristic aroma and flavor of the fresh fruit is imparted by the volatile oil containing a range of alkylmethoxypyrazines (e.g., 2-methoxy-3-isobutylpyrazine, the "earthy" flavor) and a structurally diverse group (alcohols, aldehydes, ketones, carboxylic acids, and esters of carboxylic acids) of oxygenated hydrocarbons.

Furthermore, the fresh ripe paprika contains sizable amounts (0.1%) of vitamin C (ascorbic acid). It was the Hungarian biochemist Albert Szent-Györgyi who discovered that the Hungarian paprika is a rich source of vitamin C. Later (1937) he won the Nobel Prize "for his discoveries in connection with the biological combustion processes, with special reference to vitamin C and the catalysis of fumaric acid" (Encyclopedia Britannica).

Paprikas derive their color in the ripe state mainly from carotenoid pigments, which range from bright red (capsanthin, capsorubin) to yellow (cucurbitene); the total carotenoid content in dried paprika is 0.1 to 0.5%.

2.1. Volatiles

The characteristic flavor and aroma of the fresh fruits is due to their volatile oil content. The fruits of *Capsicum* species have relative low volatile oil content, ranging from about 0.1% to 2.6% in paprika. The total volatiles are generally isolated by steam distillation. In the case of heat-sensitive compounds present, vacuum distillation-continuous solvent extraction can be used. The pure volatile oil and concentrated extracts were analyzed by GC-MS methods. Most compounds of odor significance have been tentatively identified by their mass spectra, and the identification was confirmed by checking the retention time and mass spectra of authentic reference compounds. When Buttery et al. (1969a,b) identified 3-isobutyl-2-methoxypyrazine (1) (Fig 1) as a characteristic aroma compound, the alkylmethoxypyrazines aroused great interest among flavor chemists. The alkylmethoxypyrazines have been shown to be widely distributed in vegetables and with a greenish sweet smell that possibly plays a significant role in the aroma of salad vegetables (Murray, and Whitfield, 1975).

Volatiles have been identified in fresh, homogenized, cooked and stir-fried bell peppers and the effects of ripening and tissue disruption on the composition of volatiles have been determined (Wu and Liou, 1986; Whitfield and Last, 1991; Cremer and Eichner, 2000). About 60 volatile compounds have been identified in green California bell pepper using a vacuum Liken-Nickerson (Buttery et al., 1969a,b). Luning et al. (1994a,b) have identified 64 volatile compounds in fresh bell pepper at three ripening stages (green, turning, red) with dynamic headspace. The composition of volatile compounds indicated that the majority of green related odour volatile compounds decreased or even disappeared during maturation and fruity and sweet odour were higher at the turning and red stages.

There are common aroma compounds amongst the different species of the different fresh pepper, namely, 2,3-butanedione (caramel), 1-penten-3-one (pungent/spicy), hexanal (2) (grassy, herbal), 3-carene (red bell pepper, rubbery), *trans*-beta-ocimene (rancid), octanal (fruity), *trans*-2-hexenal (3) (sweet) and 2-isobutyl-3-methoxypyrazine (1) (green bell pepper). Keller et al. (1981) reported that volatiles of fresh red Jalapeno pepper extracts had a pleasant floral aroma (3-carene). Likewise, *trans*-2-hexenal (3) and *trans*-2-hexenol (4), which have an almond, fruity and spicy odour, were found to increase during maturation.

Study by Chitwood et al. (1983) suggested that *trans*-3-hexenol, 2-*sec*-butyl-3-methoxypyrazine and 2-isobutyl-3-methoxypyrazine are responsible for the frequent use of green descriptors in the aroma descriptive analysis of three *C. annuum* cultivar (Anaheim, Jalapeno and Fresno). Based on GC-MS and sensory analysis of volatiles of three cultivars of *C. annuum – Jalapeno, Fresno*, and *Anaheim* – twelve odor significant compounds were identified that had been found in one or the other of the earlier studies: 2,3-butadienone (caramel), 1-penten-3-one (pungent/ spicy), hexanal (grassy, herbal), 3-carene (red bell pepper, rubbery), *trans*-3-hexenol (4), *trans*-3-hexenyl isopentanoate (6) (associated with green and green-fruity odors); 3-isobutyl-(1) and 3-*sec*-butyl-2-methoxypyrazine (7) (with green vegetable and green bell capsicum odors); *beta*-ionone (5) (only in Jalapeno), linalool (both with floral character); and the aromatic compounds benzaldehyde (8) and methyl salicylate (9) (with sweetish, penetrating odors) (Chitwood et al., 1983).

The analysis of volatile compounds has been a challenge to many researchers. Many different analytical methods have been developed to determine fresh and processed chilli flavour, such as solvent extraction-simultaneous distillation extraction (Chitwood et al., 1983; Wu and Liou, 1986; Korany et al., 2002) and dynamic headspace (Luning et al., 1994a,b). However, these methods are time-consuming, expensive and likely to introduce artifact resulting from sample preparation and solvent interaction steps. Moreover they cannot represent the total composition of volatile chemicals in equilibrium as found in the aroma of intact, fresh chilli. Solid phase microextraction (SPME) is a method that approaches the ideal extraction method and has been applied to the analysis of various aroma and flavour compound in samples (Peppard and Yang, 1994; Penton, 1996; Steffen and Pawliszyn, 1996; Ibanez et al., 1998; Sides et al., 2000). SPME has been recommended for the quantitative analysis of flavour and fragrance compounds (Zhang and Pawliszyn, 1993). The main advantages of SPME are simplicity, speed, solvent-free, high sensitivity, small sample volume, lower cost and simple automation (Kataoka et al., 2000).

2.2. Coloring pigments

The coloring pigments of red peppers are comprised of *carotenoids*. The term "carotenoid" encompasses not only the carotenes (C_{40} hydrocarbons), but also their oxygenated derivatives, the xanthophylls. Carotenoids are widely distributed groups of natural pigments, responsible for the yellow, orange, and red colors of fruits, roots, flowers, fish, invertebrates, and birds. Only bacteria, algae, fungi, and green plants can synthesize carotenoids, but humans incorporate them from the diet. Especially bacterial carotenoids are most diverse. Carotenoid extracts and fruits rich in carotenoids are now being used in the food industry to color foods, thus such foods are also representing carotenoid sources of the human diet. The nutritional importance of carotenoids is mostly associated with the provitamin A activity of *beta*-carotene and others. Besides its well-established provitamin A activity, research is under way to study the relationship between *beta*-carotene intake and occurrence of atherosclerosis, cardiovascular diseases, in particular degree of LDL oxidation (Poppel and von Goldbochm, 1995; Hinds et al., 1997; Rodriguez-Amaya, 1997; Woodall et al., 1997; Maillard et al., 1998; Manirakiza et al., 1999, 2003).

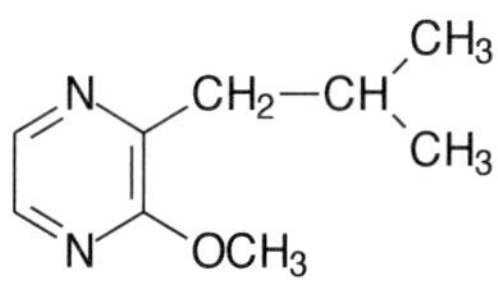

1

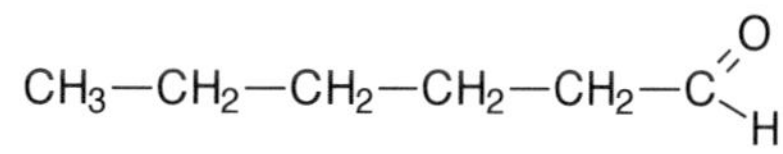

2

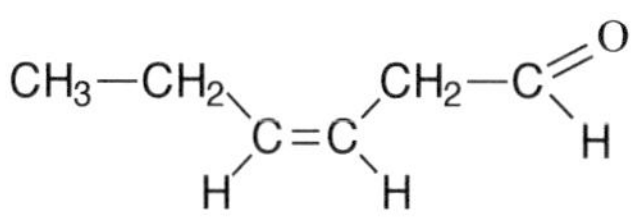

3

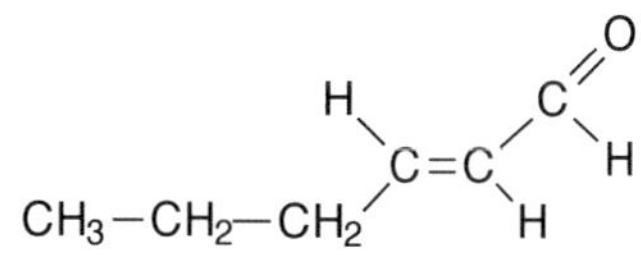

4

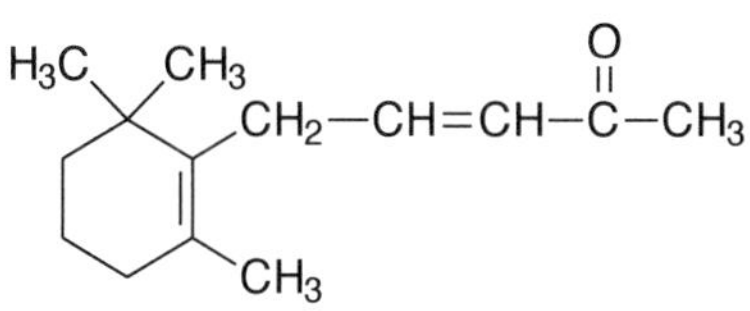

5

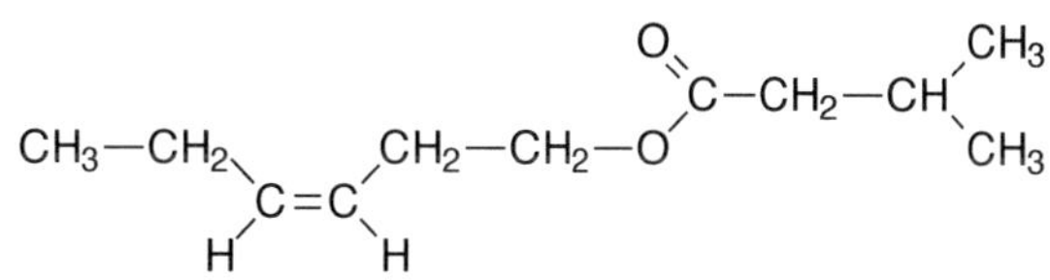

6

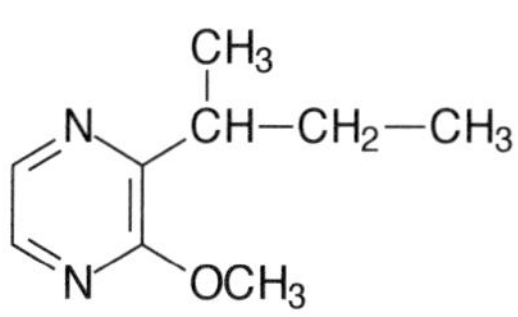

7

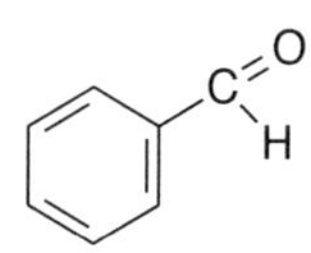

8

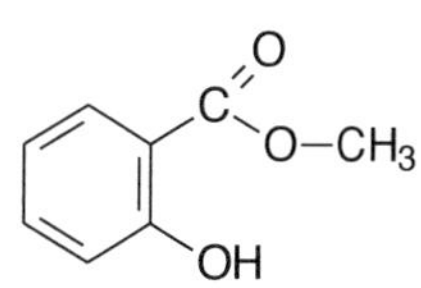

9

Figure 1. Main components of volatile oils of *Capsicum* furits.

The basic carotenoid structure is a symmetrical, linear, 40-carbon tetraterpene built from eight carbon isoprenoid units joined in such a way that the order is reversed at the center. Fig 2 shows the structure of *beta*-carotene (10), one of the most typical carotenoid components of *Capsicum* fruits.

Carotenoids were for a long time assumed being synthesized by the mevalonate pathway for isoprenoid biosynthesis. This view was prevalent up until the mid-nineties when it was discovered that the carotenoid precursor isopentenyl-pyrophosphate (IPP) was synthetized by two independent metabolic pathways in plants (Lichtenthaler et al., 1997).

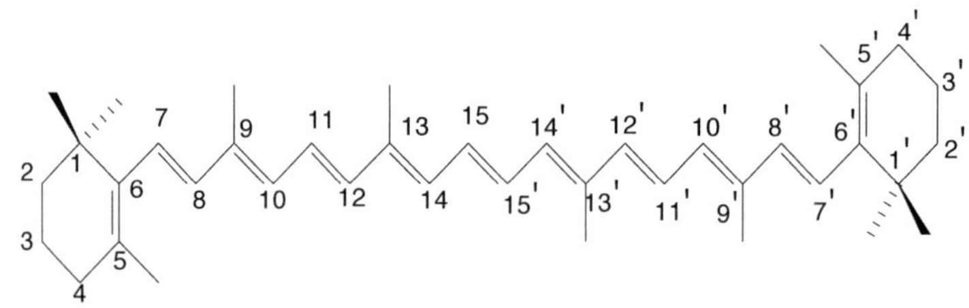

Figure 2. Structure of *beta*-carotene (10)

The first pathway occurs in the cytoplasmic compartment from mevalonic acid and gives rise to compounds such as sterols and cytokinins. In fungi, carotenoids are derived via the mevalonate biosynthetic pathway. The second pathway, effective in bacteria and plastids of plants, is responsible for biosynthesis of gibberellins, carotenoids, abscisic acid, and also contributes to the biosynthesis of tocopherols as well as chlorophyll A and B. This plastidial pathway of isoprenoid synthesis is named after its first metabolite 1-deoxyxylulose 5-phosphate (DOXP) and has pyruvate and glycerinaldehyde-3-phosphate as precursors. Further details can be obtained from a number of review articles, (Davies, 1980; Spurgeon, and Porter, 1983; Britton, 1991).

Carotenoids can be extracted from natural sources by lipid solvents. With fresh material, ethanol or acetone act both as dehydrating agent and extracting solvents. When lipids and esterified xantophylls are present (hydroxylated carotenoids generally occur as esters of fatty acids), the extracts are saponified and the free carotenoids extracted for analysis. Most carotenoids are unstable in oxygen atmosphere and light thus careful extractions and separations are generally carried out under inert atmosphere, subdued light and low temperature (Rodriguez-Amaya, 1997; Deli and Molnár, 2002). High performance liquid chromatography (HPLC) is the most powerful chromatographic technique to separate and – coupled with mass spectrometry (MS) – identify carotenoids. Recent reviews on the field provide up-to-date summary of carotenoid analysis (Rodriguez-Amaya, 1997; Wall and Bosland, 1998; Deli and Molnár, 2002; Felt et al., 2005).

The composition of carotenoid pigments produced by paprika has been investigated in detail. Some twenty carotenoids have been isolated so far with *capsanthin* (11) and *capsorubin* (12) (Figure 3) representing the most abundant (Deli and Molnár, 2002). The ripening process is marked by the disappearance of chlorophyll and a rapid rise in the colored carotenoids (Rodriguez-Amaya, 1997; Rahman, and Buckle, 1980; Hornero-Mendez et al., 2000; Gnayfeed et al., 2001; Deli and Molnár, 2002). A small number of cultivars do not produce significant amounts of carotenoids; when chlorophyll levels decrease in the last stages of ripening, these chilies develop a pale hue often referred to as "white". Due to small amounts of chlorophyll and/or yellow carotenoids, the "white" is, however, more precisely described as a pale greenish-yellow.

Some varieties of paprika contain pigments of anthocyanin type and develop dark purple, aubergine-coloured or almost black pods; in the last stage of ripening, however, the anthocyanins get decomposed, and the unusual darkness thus gives way to normal orange or red colors. The same anthocyanins cause the dark spots which are sometimes seen on unripe fruits or particularly the stems of paprika plants and which almost all paprika varieties can develop. In other *Capsicum* species, anthocyanin production is a rare phenomenon.

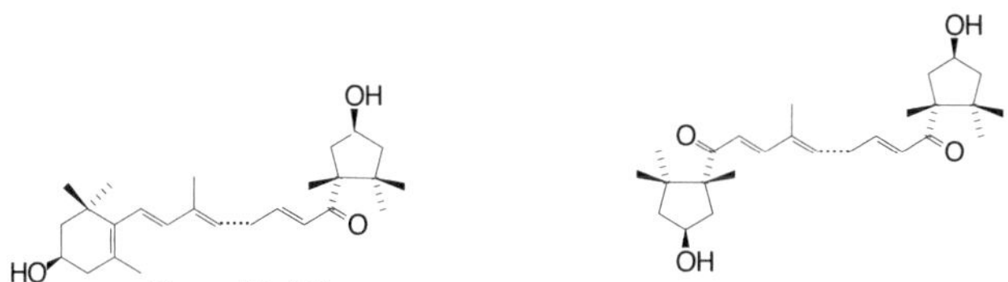

Capsanthin (**11**) Capsorubin (**12**)

Figure 3. Structure of capsanthin (11) and capsorubin (12).

2.3. Capsaicinoids

Capsicum fruits have been valued for over a thousand of years for the piquant taste they added to the flavorless foods, as well as for the therapeutic effects as a stimulant and counter irritant. These effects have been related to the components stimulating pungency.

The degree of pungency (heat or bite) is determined by the amount of compounds called capsaicinoids. These substances produce the characteristic sensations associated with ingestion of spicy cuisine as well as the agents responsible for causing severe irritation, inflammation, erythema, and transient hypo-and hyperalgesia at sites exposed to paprika extracts. Capsaicinoids are particulary irritating to the eyes, skin, nose, tongue and respiratory tract.

The nature of the causal components in the spice has been established as a mixture of acid amides of vanillylamine and C_8 to C_{13} fatty acids, which are known generally as *capsaicinoids*. The major capsaicinoids in red peppers are *capsaicin* (13), *dihydrocapsaicin* (17) and *nordihydrocapsaicin* (16) (Table 1). In commercial *Capsicums*, *capsaicin* generally comprises 33-59%, *dihydrocapsaicin* accounts for 30-51%, *nordihidrocapsaicin* is 7-15% and the remainder is less than 5% of the capsaicinoids (Reineccius, 1994).

The seven homologous branched-chain alkyl vanillylamides are *capsaicin* (13), *homocapsaicin I* (14), *homocapsaicin II* (15), *nordihydrocapsaicin* (16), *dihydrocapsaicin* (17), *homodihydrocapsaicin I* (18) and *homodihydrocapsaicin II* (19). (Hoffman et al., 1983; Reilly et al., 2001a, Karnka et al., 2002). In addition, three straight-chain analogs, octanoyl vanillylamide (20), nonoyl vanillylamide (nonivamide) (21) and decyl vanillylamide (22), have also been shown to occur in *Capsicum* fruits (Govindarajan, 1986d).

Each capsaicinoid possesses a 3-hydroxy-4-methoxybenzylamide (vanilloid) pharmacophore, but differ from *capsaicin* from their hydrophobic alkyl side chain. Differences in the side chain moiety include saturation of the carbon-carbon double bond, deletion of a methyl group, and changes in the length of the hydrocarbon chain. The structures of capsaicin as well as its homologs and analogs are given in Table 1.

Name	Structure
capsaicin (13)	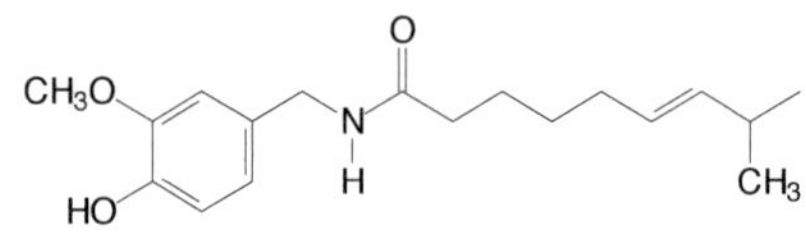
homocapsaicin I (14)	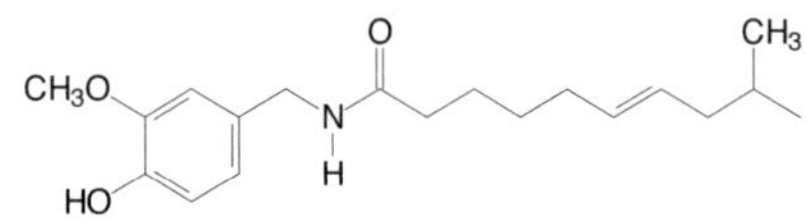
homocapsaicin II (15)	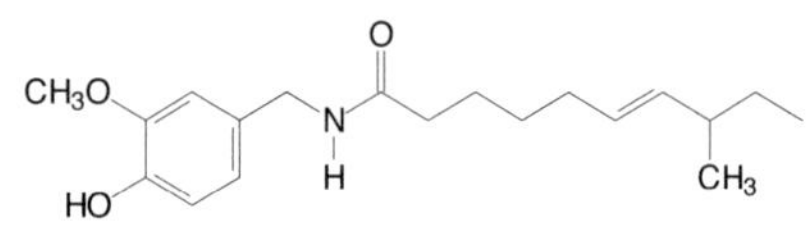
nordihydrocapsaicin (16)	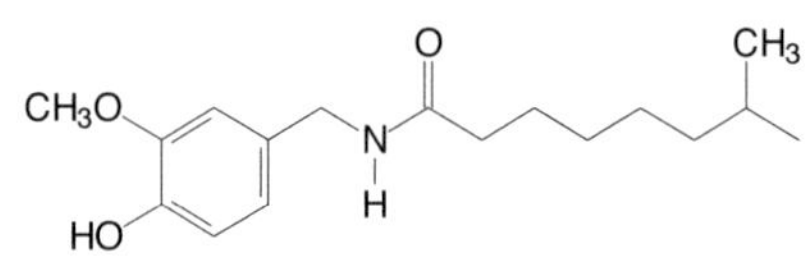
dihydrocapsaicin (17)	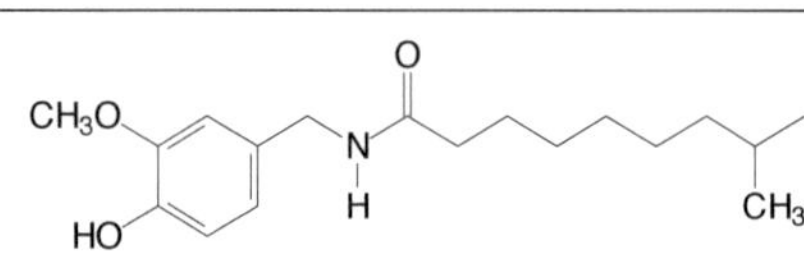
homodihydrocapsaicin I (18)	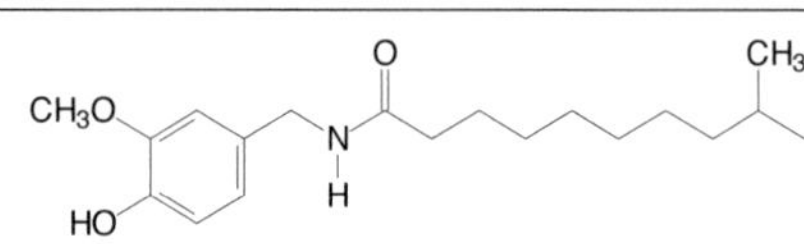
homodihydrocapsaicin II (19)	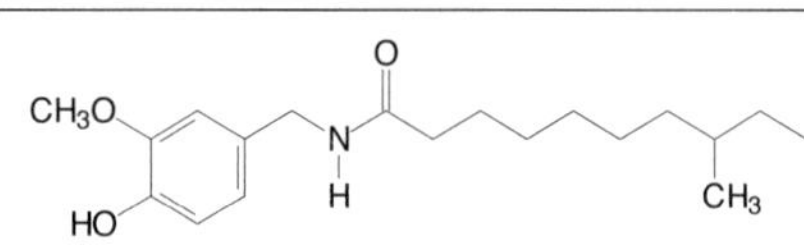
octanoyl vanillylamide (20)	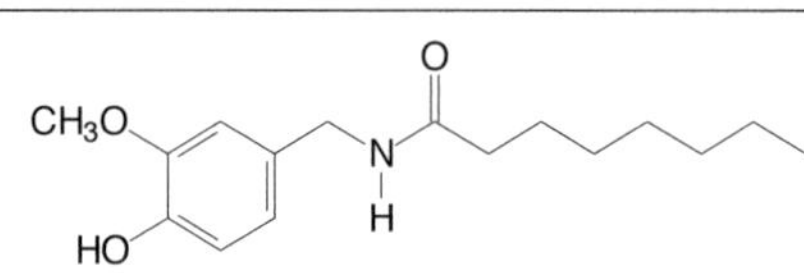
nonoyl vanillylamide (21)	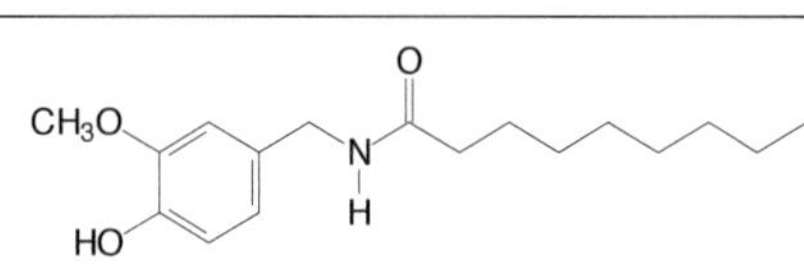
decyl vanillylamide (22)	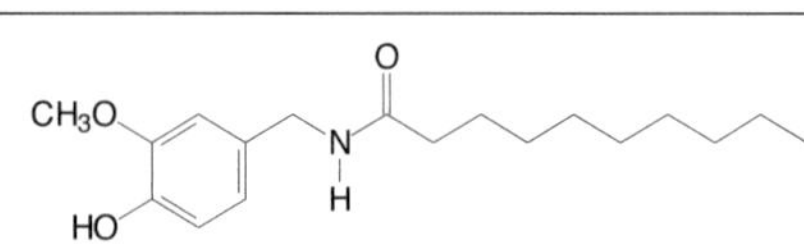

Table 1. Chemical structures of capsaicin homologs and analogs.

http://dx.doi.org/10.5772/58812

Capsaicin and its natural homologs are always found in the *trans* (*E*) form because in the *cis* (*Z*) isomer, the-$CH(CH_3)_2$ and the longer chain on the other side of the Δ6,7 carbon-carbon double bond will be too close to each other which causes strong repulsive force. This steric hindrance does not exist in the *trans* isomer, so the (*E*) form is a more stable arrangement than (*Z*) form.

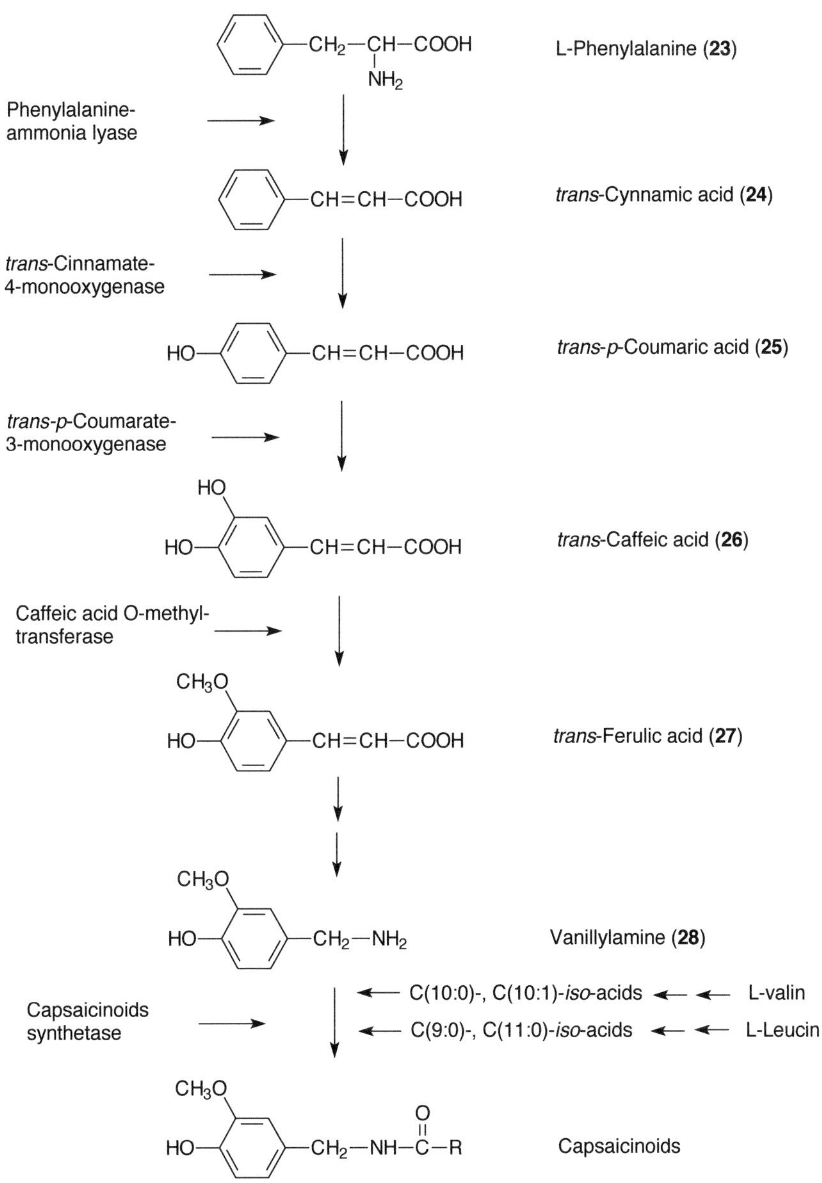

Figure 4. Simplifies biochemical pathway of synthesis of capsaicinoids.

The capsaicin biosynthetic pathway has two distinct branches, one of which utilizes L-phenylalanine (23) as the precursor of aromatic residue of capsaicinoids, presumably via *trans*-cinnamic acid (24) and its hydroxylated derivatives *trans*-caffeic acid (26) and *trans*-ferulic acid (27) following the well-established pathways in other plants (Ishikawa, 2003). Vanillylamine (28) as precursor showed a high level of incorporation into the capsaicinoids and possibly the immediate progenitor of natural capsaicinoids (Figure 4). The enzymes involved in the formation of the precursors, phenolics, and fatty acids, are similar to those studied for long in other biological systems. The second group of enzymes form the branched-chained fatty acids by elongation of deaminated valine (Figure 4). The *capsaicinoids synthetase*, however, has been found to have narrow specificity in accepting only the *iso*-C(9:0) to C(11:0) fatty acids and in the fruit system forming predominantly the vanillylamides of even-number branched fatty acids, capsaicin (13) and dihydrocapsaicin (17), in all the cultivated varieties of the *Capsicum* species (Ravishankar et al., 2003). In the isolated systems, however, the synthethase favors formation of capsaicin (13) and nordihydrocapsaicin (16), while the light induced activation of the synthase in *Capsicum annuum* cv. *grossum*, results in higher formation of nordihydrocapsaicin (16) and dihydrocapsaicin (17) (Govindarajan, 1986a,b). Synthesis of capsaicinoids by means of recent development of biotechnological methods has been reviewed in deatails (Ravishankar et al., 2003).

3. Quality control

Capsicum is now one of the two most widely used spices. Quality of food should fulfill the consumers' expectations – not necessarily the maximum of each attribute, but the optimal level and combination appropriate for each food. Thus a range of quality attributes is required to make different foods of optimal quality. Quality control which can be exercised through measurement of the physical and chemical properties of the component stimuli needs to be validated by a relationship with sensoryly perceived responses individually and in combination. It is obvious that the accuracy and reproducibility of any instrumental method meaningful for food quality measure is that which correlates with the sensoryly perceivable differences (Kramer, 1966).

Besides the sensory attributes, capsicum like other products used as foods and food additives, should also have certain functional properties for its optimal use in the industrial sectors, which also have to be considered. The standards of the importing countries are based on the requirements of the food processing industries and include additional emphasis on cleanliness, which progressively cover, in addition to insects and rodent parts, limits of chemical and microbiological contaminations, and freedom of health-hazard organisms. These specifications assure genuiness, purity and cleanliness, but they do not give information on the sensory attributes which the consumers require. In the case of some processed products, e.g., ground paprika and oleoresin, specifications for total color and capsaicinoid content are found in standards and manufacturer literature, these being the main selling factors in this increasing competitive market (Govindarajan, 1986c).

Herbs and fruits that are used as spice, active pharmaceutical ingredients of drugs, or constituents of food additives should also fulfill even more special requirements described by the Pharmacopoeias and/or other international organizations like EC, FAO, WHO, ISO, ASTA, etc., and national bodies, which guide the industry concerned in the respective activities such as manufacturing or trade. The standards are the results of conscientious efforts in standardization. In the lack of space, it is not possible to cover all such standards. Only those have been listed that are closely related to the quality of *Capsicum* and *Capsicum*-originated products that can be used for the pharmaceutical industry.

3.1. Capsicum fruits

3.1.1. Capsicum (Ph. Eur. 7.0)

The 2011 edition of the European Pharmacopoeia Edition 7.0 (Ph. Eur. 7.0) lists *Capsicum fruit* (Capsici fructus) and describes its *Definition, Identification, Nonivamid Test*, and *Assay* as follows.

DEFINITION: Dried ripe fruits of *Capsicum annuum* L. var. *minimum* (Miller) Heise and small-fruited varieties of *Capsicum frutescens* L.

CONTENT: Minimum 0,4 per cent of total capsaicinoids expressed as capsaicin ($C_{18}H_{27}NO_3$; M_r 305.4) (dried drug).

IDENTIFICATION

a. The fruit is yellowish-orange to reddish-brown, oblong conical with an obtuse apex, about 1 cm to 3 cm long and up to 1 cm in diameter at the widest part, occasionally attached to a 5-toothed inferior calyx and a straight pedicel. Pericarp somewhat shrivelled, glabrous, enclosing about 10 to 20 flat, reniform seeds 3 mm to 4 mm long, either loose or attached to a reddish dissepiment.

b. Reduce to a powder. The powder is orange. Examine under a microscope using *chloral hydrate solution R*. The powder shows the following diagnostic characters: fragments of the pericarp having an outer epicarp with cells often arranged in rows of 5 to 7, cotucle uniformly striated: parenchymatous cells frequently containing droplets of red oil, occasionally containing misrosphenoidal crystals of calcium oxalabe; endocarp with characteristic island groups of sclerenchymatous cells, the groups being separated by thin-walled parenchymatous cells. Fragments of the seeds having an episperm composed of large, greenish-yellow, sinuous-walled sclereids with thin outer walls and strongly and unevenly thickened radial and inner walls which are conspicuously pitted; endosperm parenchymatous cells with drops of fixed oil and aleurone grains 3 μm to 6 μm in diameter. Occassional fragments from the calyx having an outer epidermis with anisocytis stomata, inner epidermis with many trichomes but no stomata; trichomes glandular, with uniseriate stalks and multicellular heads; mesophyll with many idioblasts containing microsphenoidal crystals of calcium oxalate.

c. Thin-layer chromatography.

Test solution. To 0.50 g of the powdered drug (500) add 5.0 ml of *ether R,* shake for 5 min and filter.

Reference solution. Dissolve 2 mg of *capsaicin R* and 2 mg of *dihidrocapsaicin R* in 5.0 ml of ether R.

Plate: *TLC octadecylsilyl silica gel plate R. Mobile phase: water R, methanol R* (20:80 V/V).

Aplication: 20 μl, as bands.

Development: over a path of 12 cm.

Drying: in air.

Detection: spray with a 5 g/l solution of *dichloroquinonechlorimide R* in *methanol R.*

Expose the plate to ammonia vapour until blue zones appear. Examine in daylight.

Results: see below the sequence of the zones present in the chromatograms obtained with the reference solution and the test solution. Furthermore, other zones may be present in the chromatogram obtained with the test solution (Figure 5).

Top of the plate	
Capsaicin: a blue zone	A blue zone (capsaicin)
Dyhidrocapsaicin: a blue zone	A blue zone (dihydrocapsaicin)
Reference Solution	**Test solution**

Figure 5 Characterization of the top of the TLC plate (Ph. Eur. 7.0)

TESTS

Nonivamide. Liquid chromatography.

Test solution. To 2.5 g of the powdered drug add 100 ml of *methanol R.* Allow to macerate for 30 min. Place in an ultrasonic bath for 15 min. Filter into a 100 ml volumetric flask, rinse the flask and filter with *methanol R.* Dilute to 100,0 ml with *methanol R.*

Reference solution. Dissolve 20.0 mg of *capsaicin R* and 4.0 mg of *nonivamide R* in 100.0 ml of *methanol R.*

Column: *size*: l=0.25 m, ∅=4.6 mm; *stationary phase*: phenylsilyl silica gel for chromatography R (5 μm); *temperature*: 30 °C.

Mobile phase: mixture of 40 volumes of *acetonitril R* and 60 volumes of a 1 g/l solution of *phosphoric acid R.*

Flow rate: 1.0 ml/min.; *Detection:* spectrophotometer at 225 nm.; *Injection:* 10 μl.

System suitability: reference solution:

- *resolution:* minimum 3.0 between the peaks due to capsaicin and nonivamide.

Limit: calculate the percentage content of nonivamide

- *nonivamide:* maximum 5.0 per cent of the total capsaicinoid content.

ASSAY: Liquid chromatography as described in the test for nonivamide.

3.2. Capsicum extracts

Presently, virtually all commercial spice extraction is carried out by one of two methods. One the methods is solvent extraction, wich involves treating a ground dry spice with an organic solvent such as hexane, acetone, methanol, ethanol or methylene chloride. Pursuant to this method, the spice extract is recovered by removal of the solvent, usually by distillation with heat under vacuum. The spice extract recovered in this way is known as an "Oleoresin" (Eisvale, 1981; Pruthi, 2003). In the case of oleoresin from *Capsicum*, the oleoresin is further treated with polar solvent, methanol, in order to separate the pungent component *Oleoresin Capsicum* from the color component *Oleoresin paprika*. Oleoresins are used almost exclusively by the food and pharmaceutical industries as a substitute of ground spices and spice tinctures.

The composition of an oleoresin is affected by the choice of organic solvent used in the extraction, but typically will include phospholipids, oils, waxes, sterols, resins, and a range of non-volatile and volatile compounds which make up much of the aroma and flavor of the original spice. In its use as food additive, the best oleoresin of *Capsicum* is that which contains the color and flavor components and that which truly recreates, when appropriately diluted in food formulations, the sensory qualities of fresh materials (Govindarajan, 1986c).

The other commercial method of spice extraction is the aqueous distillation of the whole or ground, fresh or dried spice using either boiling water or steam. This method recovers only the steam volatile components of the spice; i.e., the "*Essential oil*" which is high in aroma and flavor compounds (Simon, 1990). Many variations of these two methods are possible. The essential oil may be prepared by distillation from the original spice, or by distillation from a previously prepared solvent extracted oleoresin.

These traditional processes have a number of disadvantages. Most organic solvents are toxic, and government food regulations dictate that their residues must be reduced in the oleoresin to very small concentrations, generally in the range of 25-30 ppm or less (Pruthi, 2003). The distillation processes used to remove the solvents, or to recover essential oils, lowers the content of the very light volatiles which contribute to aroma and flavor. Of more importance is the growing consumer demand for food ingredients which are completely natural and free of contact with synthetic chemicals.

Extraction of spices with supercritical fluid carbon dioxide has been proposed as a means of eliminating the use of organic solvents and providing the prospect of simultaneous fractionation of the extract. The use of supercritical fluids (SCF) for extraction purposes was introduced in the late nineteenth century. A supercritical fluid is a substance at temperatures and pressures beyond its critical point at which the liquid phase of the substance will not exist. At these temperatures and pressures, the supercritical fluid has properties between gas-and liquid-phase characteristics. These properties make supercritical fluids efficient extraction solvents with high mass transfer characteristics (McHugh and Krukonis, 1986;; Krukonis, 1988). Consequently, supercritical fluids are often used to selectively extract or separate specific compounds from a mixture by varying fluid density through changes in pressure and temperature. In food technology, the use of supercritical fluids is essentially limited to supercritical carbon dioxide (SCF-CO_2) extraction since carbon dioxide has the advantages of being inexpensive and nontoxic and because its critical point is easily reached.

Oleoresins have several advantages over ground spices, e.g., elimination of microbial contamination, uniformity of color and flavor strenght and optimal utilization. The Essential Oil Association of America has detailed specifications for three types of *Capsicum* oleoresins (Table 2). *Oleoresin paprika* is mainly used as food coloring in meats, dairy products, soups, sauces and snacks. *Oleoresin red pepper* is used for both coloring and pungency, mainly in canned meats, sausages, in some snacks and in a dispersed form in some drinks such as ginger ale. *Oleoresin Capsicum* is the most pungent and is used for its counter-irritant properties in plasters and some pharmaceutical preparations.

Type of oleoresin Capsicum	Botanical source	Preparation	Color value	Color discription	Scoville Heat Units
Oleoresin Capsicum (EOA No. 244)	C. frutescens or C. annuum	Solvent extraction	4,000 max	Clear red, light amber, or dark red	480,000 min
Oleoresin red pepper (EOA No. 245)	C. annuum var. lognum	Solvent extraction	20,000 max	Deep red	240,000 min
Oleoresi paprika (EOA No. 239)	C. annuum	Solvent extraction	40,000-100,000	Deep red	Nil or negligible

Table 2. Nomenclature of oleoresins of Capsicums (Essential Oils Association, 1975).

3.2.1. Capsicum Oleoresin

The 2012 edition of the United States Pharmacopoeia-National Formulary (*USP36-NF31*) lists *Capsicum Oleoresin* and describes its *Capsicum Oleoresin* as follows.

3.2.1.1. Capsicum Oleoresin (USP30-NF25)

DEFINITION: *Capsicum Oleoresin* is an alcoholic extract of the dried ripe fruits of *Capsicum annum* var. *minimum* and small fruited varieties of *C. frutescens* (Solanaceae). It contains not less than 8.0 percent of total capsaicins [capsaicin ($C_{18}H_{27}NO_3$), dihydrocapsaicin ($C_{18}H_{29}NO_3$), and nordihydrocapsaicin ($C_{17}H_{27}NO_3$)].

IDENTIFICATION: To about 0.5 g of it in a beaker add 5 mL of water and 10 mL of a mixture of water, 0.2 *M* potassium chloride, and 0.2 N hydrochloric acid, and mix. Add 5.0 mL of 0.5 *M* sodium nitrite and 5.0 mL of 0.02 *M* sodium tungstate, and mix. Heat at 55° to 60° for 15 minutes, allow to cool, and filter. To the filtrate add 10 mL of 1 N sodium hydroxide: a bright yellow color is produced (*presence of capsaicin*).

ASSAY

Mobile phase— Prepare a mixture of methanol and 2% acetic acid (56:44), filter through a 0.5-µm or finer porosity filter, and degas.

Standard preparation— Prepare a solution of *USP Capsaicin RS* in methanol having a known concentration of about 0.5 mg per mL. Filter a portion of this solution through a 0.2-µm porosity filter, and use the filtrate as the *Standard preparation.*

Assay preparation— Transfer about 1000 mg of *Capsicum Oleoresin*, accurately weighed, to a 100-mL volumetric flask, dissolve in and dilute with methanol to volume, and mix. Filter a portion of this solution through a 0.2-µm porosity filter, and use the filtrate as the *Assay preparation.*

Chromatographic system— The liquid chromatograph is equipped with a 280-nm detector and a 3.9-mm × 30-cm column that contains packing L1. The flow rate is about 2 mL per minute. Chromatograph the *Standard preparation*, and record the peak responses as directed for *Procedure:* the tailing factor is not more than 2.0; and the relative standard deviation for replicate injections is not more than 2.0%. Chromatograph the *Assay preparation*, and record the peak responses as directed for *Procedure:* the relative retention times are about 0.9 for nordihydrocapsaicin, 1.0 for capsaicin, and 1.6 for dihydrocapsaicin; and the resolution, *R*, between the nordihydrocapsaicin peak and the capsaicin peak is not less than 1.2.

Procedure— Separately inject equal volumes (about 10 µL) of the *Standard preparation* and the *Assay preparation* into the chromatograph, record the chromatograms, and measure the responses for the three major peaks. Calculate the percentage of total capsaicins in the portion of *Capsicum Oleoresin* taken by the formula:

$$(CP / W)(r_U / r_S)$$

in which

C is the concentration, in mg per mL, of *USP Capsaicin RS* in the *Standard preparation;*

P is the designated purity, in percentage, of *USP Capsaicin RS,*

W is the weight, in mg, of *Capsicum Oleoresin* taken to prepare the *Assay preparation;*

r_U is the sum of the peak responses for nordihydrocapsaicin, capsaicin, and dihydrocapsaicin obtained from the *Assay preparation*; and

r_S is the peak response obtained from the *Standard preparation.*

3.3. Quantitation of capsicum pigments

Appearance and color, the first of the percieved attributes, directly provide a basis for a decision of appropriateness. Size, shape, and maximum percentage of defects are easily measured specifications are given in standards. Color of *Capsicum* fruits is basicly determined by the nature and distribution of the above described carotenoids of which can be hidden or modified by other pigments such as chlorophylls and anthocyanins. The major coloring pigments in paprika are capsanthin and capsorubin, comprising majority of the total carotenoids. Other pigments are *beta*-carotene, zeaxanthin, violaxanthin, neoxantin and lutein (Anu and Peter, 2000). It is also worth repatedly mentioning that the relative amounts of the colored pigments are changing during the ripening period according to a rather well investigated biochemical pathways (Rodriguez-Amaya, 1997; Rahman and Buckle, 1980; Hornero-Mendez et al., 2000; Gnayfeed et al., 2001; Deli and Molnár, 2002).

It is also worth mentioning that carotenoid research in the field of plant and food chemistry is a very extensive area. The interested readers can consult recent reviews to learn the analytical methods that are currently used to analyse plant and food samples for their carotenoid contents (Rodriguez-Amaya, 1997; Wall and Bosland, 1998; Deli and Molnár, 2002; Felt et al., 2005). Some of the methods to measure coloring parameters of paprika and oleoresins currently accepted as official are summarized below.

3.3.1. The color matching method

This early method for total pigments expressed as Nesslerimeter color value used in the industry was standardized and adopted by the Essential Oils Association of America (EOA) for *Oleoresin Capsicum* (Essential Oil Association (1975): Specification of oleoresin paprika – EOA No. 239, Oleoresin Capsicum – EOA No. 244, Oleoresin red pepper – EOA No. 245, Essential Oil Association, New York). The method is based on matching the color of the properly diluted oleoresin acetone solution with that of a potasium dichromate ($K_2Cr_2O_7$) and cobaltous chloride ($CoCl_2 \times 6H_2O$) containing reference solutions.

3.3.2. Spectrophotometric methods

The alternative method uses the spectrophotometer to measure the total carotenoid pigments.

3.3.2.1. The EOA method

(Essential Oil Association (1975): Specification of oleoresin paprika – EOA No. 239, Oleoresin Capsicum – EOA No. 244, Oleoresin red pepper – EOA No. 245, Essential Oil Association, New York)

The absorbance of a 0.01% acetone solution of oleoresin is measured at 458 nm. The absorbance value is multiplied by 61,000 (an empirical factor worked out to relate the data from the color matching method) gives the total pigment as the Nesslerimeter color value.

3.3.2.2. The American Spice Trade Association (ASTA) method

By the above spectrophotometric method, results from different laboratories were not directly comparable due to differences in the spectrophotometers. In the new ASTA 20.1 Method (ASTA, 1968) a reference solution of inorganic salts (potassium dichromate and cobaltous ammonium sulfate in 1.8 M sulfuric acid solution) absorbing in the same region as the carotenoids is used to calculate an instrument factor which makes interlaboratory comparison possible. In the ASTA Method 20.1 for extractable color (pigments) in *Capsicums* absorbance of acetone extract of ground paprika and other capsicums is measured at 460 nm. The color value (in ASTA) is calculated using the determined instrument correction factor.

A direct correlation between the earlier ASTA Method 19, measuring absorbance at 450 nm, and the new Method 20.1 can not be established, an empirical factor (16.4) in the formula to give values nearly equal to those obtained by the earlier Method No. 19.

3.3.2.3. The Hungarian standard method

In Hungary, where specified grades of ground paprika are produced (*csípős, csemege, édes-nemes*), the total pigments are determined by similar absorbtion measurements. Earlier, the total pigment concentration in ground capsicums or in oleoresins was calculated by using the extinction coefficient in benzene of the major pigment capsanthin ($^{1\%}E_{477nm}$=1826). The results were expressed in grams of capsanthin per kilograms of dry matter (Hungarian Standard. Examination of Ground Paprika Spice. Determination of Pigment Content, MSZ 9681/5-76.). At present, the measurements are performed using acetone extracts similar to the ASTA Method 20.1 (MSZ 9681-5:2002)

3.4. Quantitation of pungent principles

For the major portion of *Capsicum* species pruduced and traded, pungency is the important quality attribute. The nature of the causal components in the spice has been established as a mixture of seven homologous branched-chain alkyl vanillylamides, named *capsaicinoids*. Smal amounts of three straight-chain analogues have also been shown to occure. The chemistry of these compounds has been reviewed (Suzuki and Iwai, 1984). The structures are given in Table 1.

The average composition of these related vanillylamides in the videly traded chillis (*Capsicum annuum* var. *annuum*) varieties is capsaicin 33 to 59%; dihydrocapsaicin, 30 to 51%; nordihy-drocapsaicin, 7 to 15%; and others, in the range of 0 to 5% each. Fruits of the species *Capsicum frutescens*, stimulating high pungency and mostly used in the pharmaceutical industry, have higher capsaicin (63 to 77%) and dihydrocapsaicin (20 to 32%) with other homologues and analogues making up around 10% (Jurenitsch et al., 1978). The total capsaicinoids varied greatly (0.001 to 0.01% in paprika and 0.1 to >1% in chillis), but the proportion of capsaicin and dihydrocapsain ranged from 77 to 90% int he fruits of the species *C. annuum* and from 89 to 98% in those from species *C. frutescens* (Govindarajan et al., 1987).

The pungency stimulated by the different alkyl acyl vanillylamides varied greatly, all much lower compared to capsaicin and dihydrocapsaicin, which were equal (Govindarajan et al.,

1987). Thus, the estimation of total capsaicinoids, reproducibly and accurately correlating with the determined pungency, should be sufficient for quality control. Where the minor capsaicin-related vanillylamides make up a larger portion (above 20%), however, their individual estimation could become necessary because they stimulate much lower pungency. It is also known for a long time that synthetic nonoyl vanillylamide (pelargonyl vanillylamide) has considearable pungency and heat (Kulka, 1967). and has been found in varying amounts in commercial oleoresins. Therefore, it was necessary to determine the upper limits of the straight chain analogs to determine adulteration.

3.4.1. Official methods for organoleptic determination of pungency

3.4.1.1. The Scoville method

A number of methods have been reported from time to time since 1912 for assaying the pungency or capsaicin content of *Capsicum* fruits and/or the processed fruits (Pruthi, 2003). The basic principle of pungency evaluation using an organoleptic method was eshtablished in 1912 by W. L. Scoville (Scoville, 1912). The method is based on sensory evaulation determining the amount of sugar to neutralize the heat from the pepper. A solution of the pepper extract is variably diluted with sugar solution are tested in increasing concentration. The highest dilution at wich pungency is just detected is taken as a measure of the heat value. The dilution value, in milliliters per gram has since then been called Scoville Heat Units (SHU). The SHU for pure capsaicin is reported as 16-17 x 10^6. The Scoville Heat Units of various chilli pepper varieties are shown in Table 3. The greatest weakness of the Scoville organoleptic test is its imprecision, because it relies on human subjectivity.

Type	Heat rating (in Scoville Heat Units)
Habanero	200,000-300,000
Tabasco	30,000-50,000
Cayenne	35,000
Serrano	7,000-25,000
Jalapeno	3,500-4,500
Anaheim	1,000-1,400
Bell & Pimento	0

Table 3. The Scoville Heat Units of various chilli pepper varieties.

3.4.1.2. The EOA method

This method (Essential Oil Association (1975): Specification of oleoresin paprika – EOA No. 239, Oleoresin Capsicum – EOA No. 244, Oleoresin red pepper – EOA No. 245, Essential Oil Association, New York) is the codification of the procedure that was in use by the spice processing industry to check the constancy of pungency of a usual trade variety and source.

The method, based on the approach of the original Scoville method, specified for oleoresins of capsicum as follows.

A standard solution for testing is made by diluting a stock alcoholic solution of the oleoresin and it is tested by five trained panelists. If three of the five on a panel agree on just perceptible pungency at the given dilution (which is equivalent to 240,000 ml/g), this value is called the SHU of pungency of the sample. If the pungency response is strong, this first diluted standard is further diluted and the panel testing is repeated to find the dilution at which three of the five judge the pungency just perceptible. The Scoville test run shows a rather high correlation to total capsaicinoids content (1,500,000 Scoville units=1% capsaicin).

3.4.1.3. The British standard method

The British Standard Institution adapted the above industry procedure except that dilutions were rationalized in more convenient volumes (British Standards Institution (1979): Methods for testing spices and condiments: Determination of Scoville index of chillies, BS 4548 (Part 7), BSI, London)

3.4.1.4. The International Standard Organization (ISO) method

The British Standard Method adopted and improved by the International Standards Organization (ISO) requires the testing of a series of dilutions around the anticipated value by individuals experienced in recognizing pungency (International Standards Organization (1997): Spices and condiments – chillies: Determination of Scoville index, ISO 3513:1977E, ISO, Geneva). Testing of dilutions should be done from the weekest to the strongest until a level at which three of five panelists agree on recognition pungency. There is no published reports on the extensive use and efficiency of these latter two methods, except a few which reported comparison of experimentally determined SHU values with that of calculated based on capsaicinoid content of oleoresin capsicum samples. (Suzuki et al., 1957).

3.4.1.5. The ASTA method

The ASTA adopted as early as 1968 Method No. 21.0 as an official method for pungency evaluation which took care of many variables that were to be controlled for good reproducibility (ASTA (1968): Method 21.0, Pungency of capsicum spices and oleoresins (Scoville heat test), In: Official Analytical Methods, ASTA, Englewood Cliffs, N.J.). The procedure followed in the industry and EOA was thoroughly revised by designing it as a general method applicable to samples of a large range of capsaicinoids content by careful steps for determining the recognition threshold using an ascending concentration series.

3.5. Quantitation of capsaicinoids

In addition to pungency, as a bulk characteristics of total capsaicinoids, estimation of individual level of each capsaicinoid is also an important quality attribute of *Capsicum* fruits. There are over a hundred papers published on the estimation of total capsaicinoids in *Capsicum* fruits, the oleoresins and products containing their extracts. The methods can be grouped into four sets as follows:

3.5.1. Early direct and methods

As early as 1931, von Fodor used vanadium oxytrichloride or ammonium vanadate and hydrochloric acid to react with the phenolic hydroxyl group of capsaicinoids and measured the blue color formed. The accuracy of determinations based on color formation reactions of the phenolic moiety could be conveniently used when the color produced with the chromogenic reagent had absorption maxima far removed from the absorption range (300 to 550 nm) of the red and yellow carotenoids of *Capsicum* fruits. Thus the blue colors formed when the phenolic moiety of the capsaicinoids reacted with reagents such as vanadium oxychloride (Palacio, 1977) and phosphomolybdic or phosphotungstic reagents (Jentzsch et al., 1969) had their absorption maxima around 725 nm. On the other and, the chromophore produced by the more specific 2,6-dichloro-*p*-benzoquinone-4-chlorimide (Gibb's phenol reagent), depending on the reaction conditions, absorbed maximally at 590 or 615 nm (Jentzsch et al., 1969; Rajpoot and Govindarajan, 1981). The extinction coefficients for the blue colours using different reagents varied greately and affected sensitivity. There are also reports using potassium ferricianide plus ferric chloride (Spanyar and Blazovich, 1969) sodium nitrite molybdate reagent (Bajaj, 1980) and Folin-Ciocalteu reagent (Kosuge and Inagaki, 1959) as chromogenic reagents for determination of total capsaicinoids. It is worth mentioning that the color reactions could also be applied for visualization of thin layer chromatography (TLC) spots of separated capsaicinoids.

3.5.2. Methods based on separation of capsaicinoids

The specificity and accuracy of determination of capsaicinoids were improved by a preliminary separation of interfering pigments and other substances. In the early methods separation of capsaicinoids from the pigments was accomplished by solvent partition. Several combination of partition system has been found in the literature (Spanya et al., 1957; Benedek, 1959; Chem. Abstr. 1963a; Tirimanna, 1972) none of the methods, however, was validated by pungency tests, without which the accuracy of the determination can not be ascertained.

There have been several methods developed for preliminary separation of capsaicinoids from the *Capsicum* pigments using short column clean-up methods. The purified capsaicinoids were quantitated by colorimetry after reacting with chromogenic reagents (Hollo et al., 1957, Chem. Abstr., 1958; Bajaj, 1980) or directly at the absorption maxima (282 nm) of pure capsaicin (Suzuki et al., 1957; Brawer and Schoen, 1962; Chem. Abstr., 1963b). Suzuki et al. determined pungency values for a number of chilli and oleoresin samples by threshold testing and validated the capsaicinoids values determined by the proposed method (Suzuki et al., 1957). After several reviews, the Joint committe (Pharmaceutical Society/Society of Analytical Chemistry) recommended the diethyl ether-alkali partition method for separation and the spectrophotometric difference method or the method using the Gibb's reagent for measurement (Joint Committee (PS/SAC) 1964). The method has been adopted by both the British

Standards (BS) and International Standards Institutions (ISO) for estimation of capsaicinoids (International Standards Organization, 1981).

3.5.2.1. Thin layer chromatography

As newer separation methods emerged (e.g., paper chromatography and TLC) which gave rapid and more efficient separation, they were quickly used in the determination of total and later the individual capsaicinoids. The main body of papers in the 1960s practically relegated the earlier solvent partition and column methods to the past and published reliable, rapid micromethods. Most of the early thin layer chromatography (TLC) methods used silica gel plates with a wide range of variations in the developing solvents. The versatility of TLC method for separation of complex mixture of compounds could be further improved, however, by using reversed-phase plates and polar developing solvents containing silver nitrate (Todd et al., 1975). Methods of visualization applied UV light or chromogenic reagents. The estimation method also varied: visual comparison of size and intensity of spots, direct densitometry on the plate, collection of the marked spot into a tube, development of color with a chromogenic reagent and absorption measurements. Quantitation was by reference to a standard curve using pure capsaicinoids treated under the same conditions. A comprehensive listing of the methods can be found in some reviews on capsaicinoids (Suzuki, and Iwai, 1984; Govindarajan et al., 1987).

3.5.2.2. Gas chromatography

Gas chromatography (GC) was early used to detect adulteration of capsaicinoids with synthetic vanillylamides and individual components in crystalline capsaicinoids through the analysis of methyl esters of fatty acids derived from them (see Table 2). As early as 1967, Morrison demonstrated that capsaicinoids can be analyzed by gas chromatography without derivatization (Morrison, 1967). In order to improve peak symmetry, prevent degradation of column and improve reproducibility of measurements, however, most of the GC methods need derivatization step to increase volatility of the capsaicinoids, and, furthermore, an efficient clean-up step is necessary (Todd et al., 1977; Iwai et al., 1979; Krajewska and Powers, 1987; Manirakiza et al., 1999). Two types of derivatization procedures have been reported: trimethylsilylation of capsaicinoids (Lee et al., 1976; Todd et al., 1977; Iwai et al., 1979; Fung et al., 1982) and hydrolysis of capsaicinoids to yield fatty acids and subsequent esterification (Jurenitsch et al., 1978; Jurenitsch and Leinmueller, 1980). To overcome the problem of tailing peaks and to avoid the use of derivatization step, Thomas et al. (Thomas et al., 1998) and Hawer et al. (Hawer et al., 1994) have recognized the use of polar capillary column for interaction with polar functional group of the molecules. In an earlier work Di Cecco also used stable polar analytical column (Carbowax-Teflon) to analyse column purified capsaicinoids from ground capsicum (Di Cecco, 1976). Furthermore, the use of a thermoionic selective detector (TSD) instead of flame ionization detection allowed the elimination of sample clean-up (Thomas et al., 1998)

Although direct analysis of capsaicinoids could be disandvantageous direct GC-MS analysis of commercially available natural capsainoids has been proved to be a proper method to separate the main capsaicinoids and quantitate capsaicin and dihydrocapsaicin in *Capsicum* extracts as well (Kuzma et al., 2006) A typical gas chromatogram of a commercially available natural capsaicin is shown on Figure 6.

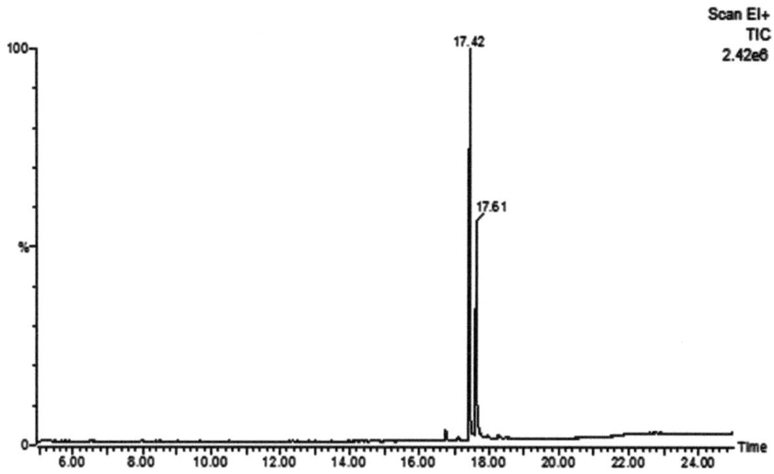

Figure 6. Gas chromatogram of a commercially available natural capsaicin preparation (Mózsik et al., 2009). Retention times: 16.8 min (not shown): nordihydrocapsaicin; 17.4 min capsaicin; 17.6 min: dihydrocapsaicin.

Lee et al. (Lee et al., 1976) used selective ion monitoring to identify and quantify individual capsaicinoids at the nanogram level in partially or fully separated and even mixed peaks from GC of trimethylsylilated capsaicinoids. Aliquots of fruit extracts were subjected to TLC or reversed phase (RP) HPLC to separate the capsaicinoids from other components of the extracts. Iwai et al. (Iwai et al, 1979) developed a similar method for determining all homologs in total extracts of *Capsicum* fruits. By this analysis, similar to other GC-MS methods (Fung et al., 1982; Reilly et al., 2001a, b) the straight-chain homologs (octanoyl, nonoyl and decyl vanillylamides – identified in minor amounts in other analyzes (Jurenitsch et al., 1978; Jurenitsch and Leinmueller, 1980) – were not found in any of the samples. This was the case because the analysis was based on selected *m/e* values but not on monitoring the mass of octanoyl vanillylamide, and the method could not differentiate between nonoyl vanillylamide and nordihydrocapsaicin eluting in the same area. Pena-Alvarez et al. (Pena-Alvarez et al., 2009) used solid phase microextraction (SPME)–gas chromatography–mass spectrometry for the analysis of capsaicin and dihydrocapsaicin in peppers and pepper sauces. In addition to capsaicin and dihydrocapsaicin, the method could differentiate several straight-chain analogs (e.g. nordihydrocapsaicin, nonoyl vanillylamide, homodihydrocapsaicin I and homodihydrocapsaicin II) in the different peppers and pepper sauces.

3.5.2.3. High performance liqiud chromatography

This chromatographic technique has superior and rapid separation capabilities arising from the use of very fine and highly uniform particles, newer solid phases, and high pressure to

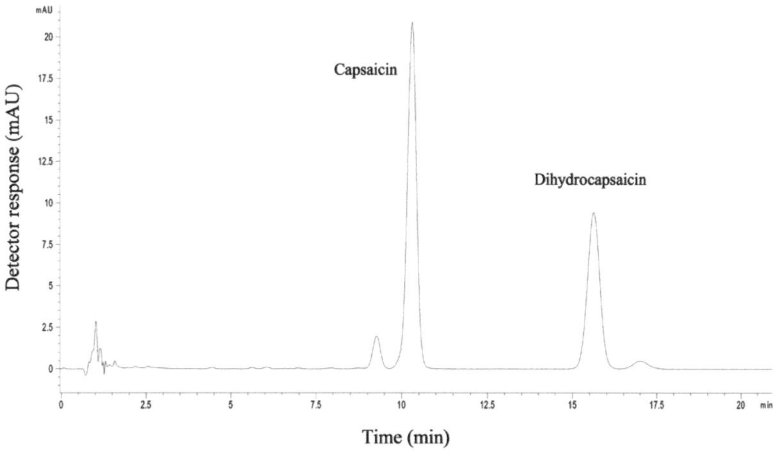

Figure 7. HPLC chromatogram of a commercially available capsaicin preparation (Mózsik et al., 2009). Retention times: 9.3 min: nordihydrocapsaicin; 10.3 min: capsaicin; 15.6 min: dihydrocapsaicin; 17.0 min: homocapsaicin.

move the eluting solvent and fractions. With all its advantages, high performance liquid chromatographic analysis is being increasingly used for routine analyses in both industrial and research laboratories. HPLC has superior separation capabilities for closely related compounds typically occuring in the case of extract of natural sources. Combined with additional operational parametres, e.g., reversed-phase systems, silver-ion complexing of olefinic compounds, optical as well as mass selective detectors, the separation efficiency, sensitivity, and quantification at submicrogram levels of capsaicinoids have been demonstrated in the recent years.

There has been published several HPLC methods for determination of capsaicin homologs and analogs. Since there is no space to summarize all the methods published so far, attention of interested readers is drawn to recent reviews to get a comprehensive knowledge on the field (e.g., Govindarajan et al., 1987; Wall and Bosland, 1998; Pruthi, 2003; Manirakiza et al., 2003). Here only selective papers are summarized with data obtained. A typical HPLC chromatogram of a commercially available natural capsaicin is shown on Figure 7.

Lee et al (Lee et al., 1976) and Iwai and colleagues (Iwai et al., 1979) early used HPLC for separation of capsaicinoids in one or two fractions from total extracts for the subsequents analysis by mass spectrometry. Sticher et al. (Sticher et al., 1978) reported separation of four homologs of capsaicin in purified capsaicinoids using a reversed-phase system. Jurenitsch at al. (Jurenitsch et al., 1979a,b) accomplished separation of the capsaicin homologs and analogs directly from ground fruit extracts on a reversed-phase system. Detection and quantitation were done by absorbance at 280 nm. Four samples of *Capsicum* fruits were analyzed by this HPLC method and also by the TMS-GC method earlier used by the group (Jurenitsch et al., 1978) for comparison.

Nonoyl vanillyamide content has assumed importance since more than 3 to 4% of this analog in a natural sample is considered adulteration unless declared. The method developed by

Jurenitsch et al. (1979a,b) was modified with the inclusion of silver nitrate in the mobile phase to selectively shorten the retention time of capsaicin, thus separating it from the coeluting nonoyl vanillylamide (Jurenitsch and Kampelmuehler, 1980). Constant and coworkers (Constant et al., 1995) also used complexation chromatography ($AgNO_3$) to separate norcapsaicin, zucapsaicin (civamide), capsaicin, nordihydrocapsaicin, nonivamide, homocapsaicin, dihydrocapsaicin and homodihydrocapsaicin-I.

Kawada et al. performed microdetermination of capsaicin by high-performance liquid chromatography with electrochemical detection (Kawada et al., 1985). Karnka et al. has reported an optimized HPLC method for sample preparation, separation, detection and identification of the major capsaicinoid compounds in various capsicum samples (Karnka et al., 2002). Isocratic reversed phase HPLC analysis performed in the author's laboratory allowed separation of five main capsaicinoids of a commercially available capsaicin preparation. The validated analytical method has been successfully applied to quantitate capsaicin and dihydrocapsaicin in industrial *Capsicum* extracts (Kuzma et al., 2014). Isocratic HPLC method with fluorimetric detection was used to determine capsaicin in rat tissues after acetone extraction (Saria et al., 1981).

HPLC analysis has made possible the accurate determination of the homologs and analogs of capsaicin and, combined with mass spectral analysis, has led to identification of structural isomers of some minor components (Govindarajan, 1986b; Reilly et al., 2001; Schweiggert et al., 2006; Singh et al., 2009; González-Zamora et al., 2013) and has made possible determination of nanogram levels of the individual capsaicinoids as is required in biosynthetic and metabolic studies (Reilly et al., 2002; Kozukue et al., 2005; Thompson et al., 2005; Zhang et al., 2010). The use of HPLC-MS (Reilly et al., 2001a) has been reported to differentiate nonivamide and capsaicin by mass-to-charge (*m/e*) ratio. The same authors have reported the use of LC-MS-MS with electrospray ionization source operating at selective ion monitoring mode (Reilly et al., 2001b). The quantification of capsaicinoids using LC-MS-MS was more sensitive (in the ng/ml range) and exhibited greater accuracy, even at low analyte concentrations. HPLC coupled with atmospheric pressure chemical ionization masss spectrometry has been reported to be a method of choice for separation and identification of the three groups of capsaicinoids: capsaicins possessing a methyl branched acyl residue with a carbon-carbon double bond, dihydrocapsaicins analogous to the previous class, but beeing saturated compounds, and capsaicin analogs (N-vanillyl-N-acylamides) composed of saturated, unbranched alkyl chains (Schweiggert et al., 2006).

In summary, HPLC analysis for total capsaicinoids or individual capsaicinoids is certainly rapid, reproducible, sensitive, and convenient for analysis of capsaicinoids in various capsaicinoid containing matrices.

3.5.3. Official methods for determination of capsaicinoids

3.5.3.1. The ASTA method for determination of capsaicinoids

In the 1980's it became clear that a more accurate and reproducible method of determining "heat" in peppers and pepper products was necessary. Under the auspices of the American

Spice Trade Association (ASTA), a new High Pressure Liquid Chromatography (HPLC) Method was adopted as ASTA Method 21.1. The HPLC measurement of capsaicin has evolved over the years as new and better instrumentation has allowed of greater accuracy of analysis. In 1996 AOAC issued Method 995.03: Capsaicinoids in Capsicums and their Extractives. In 1998, in a collaborative effort with AOAC, ASTA issued a revised method of analysis, ASTA Method 21.3 (HPLC Method). Using the revised method, the accepted pungency of pure capsaicin was re-stated from 15,000,000 to 16,000,000 SHU. AOAC revised its method to coincided with ASTA Method 21.3, in 1999, and in 2003 AOAC revised the method once more.

3.5.3.2. The United States Pharmacopoeia (USP) method

The 2012 edition of the USP36-NF31 lists *Capsaicin* and describes its Definition, Identification, Melting range, and Content of capsaicin, dihydrocapsaicin, and other capsaicinoids as follows.

Chemical name: 6-Nonenamide, (*E*)-N-[(4-Hydroxy-3-methoxy-phenyl)methyl]-8-methyl

Formula: $C_{18}H_{27}NO_3$

Molecular weight: 305.41

(*E*)-8-Methyl-N-vanillyl-6-nonenamide CAS-number: 404-86-4

Capsaicin contains not less than 90.0 percent and not more than 110.0 percent of the labeled percentage of total capsaicinoids. The content of capsaicin ($C_{18}H_{27}NO_3$) is not less than 55 percent, and the sum of the contents of capsaicin and dihydrocapsaicin ($C_{18}H_{27}NO_3$) is not less than 75 percent, and the content of other capsaicinoids is not more than 15 percent, all calculated on the dried basis.

Packaging and storage— Preserve in tight containers, protected from light, and store in a cool place

Caution—Handle *Capsaicin* with care. Prevent inhalation of particles of it and prevent its contact with any part of the body.

Solubility – It does not dissolve in water. It well dissolves in alcohols (methanol, ethanol 96%), ethylacetate and acetonitrile.

IDENTIFICATION: Prepare a test solution of *Capsaicin* in methanol containing 1 mg per mL. Prepare a Standard solution of *USP Capsaicin RS* in methanol containing 1 mg per mL. Separately apply 10-µL portions of the test solution and the Standard solution to a thin-layer chromatographic plate coated with a 0.25-mm layer of chromatographic silica gel mixture. Develop the chromatograms in a solvent system consisting of a mixture of ether and methanol (19:1) until the solvent front has moved about three-fourths of the length of the plate. Remove the plate from the chamber, and allow it to air-dry. Spray the plate with a 0.5% solution of 2,6-dibromoquinone-chlorimide in methanol, allow to stand in a chamber containing ammonia fumes, and examine the chromatograms: the blue color and the R_f value of the principal spot obtained from the test solution correspond to those properties of the principal spot obtained from the Standard solution.

Melting range: between 57° and 66°, but the range between beginning and end of melting does not exceed 5°.

3.5.3.3. Content of capsaicin, dihydrocapsaicin and other capsaicinoids

Mobile phase— Prepare a mixture of diluted phosphoric acid (1 in 1000) and acetonitrile (600:400). Filter through a filter having a porosity of 0.5 µm or finer, and degas.

Standard capsaicin solution— Dissolve an accurately weighed quantity of *USP Capsaicin RS* quantitatively in methanol to obtain a solution having a known concentration of about 0.1 mg per mL.

Standard dihydrocapsaicin solution— Dissolve an accurately weighed quantity of *USP Dihydrocapsaicin RS* quantitatively in methanol to obtain a solution having a known concentration of about 0.025 mg per mL.

Test solution— Transfer about 25 mg of *Capsaicin*, accurately weighed, to a 250-mL volumetric flask, dilute with methanol to volume, and mix.

Chromatographic system— The liquid chromatograph is equipped with a 281-nm detector and a 4.6-mm × 25-cm column that contains 5-µm packing L11 and is maintained at a constant temperature of about 30°. Adjust the flow rate to obtain a retention time of about 20 minutes for the main capsaicin peak. Chromatograph the *Standard capsaicin solution*, and record the peak responses as directed for *Procedure:* the relative standard deviation for replicate injections is not more than 2%.

Procedure— Separately inject equal volumes (about 20 µL) of the *Standard capsaicin solution*, the *Standard dihydrocapsaicin solution*, and the *Test solution* into the chromatograph, record the chromatogram for a period of time that is twice that of the retention time of capsaicin, and measure the areas of the responses for all of the peaks.

Calculate the percentage of capsaicin ($C_{18}H_{27}NO_3$) in the portion of *Capsaicin* taken by the formula:

$25{,}000(C / W)(r_U / r_S)$

in which

C is the concentration, in mg per mL, of *USP Capsaicin RS* in the *Standard capsaicin solution*,

W is the weight, in mg, of *Capsaicin* taken to prepare the *Test solution*, and

r_U and r_S are the capsaicin peak responses obtained from the *Test solution* and the *Standard capsaicin solution*, respectively.

Not less than 55% is found.

Calculate the percentage of dihydrocapsaicin ($C_{18}H_{29}NO_3$) in the portion of *Capsaicin* taken by the formula:

$25{,}000(C / W)(r_U / r_S)$

in which

C is the concentration, in mg per mL, of *USP Dihydrocapsaicin RS* in the *Standard capsaicin solution,*

W is the weight, in mg, of Capsaicin taken to prepare the *Test solution,* and

r_U and r_S are the dihydrocapsaicin peak responses obtained from the *Test solution* and the *Standard dihydrocapsaicin solution,* respectively.

The sum of the percentage of capsaicin found and of the percentage of dihydrocapsaicin found is not less than 75%. Using the chromatograms obtained from the *Standard capsaicin solution* and the *Test solution,* calculate the percentage of other capsaicinoids in the portion of *Capsaicin* taken by the formula

$$25{,}000(C / W)(r_T / r_S)$$

in which

C is the concentration, in mg per mL, of *USP Capsaicin RS* in the *Standard capsaicin solution,*

W is the weight, in mg, of *Capsaicin* taken to prepare the *Test solution,*

r_T is the sum of the peak responses of the capsaicinoids other than capsaicin and dihydrocapsaicin in the chromatogram obtained from the *Test solution,* and

r_S is the capsaicin peak response obtained from the *Standard capsaicin solution.*

Not more than 15% of other capsaicinoids is found.

4. Pesticide control

Quality is a mandatory requirement in the materials to accomplish the Pharmaceutical Good Manufacturing Practices. Nowadays, the presence of pesticides in animal and vegetal (herbal) commodities is a topic of public concern for the potential health hazards derived from them (WHO, 1998). The presence of pesticide residues in vegetal raw materials can be originated in agricultural practices, environmental contamination or cross contamination.

Table 1 shows examples of potentially hazardous contaminants and residues that may occur in herbal products (WHO, 1998). The summary table includes information on possible sources of contaminants and residues, as well as the manufacturing stages at which they may be detectable. Some of them are considered as unavoidable contaminants or residues of herbal medicines.

4.1. Classification of contaminants

Contaminants in herbal medicines are classified into *chemical contaminants* and *biological contaminants*. A variety of *agrochemical agents* and some *organic solvents* may be important residues in herbal medicines (WHO, 1998).

4.1.1. Chemical contaminants

4.1.1.1. Toxic metals and non-metals

Contamination of herbal materials with toxic substances such as arsenic can be attributed to many causes. These include environmental pollution (i.e. contaminated emissions from factories and leaded petrol and contaminated water including runoff water which finds its way into rivers, lakes and the sea, and some pesticides), soil composition and fertilizers. This contamination of the herbal material leads to contamination of the products during various stages of the manufacturing process.

4.1.1.2. Persistent organic pollutants

Persistent organic pollutants include organic chemicals, such as the synthetic aromatic chlorinated hydrocarbons, which are only slightly soluble in water and are persistent or stable in the presence of sunlight, moisture, air and heat. In the past, they were extensively used in agriculture as pesticides. The use of persistent pesticides, such as DDT and benzene hexa-chloride (BHC), in agriculture has been banned for many years in many countries. However they are still found in the areas where they were previously used and often contaminate medicinal plants growing nearby.

4.1.1.3. Radioactive contamination

A certain amount of exposure to ionizing radiation is unavoidable because many sources, including of radionuclides occur naturally in the ground and the atmosphere. Dangerous contamination may be the consequence of a nuclear accident or may arise from other sources. WHO, in close collaboration with several other international organizations, has developed guidelines for use in the event of widespread contamination by radionuclides resulting from a major nuclear accident.

4.1.1.4. Mycotoxins

The presence of mycotoxins in plant material can pose both acute and chronic risks to health.. Mycotoxins produced by species of fungi including *Aspergillus*, *Fusarium* and *Penicillium* are the most commonly reported. Mycotoxins comprise four main groups, namely, *aflatoxins*, *ochratoxins*, *fumonisins* and *tricothecenes*, all of which have toxic effects. Aflatoxins have been extensively studied and are classifi ed as Group 1 human carcinogens by the International Agency for Research on Cancer.

4.1.2. Biological contaminants

4.1.2.1. Microbiological contaminants

Herbs and herbal materials normally carry a large number of bacteria and moulds, often originating in soil or derived from manure. While a large range of bacteria and fungi form the naturally occurring microflora of medicinal plants, aerobic spore-forming bacteria frequently predominate.. The presence of Escherichia coli, Salmonella spp. and moulds may indicate poor quality of production and harvesting practices.

4.1.2.2. Parasitic contamination

Parasites such as protozoa and nematoda, and their ova, may be introduced during cultivation and may cause zoonosis, especially if uncomposted animal excreta are used. Contamination with parasites may also arise during processing and manufacturing if the personnel carrying out these processes have not taken appropriate personal hygiene measures.

4.1.3. Agrochemical residues

The main agrochemical residues in herbal medicines are derived from pesticides and fumigants.

Pesticides may be classified on the basis of their intended use, for example as follows:

- insecticides;
- fungicides and nematocides;
- herbicides; and
- other pesticides (e.g. ascaricides, molluscicides and rodenticides).

Examples of fumigants include ethylene oxide, ethylene chlorohydrin, methyl bromide and sulfur dioxide.

4.1.3.1. Pesticide residues

Medicinal plant materials may contain pesticide residues, which accumulate as a result of agricultural practices, such as spraying, treatment of soils during cultivation and administration of fumigants during storage. It is therefore recommended that every country producing medicinal plant materials should have at least one control laboratory capable of performing the determination of pesticides using a suitable method.

4.1.3.2. Classification of pesticides

Different classifications of pesticides exist. A classification based on the chemical composition or structure of the pesticide is the most useful for analytical chemists, for example:

- *chlorinated hydrocarbons* and related pesticides: hexachlorocyclohexane (HCH) or benzene hexachloride (BHC), lindane, methoxychlor
- *chlorinated phenoxyalkanoic acid* herbicides: 2,4-D, 2,4,5-T
- *organophosphorus* pesticides: carbophenothion (carbofenotion), chlorpyrifos and methyl-chlorpyrifos, coumaphos (coumafos), demeton, dichlorvos, dimethoate, ethion, fenchlorphos (fenclofos), malathion, methyl parathion, parathion
- *carbamate* insecticides: carbaryl (carbaril)

- *carbamoyl benzimidazoles*: benomyl, carbendazim
- *dithiocarbamate* fungicides: ferbam, maneb, nabam, thiram, zineb, ziram
- *amino acid* herbicides: glyphosate
- *inorganic* pesticides: aluminium phosphide, calcium arsenate
- *miscellaneous*: bromopropylate, chloropicrin, ethylene dibromide, ethylene oxide, methyl bromide, sulfur dioxide
- pesticides of plant origin: tobacco leaf extract, pyrethrum flower, and pyrethrum extract; derris and Lonchocarpus root and rotenoids.

Only the chlorinated hydrocarbons and related pesticides (e.g. HCH) and a few organophosphorus pesticides (e.g. carbophenothion) have a long residual action. Although the use of many persistent pesticides has been widely discontinued, residues may still remain in the environment (e.g. DDT). Thus the recording of all pesticide usage in countries should be strongly encouraged so as to enable cost-effective quality control of medicinal plants and of their products. The Stockholm Convention on Persistent Organic Pollutants currently includes DDT and 11 other POPs including dioxin (a potent carcinogen), aldrin, chlordane, dieldrin, endrin, heptachlor, mirex, toxaphene and hexachlorobenzene.

Most other pesticides have very short residual actions. Therefore it is suggested that, where the length of exposure to pesticides is unknown, the herbal materials should be tested for the presence of organically bound chlorine and phosphorus as a preliminary screening method which can be useful in predicting where a pesticide might be used.

4.1.4. Residual solvents

A range of organic solvents are used for manufacturing herbal medicines, and can be detected as residues of such processing in herbal preparations and finished herbal products. They should be controlled through GMP and quality control.

Solvents are classifi ed by ICH (Q3C (R5), according to their potential risk, into:

- class 1 (solvents to be avoided such as benzene);
- class 2 (limited toxic potential such as methanol or hexane); and
- class 3 (low toxic potential such as ethanol).

4.2. Pesticide analysis

One area of chemical testing of growing concern is pesticide analysis. Pesticides and their degradation products migrate from their intended point of application and spread through the air, water, soil, plants, microorganisms, and animals, including birds and fish. While many of the chemicals used in pesticide formulations are harmless, others may have toxic properties or could even form toxic by-products, potentially causing risks to human and animal health and/or environmental damage.There are over 1,000 pesticides available for use, many of which are regulated by government agencies. As a result, powerful and rapid analytical methods are needed to detect very low concentrations of pesticides and their degradation products in diverse sample matrices.

4.2.1. Analytical advances

Scientific advances in the field of application of natural products with pharmaceutical relevance has been focused on analysis of (a) the actice constituents, and (b) the potentially hazardous contaminats. Methods for quantitative determination of the above mentioned contaminations varies for different classes of contaminants. Comprehensive review of the different methodologies is out of scope ofthe present monograph. Since pesticide residue analysis has been appeared as the most seriuus issue in connection with our *Capsicum extracts*, here we concentrate on regulatory requirements on this class of possible hasardous contaminants of herbal products.

Several modern *multiresidue precedures* employing different (a) *extraction methods*, (b) *clean-up techniques* and (c) a variety of *determination methods* have been reported for quantitation of pesticide residues in natural products with pharmaceutical applications. One of the cruitial point of these methods is to extract and isolate the target pesticides from the matrix. The optimal sample treatment hevealy depends on the complexicity of the matrix.

Not going into details, the most imortant ad frequntly used extraction techniques as follows:

- Liquid phase extraction,
- Solid phase extraction,
- Solid phase micro extraction,
- Microvawe assisted solvent extraction, and
- Supercritical fluid extraction

During extraction, the solvent comes in contact with the substrate matrix, to enable extraction of the pesticide along with some of the constituents of the substrate matrix also get solubilized. The extract not only contains pesticide residues but also other constituents, which are called co-extractives. The removal of interfering co-extractives from extract is called *clean up*. After removal of moisture, the other coextractives are removed by using various separation techniques.

The most imortant ad frequntly used clean-up techniques as follows:

- Liquid-liquid partitioning
- Chemical treatments
- Chromatographic techniques
- Thin layer chromatography
- Ion exchange chromatography

- Gel permeation chromatography, and
- Adsorption column chromatography

In accordance to the official methodologies, capillary gas-liquid chromatography (GC) is the most used separation technique in residue analysis of non-polar and semi-polar pesticides. Majos attantion has paid for determination of organochlorine, organophosphorus and pyrethroid pesticides. Most reports focuses on selective detection of pesticied using electron capture (ECD), nitrogen-phosphorous (NPD), thermal conductivity (TCD) and flame photometric (FPD) detectors. In spite of the increased selectivity and sensitivity of the GC-coupled detectors, the use of mass spectrometry is being compulsory induced in order to obtain relaible identification and confirmation of residues.

As a result of searching for non-persistent and biodegradable pesticides, which kill both detrimental and beneficial insects, introduction of more polar (and less volatile) agrochemical has been recognized. Such compounds have promted the use of high presuure liquid chromatography coupled with mass spectrometry (HPLC-MS), which at the moment is a widely accepted technique for monitoring of polar and most semipolar pesticeds as well as for regulatory isuues.

Recent advances of modern multiresidue precedures including application of different GC- and HPLC-based methodologies have been summarized in several review articles. Readers interested in the field can consult this literature (Hirahara et al., 2005, Abd El-Moneim et al., 2010, Perez-Parada et al., 2011, Niell et al., 2014).

4.2.2. Regulatory methods for pestice analysis of herbal products of pharmaceutical use

4.2.2.1. The European Pharmacopoeia (Ph.Eur.)

In the seventh edition of the European Pharmacopoeia (Ph. Eur. 7.0) pesticide residues are described under chapter 02 „Methods of analysis". The Ph.Eur. Monograph „2.8.13. Pesticide residues" contains „Definition", „Limits", „Sampling" and „Qualitative and quantitative analysis of pesticide residues" of herbal drugs. The requirements for "Herbal Drugs" and "Extracts", as well as "Herbal Drugs for Homoeopathic Preparations" and "Mother Tinctures for Homoeopathic Preparations" are refered within the scope of their monographs in chapter 05 „General texts":

For the purposes of the European Pharmacopoeia Pharmacopoeia, a pesticide is any substance or mixture of substances intended for preventing, destroying or controlling any pest, unwanted species of plants or animals causing harm during or otherwise interfering with the production, processing, storage, transport or marketing of vegetable drugs. The item includes substances intended for use as growth-regulators, defoliants or desiccants and any substance applied to crops either before or after harvest to protect the commodity from deterioration during storage and transport.

4.2.2.1.1. Limits

Unless otherwise indicated in the monograph, the drug to be examined at least complies with the limits indicated in Table 4. The limits applying to pesticides that are not listed in the table and whose presence is suspected for any reason comply with the limits set by European Community directives 76/895 and 90/642, including their annexes and successive updates. Limits for pesticides that are not listed in Table 4 nor in EC directives are calculated using the following expression:

$$\frac{ADI\ x\ M}{MDD\ x\ 100}$$

where

ADI=acceptable daily intake, as published by FAO-WHO, in milligrams per kilogram of body mass,

M=body mass in kilograms (60 kg),

MDD=daily dose of the drug, in kilograms.

If the drug is intended for the preparation of extracts, tinctures or other pharmaceutical forms whose preparation method modifies the content of pesticides in the finished product, the limits are calculated using the following expression:

$$\frac{ADI\ x\ M\ x\ E}{MDD\ x\ 100}$$

where

E=extraction factor of the method of preparation, determined experimentally, and

ADI, *M*, and *MDD* are as defined above.

Higher limits can also be authorised, in exceptional cases, especially when a plant requires a particular cultivation method or has a metabolism or a structure that gives rise to a higher than normal content of pesticides. The competent authority may grant total or partial exemption from the test when the complete history (nature and quantity of the pesticides used, date of each treatment during cultivation and after the harvest) of the treatment of the batch is known and can be checked precisely.

Substance	**Limit (mg/kg)**
Alachlor	0.02
Aldrin and Dieldrin (sum of)	0.05
Azinphos-methyl	1.0
Bromopropylate	3.0
Chlordane (sum of *cis*-, *trans*- and Oxythlordane)	0.05

Substance	**Limit (mg/kg)**
Chlorfenvinphos	0.5
Chlorpyrifos	0.2
Chlorpyrofos-methyl	0.1
Cypermethrin (and isomers)	1.0
DDT (sum of *p,p'*-DDT, *o,p'*-DDT, *p,p'*-DDE and *p,p'*-TDE)	1.0
Deltamethrin	0.5
Diazinon	0.5
Dichlorovos	1.0
Dithiocarbamates (as CS_2)	2.0
Endosulfan (sum of isomers and Endosulfan sulphate)	3.0
Endrin	0.05
Ethion	2.0
Fenitrothion	0.5
Fenvalerate	1.5
Fenofos	0.05
Heptachlor (sum of Heptachlor and Heptachlorepoxide)	0.05
Hexachlorobenzene	0.1
Hexachlorocyclohexane isomers (other than γ)	0.3
Lindane (γ-Hexachlorocyclohexane)	0.6
Malathion	1.0
Methidathion	0.2
Parathion	0.5
Parathion-methyl	0.2
Permethrin	1.0
Phosalone	0.1
Piperonyl butoxide	3.0
Pirimiphos-methyl	4.0
Pyrethrins (sum of)	3.0
Quintozene (sum of quintozene, pentachloroaniline and methyl pentachlorophenyl sulphide)	1.0

Table 4. Limits for pesticide residues (Ph. Eur. 7.0).

http://dx.doi.org/10.5772/58812

4.2.2.1.2. Qualitative and quantitative analysis of pesticide residues

The analytical procedures used are validated according to the regulations in force. In particular, they satisfy the following criteria:

- the chosen method, especially the purification steps, are suitable for the combination pesticide residue/substance to be analysed, and not susceptible to interference from co-extractives; the limits of detection and quantification are measured for each pesticide-matrix combination to be analysed,
- between 70 per cent to 110 per cent of each pesticide is recovered,
- the repeatability of the method is not less than the values indicated in Table 5,
- the reproducibility of the method is not less than the values indicated in Table 5,
- the concentration of test and reference solutions and the setting of the apparatus are such that a linear response is obtained from the analytical detector.

Concentration of the pesticide (mg/kg)	Repeatability (difference, ± mg/kg)	Reproducibility (difference, ± mg/kg)
0.010	0.005	0.01
0.100	0.025	0.05
1.000	0.125	0.25

Table 5. Repeatibility and reproducibility limits of determination of pesticides (Ph. Eur. 7.0).

Detailed description of qualitative and quantitative determination of organochlorine, organophosphorus and pyrethroid insecticides is divided into three sections:

- Extraction;
- Purification; and
- Quantitative analysis.

4.2.2.1.3. Extraction

To 10 g of the substance being examined, coarsely powdered, add 100 ml of *acetone R* and allow to stand for 20 min. Add 1 ml of a solution containing 1.8 µg/ml of *carbophenothion R* in *toluene R*. Homogenise using a high-speed blender for 3 min. Filter and wash the filter cake with two quantities, each of 25 ml, of *acetone R*. Combine the filtrate and the washings and heat using a rotary evaporator at a temperature not exceeding 40 °C until the solvent has almost completely evaporated. To the residue add a few millilitres of *toluene R* and heat again until the acetone is completely removed. Dissolve the residue in 8 ml of *toluene R*. Filter through a membrane filter (45 µm), rinse the flask and the filter with *toluene R* and dilute to 10.0 ml with the same solvent (solution A).

4.2.2.1.4. Purification

4.2.2.1.4.1. Organochlorine, organophosphorus and pyrethroid insecticides

Purificationis to be accomplished by means of size-exclusion chromatography.

The chromatographic procedure may be carried out using:

- a stainless steel column 0.30 m long and 7.8 mm in internal diameter packed with *styrene-divinylbenzene copolymer R* (5 µm),
- as mobilephase *toluene R* at a flow rate of 1 ml/min.

Performance of the column. Inject 100 µl of a solution containing 0.5 g/l of *methyl red R* and 0.5 g/l of *oracet blue2R R* in *toluene R* and proceed with the chromatography. The column is not suitable unless the colour of the eluate changes from orange to blue at an elution volume of about 10.3 ml. If necessary calibrate the column, using a solution containing, in *toluene R*, at a suitable concentration, the insecticide to be analysed with the lowest molecular mass (for example, dichlorvos) and that with the highest molecular mass (for example, deltamethrin). Determine which fraction of the eluate contains both insecticides.

Purification of the test solution. Inject a suitable volume of solution A (100 µl to 500 µl) and proceed with the chromatography. Collect the fraction as determined above (solution B). Organophosphorus insecticides are usually eluted between 8.8 ml and 10.9 ml. Organochlorine and pyrethroid insecticides are usually eluted between 8.5 ml and 10.3 ml.

4.2.2.1.4.2. Organochlorine and pyrethroid insecticides

In a chromatography column, 0.10 m long and 5 mm in internal diameter, introduce a piece of defatted cotton and 0.5 g of silica gel treated as follows : heat *silica gel for chromatography R* in an oven at 150 °C for at least 4 h. Allow to cool and add dropwise a quantity of *water R* corresponding to 1.5 per cent of the mass of silica gel used; shake vigorously until agglomerates have disappeared and continue shaking for 2 h using a mechanical shaker. Condition the column using 1.5 ml of *hexane R*. Prepacked columns containing about 0.50 g of a suitable silica gel may also be used provided they are previously validated. Concentrate solution B in a current of *helium for chromatography R* or *oxygen-free nitrogen R* almost to dryness and dilute to a suitable volume with *toluene R* (200 µl to 1 ml according to the volume injected in the preparation of solution B). Transfer quantitatively onto the column and proceed with the chromatography using 1.8 ml of *toluene R* as the mobile phase. Collect the eluate (solution C).

4.2.2.1.5. Quantitative analysis

4.2.2.1.5.1. Organophosphorus insecticides

Quantitative determination to be accomplished by means of gas chromatography, using *carbophenothion R* as internal standard. It may be necessary to use a second internal standard to identify possible interference with the peak corresponding to carbophenothion.

Test solution. Concentrate solution B in a current of *helium for chromatography R* almost to dryness and dilute to 100 µl with *toluene R*.

Reference solution. Prepare at least three solutions in *toluene R* containing the insecticides to be determined and carbophenothion at concentrations suitable for plotting a calibration curve.

The chromatographic procedure may be carried out using:

- a fused-silica column 30 m long and 0.32 mm in internal diameter the internal wall of which is covered with a layer 0.25 µm thick of *poly(dimethyl)siloxane R*,
- *hydrogen for chromatography R* as the carrier gas. Other gases such as *helium for chromatography R* or *nitrogen for chromatography R* may also be used provided the chromatography is suitably validated.
- a phosphorus-nitrogen flame-ionisation detector or a atomic emission spectrometry detector, maintaining the temperature of the column at 80 °C for 1 min, then raising it at a rate of 30 °C/min to 150 °C, maintaining at 150 °C for 3 min, then raising the temperature at a rate of 4 °C/min to 280 °C and maintaining at this temperature for 1 min, and maintaining the temperature of the injector port at 250 °C and that of the detector at 275 °C. Inject the chosen volume of each solution. Calculate the content of each insecticide from the peak areas and the concentrations of the solutions.

4.2.2.1.5.2. Organochlorine and pyrethroid insecticides

Quantitative determination to be accomplished by means of gas chromatography, using *carbophenothion R* as internal standard. It may be necessary to use a second internal standard to identify possible interference with the peak corresponding to carbophenothion.

Test solution. Concentrate solution C in a current of *helium for chromatography R* or *oxygen-free nitrogen R* almost to dryness and dilute to 500 µl with *toluene R*.

Reference solution. Prepare at least three solutions in *toluene R* containing the insecticides to be determined and carbophenothion at concentrations suitable for plotting a calibration curve

The chromatographic procedure may be carried out using:

- a fused silica column 30 m long and 0.32 mm in internal diameter the internal wall of which is covered with a layer 0.25 µm thick of *poly(dimethyl)(diphenyl)siloxane R*,
- *hydrogen for chromatography R* as the carrier gas. Other gases such as *helium for chromatography R* or *nitrogen for chromatography R* may also be used, provided the chromatography is suitably validated,
- an electron-capture detector,
- a device allowing direct cold on-column injection, maintaining the temperature of the column at 80 °C for 1 min, then raising it at a rate of 30 °C/min to 150 °C, maintaining at 150 °C for 3 min, then raising the temperature at a rate of 4 °C/min to 280 °C and maintaining at this temperature for 1 min, and maintaining the temperature of the injector port at 250 °C and that of the detector at 275 °C. Inject the chosen volume of each solution. Calculate the content of each insecticide from the peak areas and the concentrations of the solutions.

4.2.2.2. United States Pharmacopoea-National Formulary (USP-NF)

In the 2012 edition of the United States Pharmacopoea-National Formulary (USP36–NF31) pesticide residues are described under General Chapters „<561> Articles of Botanical Origin USP". The „General Method for Pesticide Residues Analysys" section of the USP Monograph „„<561> Articles of Botanical Origin USP" contains „Definition", „Limits", „Qualitative and quantitative analysis of pesticide residues" and „Test for Pesticides" of herbal drugs.

For the purposes of the United States Pharmacopoea the designation pesticide applies to any substance or mixture of substances intended to prevent, destroy, or control any pest, unwanted species of plants or animals causing harm during or otherwise interfering with the production, processing, storage, transport, or marketing of pure articles. The designation includes substances intended for use as growth regulators, defoliants, or desiccants, and any substance applied to crops before or after harvest to protect the product from deterioration during storage and transport.

4.2.2.2.1. Limits

Within the United States, many botanicals are treated as dietary supplements and are subject to the statutory provisions that govern foods but not drugs in the Federal Food, Drug, and Cosmetic Act. Limits for pesticides for foods are determined by the Environmental Protection Agency (EPA) as indicated in the Code of Federal Regulations (40 CFR Part 180) or the Federal Register (FR). For pesticide chemicals without EPA-established tolerance levels, the limits should be below the detection limit of the specified method. Result less than the EPA detection limits are considered zero values. The limits contained in the USP, therefore, are not applicable in the United States when articles of botanical origins are labeled for food purposes. The limits, however, may be applicable in other countries where the presence of pesticide residues is permitted.

Unless otherwise indicated in the monograph, the article to be examined complies with the limits indicated in Table 6. The limits for suspected pesticides that are not listed in Table 6 must comply with the regulations of the EPA. For instances in which a pesticide is not listed in Table 6 or in EPA regulations, calculate the limit by the formula:

$$\frac{A \; x \; M}{100 \; x \; B}$$

where

A is the acceptable daily intake (ADI), as published by FAO-WHO, in mg/kg of body weight;

M is body weight, in kg (60 kg); and

B is the daily dose of the article, in kg.

If the article is intended for the preparation of extracts, tinctures, or other pharmaceutical forms of which the preparation method modifies the content of pesticides in the finished product, calculate the limits by the formula:

$$\frac{A \; x \; M \; x \; E}{100 \; x \; B}$$

where

E is the extraction factor of the preparation method, determined experimentally; and

A, *M*, and *B* are as defined above.

A total or partial exemption from the test may be granted when the complete history (nature and quantity of the pesticides used, date of each treatment during cultivation and after harvest) of the treatment of the batch is known and can be checked precisely according to good agricultural and collection practice (GACP).

Substance	Limit(mg/kg)
Aceohate	0.1
Alachlor	0.05
Aldrin and dieldrin (sum of)	0.05
Azinphos-ethyl	0.1
Azinphos-methyl	1
Bromide, inorganic (calculated as bromide ion)	50
Bromophos-ethyl	0.05
Bromophos-methyl	0.05
Bromopropylate	3
Chlordane (sum of *cis*-, *trans*-, and oxychlordane)	0.05
Chlorfenvinphos	0.5
Chlorpyriphos-ethyl	0.2
Chlorpyriphos-methyl	0.1
Chlorthal-dimethyl	0.01
Cyfluthrin (sum of)	0.1
λ-Cyhalothrin	1
Cypermethrin and isomers (sum of)	1
DDT (sum of *o,p′*-DDE, *p,p′*-DDE, *o,p′*-DDT, *p,p′*-DDT, *o,p′*-TDE, and *p,p′*-TDE)	1
Deltamethrin	0.5
Diazinon	0.5
Dichlorofluanid	0.1
Dichlorovos	1
Dicofol	0.5
Dimethoate and omethoate (sum of)	0.1
Dithiocarbamates (expressed as CS_2)	2

Substance	Limit(mg/kg)
Endosulfan (sum of isomers and endosulfan sulphate)	3
Endrin	0.05
Ethion	2
Etrimphos	0.05
Fenchlorophos (sum of fenchlorophos and fenchlorophos-oxon)	0.1
Fenitrothion	0.5
Fenpropathrin	0.03
Fensulfothion(sum of fensulfothion, fensulfothion-oxon, fensulfothion-oxonsulfon, and fensulfothion-sulfon)	0.05
Fenthion (sum of fenthion, fenthion-oxon, fenthion-oxon-sulfon, fenthion-oxon-sulfoxid, fenthion-sulfon, and fenthion-sulfoxid)	0.05
Fenvalerate	1.5
Flucytrinate	0.05
τ-Fluvalinate	0.05
Fonophos	0.05
Heptachlor (sum of heptachlor, *cis*-heptachloroepoxide, and *trans*-heptachloroepoxide)	0.05
Hexachlorobenzene	0.1
Hexachlorocyclohexane (sum of isomers α-, β-, δ-, and ε-)	0.3
Lindan (γ-hexachlorocyclohexane)	0.6
Malathion and malaoxon (sum of)	1
Mecarbam	0.05
Methacriphos	0.05
Methamidophos	0.05
Methidathion	0.2
Methoxychlor	0.05
Mirex	0.01
Monocrotophos	0.1
Parathion-ethyl and Paraoxon-ethyl (sum of)	0.5
Parathion-methyl and Paraoxon-methyl (sum of)	0.2
Pendimethalin	0.1
Pentachloranisol	0.01
Permethrin and isomers(sum of)	1
Phosalone	0.1

Substance	Limit(mg/kg)
Phosmet	0.05
Piperonyl butoxide	3
Pirimiphos-ethyl	0.05
Pirimiphos-methyl (sum os pirimiphos-methyl and N-desethyl-pirimiphos-methyl)	4
Procymidone	0.1
Profenophos	0.1
Prithiophos	0.05
Pyrethrum (sum of cinerin I, cinerin II, jasmolin I, jasmolin II, pyrethrin I, and pyrethrin II)	3
Quinalphos	0.05
Quintozene (sum of quintozene, pentachloraniline, and methyl pentachlorphenyl sulfide)	1
S-421	0.02
Tecnazene	0.05
Tetradifon	0.3
Vinclozolin	0.4

Table 6. Limits for pesticide residues (USP36–NF31).

4.2.2.2.2. Qualitative and quantitative analysis of pesticide residues

Use validated analytical procedures (e.g., FDA Pesticide Analytical Manual (PAM) [http://www.fda.gov/Food/FoodScienceResearch/LaboratoryMethods/ucm2006955.htm], or other analytical procedures validated in accordance with EU guideline [Document No. SANCO/10684/2009, http://ec.europa.eu/food/plant/protection/resources/qualcontrol_en.pdf] or the USP Validation of Compendial Procedures <1225>) that satisfy the following criteria:

- the method, especially with respect to its purification steps, is suitable for the combination of pesticide residue and substance under test, and is not susceptible to interference from co-extractives;
- the limits of detection and quantification for each pesticide matrix combination to be analyzed;
- the method is shown to recover between 70% and 110% of each pesticide;
- the repeatability and reproducibility of the method are NLT the appropriate values indicated in Table 7; and
- the concentrations of test and reference solutions and the setting of the apparatus are such that a linear response in obtained from the analytical detector.

Concentration Range of the Pesticide (mg/kg)	Repeatability(RSD) (%)	Reproducibility(RSD) (%)
0.001-0.01	30	60
>0.01-0.1	20	40
>0.1-1	15	30
>1	10	20

Table 7. Repeatibility and reproducibility limits of determination of pesticides (USP36–NF31).

4.2.2.2.3. Test for pesticides

Unless otherwise specified in the individual monograph, the following methods may be used for the analysis of pesticides. Depending on the substance being examined, it may be necessary to modify, sometimes extensively, the procedure described hereafter. Additionally, it may be necessary to perform another method with another (e.g. mass spectrometry), or a different method (e.g. immunochemical method) to confirm the results.

Description of qualitative and quantitative determination of organochlorine, organophosphorus and pyrethroid insecticides is divided into three sections:

- Extraction;
- Purification; and
- Quantitative analysis.

4.2.2.2.4. Extraction

To 10 g of the coarsely powdered substance under test add 100 ml of acetone, and allow to stand for 20 min. add 1 ml of a solution in toluene containing 1.8 μg of carbophenothion per ml. Mix in a high-speed blender for 3 min. Filter this solution, and wash the residue with two 25-ml portions of acetone. Combine the filtrate and the washings, and heat, in a rotary evaporator, maintaining the temperature of the bath below 40° until the solvent has almost completely removed. Dissolve the residue in 8 ml of toluene. Pass through a membrane filter of 45 μm pore size, rinse the flask and the filter with toluene, dilute with toluene to 10 ml (*Solution A*), and mix. [NOTE – Use the above procedure for the analysis of samples of articles having a water content of less than 15%. Samples having a higher water content may be dried, provided that the drying procedure does not significantly affect the pesticide content.]

4.2.2.2.5. Purification

4.2.2.2.5.1. Organochlorine, organophosphorus, and pyrethroid

Purification is to be accomplished by means of size-exclusion chromatography. The size-exclusion chromatograph is equipped with a 7.8 mm x 30 cm stainless steel column containing 5 μm packing L21. Toluene is used as the mobile phase at a flow rate of about 1 ml/min.

Performance of the Column – Inject 100 µl of a solution in toluene containing, in each ml, 0.5 mg of methyl red and 0.5 mg of oracet blue or equivalent. The column is not suitable unless the color of the eluate changes from orange to blue at an elution volume of about 10.3 ml. If necessary, calibrate the column, using a solution in toluene containing suitable concentrations of the pesticide of interest having the lowest molecular weight (for example, dichlorvos) and that having the highest molecular weight (for example, deltamethrin). Determine which fraction of the eluate contains both pesticides.

Purification of the Test Solution – Inject a suitable volume (100 to 500 µl) of *Solution A* into the chromatograph. Collect the fraction (*Solution B*) as determined above under *Performance of the Column*. Organophosphorus pesticide elute between 8.8 and 10.9 ml. Organochlorine and pyrethroid pesticides elute between 8.5 and 10.3 ml.

Organochlorine and Pyrethroid Insecticides – Into a 5 mm x 10 cm chromatographic column, introduce a piece of fat-free cotton and 0.5 g of silica gel treated as follows. Heat chromatographic silica gel in oven 150° for at least 4 h. Allow to cool, and add dropwise a quantity of water corresponding to 1.5% of the weight of silica gel used. Shake vigorously until agglomerates have disappeared, and continue shaking by mechanical means for 2 h. Condition the column with 1.5 ml of hexane. [NOTE – Prepacked columns containing about 0.50 g of suitable silica gel may also be used, provided they have been previously validated.] Concentrate *Solution B* almost to dryness, with the aid of a stream of helium or oxygen-free nitrogen, and dilute with toluene to a suitable volume (200 µl to 1 ml, according to the volume injected in the preparation of *Solution B*). Quantitatively transfer this solution to the column, and proceed with the chromatography, using 1.8 ml of toluene as the mobile phase. Collect the eluate (*Solution C*).

4.2.2.2.6. *Quantitative analysis*

4.2.2.2.6.1. *Quantitative analysis of organophosphorus insecticides*

Test Solution – Concentrate *Solution B* almost to dryness, with the aid of a stream of helium, dilute with toluene to 100 µl, and mix.

Standard Solution – Prepare at least three solutions in toluene containing each of the pesticides of interest and carbophenothion at concentrations suitable for plotting a calibration curve.

Chromatographic System-The gas chromatograph is equipped with an alkali flame-ionization detector or flame photometric detector and a 0.32 mm x 30 m fused silica column coated with a 0.25 µm layer of phase G1. Hydrogen is used as the carrier gas. Other gases, such as helium or nitrogen, may also be used. The injection port temperature is maintained at 250°, and the detector is maintained at 275°. The column temperature is maintained at 80° for 1 min, then increased to 150° at a rate of 30°/min, maintained at 150° for 3 min, then increased to 280° at a rate of 4°/min, and maintained at this temperature for 1 min. Use carbophenothion as the internal standard. [NOTE – If necessary, use a second internal standard to identify any possible interference with the peak corresponding to carbophenothion.] inject the chosen volume of each solution, record the chromatograms, and measure the peak responses. Calculate the content of each pesticide from the peak areas and the concentrations of the solution.

4.2.2.2.6.2. Quantitative analysis organochlorine and pyrethroid insecticides

Test solution – Concentrate Solution C almost to dryness, with the aid of a stream of helium or oxygen-free nitrogen, dilute with toluene to 500 μl, and mix.

Standard Solution – Prepare at least three solutions in toluene containing each of the pesticides of interest and carbophenothion at concentrations suitable for plotting a calibration curve.

Chromatographic System – The gas chromatograph is equipped with an electron-capture detector, a device allowing direct on-column cold injection, and a 0.32 mm x 30 m fused silica column coated with a 0.25 μm layer of phase G1. Hydrogen is used as the carrier gas. Other gases, such as helium or nitrogen, may also be used. The injection port temperature is maintained at 275°, and the detector is maintained at 300°. The column temperature is maintained at 80° for 1 min, then increased to 150° at a rate of 30°/min, maintained at 150° for 3 min, then increased to 280° at a rate of 4°/min, and maintained at this temperature for 1 min. Use carbophenothion as the internal standard. [NOTE – If necessary, use a second internal standard to identify any possible interference with the peak corresponding to carbophenothion.] Inject the chosen volume of each solution, record the chromatograms, and measure the peak responses. Calculate the content of each pesticide from the peak areas and the concentrations of the solutions.

Acknowledgements

The study was supported by the grants of the National Office for Research and Technology, "Pázmány Péter program" (RET-II 08/2005), and that of the Faculty of Medicine, University of Pécs (AOK-PA-2014/1).

Author details

Mónika Kuzma[1], Tibor Past[2], Gyula Mózsik[2] and Pál Perjési[1]

*Address all correspondence to: pal.perjesi@aok.pte.hu

1 Institute of Pharmaceutical Chemistry, University of Pécs, Hungary

2 First Department of Medicine, Medical and Health Center, University of Pécs, Hungary

References

[1] Anu, A., Peter K.V. (2000): The chemistry of Paprika. Indian Species 37: 15–18.

[2] ASTA (1968): Method No 20, Extractable color in paprika, In: Official Anal. Meth. Englewood Cliffs, N.J.

[3] Bajaj, K.L. (1980): Colorimetric determination of capsaicin in Capsicum fruits, J. Assoc. Off. Anal. Chem. 63: 1314–1320

[4] Benedek, L. (1959): Determination of capsaicin in red peppers (paprika), Kísérletügyi Közl. C. Kertész, 52: 33; Chem. Abstr. (1963) 59: 8055b

[5] Bosland, P.W. (1994): Chiles: history, cultivation, and uses. In: Charalambous, G. (ed): Spices, Herbs, and Edible Fungi. Elsevier Publ., New York pp. 347–366.

[6] Brash, A.R., Baertschi, S.W., Ingram, C.D., Harris, T.M. (1988): Isolation and characterization of natural allene oxides: unstable intermediates in the metabolism of lipid hydroperoxides. Proc. Natl. Acad. Sci. USA 85: 3382–3386.

[7] Brawer, O., Schoen, J. (1962): Determination of flavour constituents of paprika, Angew. Botan. 36: 25–30.

[8] British Standards Institution (1979): Methods for testing spices and condiments: Determination of Scovill index of chillies, BS 4548 (Part 7), BSI, London

[9] Britton, G. (1991): The biosynthesis of carotenoids: a progress report. Pure Appl. Chem. 63: 101–108.

[10] Buttery, R.G., Seifert, R.M., Guadagni, D.G., Ling, L.C. (1969a). Characterisation of some volatile constituents of bell peppers, J. Agric. Food Chem. 17: 1322–1327.

[11] Buttery, R.G., Seifert, R.M., Lundin, R.E., Guadagni, D.G., Ling, L.C. (1969b): Characterisation of an important aroma component of bell peppers, Chem. Ind. 490

[12] Chem. Abstr. (1958): 52: 20903

[13] Chem. Abstr. (1963a) 59: 8055

[14] Chem. Abstr. (1963b): 58: 11166

[15] Chitwood, RL, Pangborn, RM, Jennings, W. (1983): GC-MS and sensory analysis of volatiles from three cultivars of Capsicum. Food Chem. 11: 201–216.

[16] Constant, H.L., Cordell, G.A., West, P.D., Johnson, J.H. (1995): Separation and quantification of capsaicinoids using complexation chromatography. J. Nat. Prod. 58: 1925–1928.

[17] Cremer, D.R., Eichner, K. (2000): Formation of volatile compounds during heating of spice paprika (Capsicum annuum) powder. Journal of Agricultural and Food Chemistry 48, 2454–2460

[18] Davies, B.H. (1980): Carotenoid biosynthesis, In: Czygan, F.C. (ed): Pigments in Plants, 2nd Ed. Gustav Fischer, Stuttgart. pp. 31–56.

[19] Deli, J., Molnár, P. (2002): Paprika Carotenoids: Analysis, Isolation, Structure Elucidation, Curr. Org. Chem. 6: 1197–1219.

[20] Di Cecco, J.J. (1976): Gas-liquid chromatographic determination of capsaicin, J. Assoc. Off. Anal. Chem. 59: 1–9.

[21] Abd El-Moneim M. R. Afify, Mohamed, M.A., El-Gammal, H.A., Attallah E.R. (2010) Multiresidue method of analysis for determination of 150 pesticides in grapes using quick and easy method (QuEChERS) and LC-MS/MS determination. Journal: Food, Agriculture and Environment (JFAE) 8: 602-606.

[22] Eisvale, R.J. (1981): Oleoresins Handbook, 3rd Edition, Dodge and Elcott, Inc., New York, NY, USA

[23] Essential Oil Association (1975): Specification of oleoresin paprika – EOA No. 239, New York

[24] Essential Oil Association (1975): Oleoresin Capsicum – EOA No. 244, New York

[25] Essential Oil Association (1975): Oleoresin red pepper – EOA No. 245, New York

[26] European Pharmacopoeia (2007): Fifth Edition, Council of Europe, Strassbourg (Ph. Eur. 6.0)

[27] Felt, L., Pacakova, V., Stulik, K., Volka, K. (2005): Reliability of carotenoid analyses: A review. Curr. Anal. Chem. 1: 93–102.

[28] Fung, T, Jeffery, W, Beveridge, A.D. (1982): The identification of capsaicinoids in tear-gas spray. J. Forensic Sci. 27: 812–821.

[29] Gnayfeed, M.H., Daood, H.G., Biacs, P.A., Alcaraz, C.F. (2001): Content of bioactive compounds in pungent spice red pepper (paprika) as affected by ripening and genotype, J. Sci. Food Agric. 81: 1580–1585.

[30] González-Zamora, A., Sierra-Campos, E., Luna-Ortega, J.G., Pérez-Morales, R., Rodríguez Ortiz, J.C., García-Hernández, J.L. (2013): Characterization of Different Capsicum Varieties by Evaluation of Their Capsaicinoids Content by High Performance Liquid Chromatography, Determination of Pungency and Effect of High Temperature, Molecules 18: 13471-13486.

[31] Govindarajan, V.S. (1986a): Capsicum – Production, technology, chemistry, and quality – Part II: Processed products, standards, world production and trade. CRC, Critical Rev. Food Sci. Nutr. 23: 207–288.

[32] Govindarajan, V.S. (1986b): Capsicum – Production, technology, chemistry, and quality – Part III: Chemistry of the color, aroma, and pungency stimuli. CRC, Critical Rev. Food Sci. Nutr. 24: 245–355.

[33] Govindarajan, V.S. (1986c): Capsicum – Production, technology, chemistry and quality. Part II. Processed products, standards, world production, and trade. In: Furia, T.E. (ed): CRC Crit. Rev. Food Sci. Nutr., CRC Press, Boca Raton, 23: 207

[34] Govindarajan, V.S. (1986d): Capsicum – Production, technology, chemistry, and quality – Part III: Chemistry of the color, aroma, and pungency stimuli. CRC, Critical Rev. Food Sci. Nutr. 24: 327–330.

[35] Govindarajan, V.S., Rajalakshmi, D., Chand, N. (1987): Capsicum – Production, technology, chemistry, and quality – Part IV: Evaluation of quality. CRC, Critical Rev. Food Sci. Nutr. 25: 266

[36] Hartman, K.T. (1970): A rapid gas-liquid chromatograpphic determination for capsaicin in capsicum species. J. Food Sci. 35: 543–574.

[37] Hawer, W.S., Ha, J., Hwang, J., Nam, Y. (1994): Effective separation and quantitative analysis of major heat principles in red pepper by capillary gas chromatography. Food Chem. 49: 99–103.

[38] Hinds, T.S., West, W.L., Knight, E.M. (1997): Carotenoids and retinoids: a review of research, clinical, and public health applications, J. Clin. Pharmacol. 37: 551–558.

[39] Hirahara, Y., Kimura, M., Inoue, T., Uchikawa, S., Otani, S., Haganuma, A., Matsumoto, N., Hirata, A., Maruyama, S., Iizuka, T., Ukyo, M., Ota, M., Hirose, H., Suzuki, S., Uchida, Y. (2005): Validation of Multiresidue Screening Methods for the Determination of 186 Pesticides in 11 Agricultural Products Using Gas Chromatography (GC). Journal of Health Science, 51: 617–627.

[40] Hoffman, P.G., Lego, M.C., Galetto, W.G. (1983): Separation and quantitation of red pepper major haet principles by reverse-phase high pressure liquid chromatography. J. Agric. Food Chem. 31: 1326–1330.

[41] Hollo, J., Gal, I., Suto, J. (1957): Chromatographic determination of capsaicin in paprika oil and paprika products. Fette Seifen Anstrichm. 59: 1048–1055.

[42] Hornero-Mendez, D., Gomez-Ladron, R., Minguez-Mosquera, M.I. (2000): Carotenoid biosynthesis changes in five red pepper (Capsicum annuum L.) cultivars during ripening. Cultivar selection for breeding. J. Agric. Food Chem. 48: 3857–3864.

[43] Ibanez, E., Lopez, S.S., Ramos, E., Tabera, J., Reglero, G., (1998). Analysis of volatile fruit components by headspace solid phase microextraction. Food Chemistry. 63 (2), 281–286.

[44] ICH Harmonized Tripartite Guideline Topic Impurities: Guidelines for Residual Solvents. (Q3C (R5). www.ich.org.

[45] International Standards Organization (1981): Spices and condiments – chillies: Determination of capsaicinoids content, draft proposal DP 7543, ISO, Geneva

[46] International Standards Organization (1997): Spices and condiments – chillies: Determination of Scoville index, ISO 3513:1977E, ISO, Geneva)

[47] Ishikawa, K. (2003): Biosynthesis of capsaicinoids in *Capsicum*, Chapter 5, In: De AK (ed): Capsicum The genus of Capsicum, Taylor and Francis, London, New York pp. 87–95.

[48] Iwai, K., Suzuki, T., Fujiwake, H., Oha, S. (1979): Simultaneous microdetermination of capsaicin and its four analogues by using high-performance liquid chromatography and gas chromatography-mass spectrometry. J. Chromatogr. 172: 303–311.

[49] Jentzsch, K., Kubelka, W., Pock, H. (1969): A method for determination of capsaicinoids content in capsicum fruits and preparations (in German) Sci. Pharm. 37: 153–162.

[50] Jurenitsch, J., Bingler, E., Becker, H., Kubelka, W (1979a): Simple HPLC method for determination of total and single capsaicinoids in Capsicum-fruits (in German), Plant. Med. 36: 54-60.

[51] Jurenitsch, J., David, M., Heresch, F., Kubelka, W. (1979b): Detection and identification of new pungent compounds in fruits of *capsicum*. Planta Med. 36: 61–67.

[52] Jurenitsch, J., Kampelmuehler, I. (1980): Rapid determination of nonylic acid vanillylamide and other capsaicinoids in capsicum fruit extracts by means of Ag+ complexation high performance liquid chromatography (in German), J. Chromatogr. 193: 101–110.

[53] Jurenitsch, J., Kubelka, W., Jentzsch, K. (1978): Gas chromatographic determination of the content of individual and total capsaicinoids in *Capsicum* fruits after thin-layer chromatographic separation (in German), Sci. Pharm. 46: 307–318.

[54] Jurenitsch, J., Leinmueller, R. (1980): Quantification of nonylic acid vanillylamide and other capsaicinoids in the pungent principle of Capsicum fruits and preparations by gas-liquid chromatography on glass capillary columns (in German), J. Chromatogr. 189: 389–397.

[55] Karnka, R., Rayanakorn, M., Wtanesk, S., Vaneesorn, Y. (2002): Optimization of high-performance liquid chromatographic parameters for the determination of capsaicinoid compounds using the simplex method. Anal. Sci. 18: 661–665.

[56] Kataoka, H., Lord, H., Pawliszyn, J., 2000. Application of solid phase microextraction in food. Journal of Chromatography A 880 (1-2), 35–62.

[57] Kawada, T., Watanabe, T., Katsura, K., Takami, H., Iwai, K. (1985): Formation and metabolism of pungent principle of Capsiucum Fruits. XV. Microdetermination of capsaicin by high-performance liquid chromatography with electrochemical detection, J. Chromatogr. 329: 99-105.

[58] Keller, U., Flath, R.A., Mon, R.A., Teranishi, R. (1981): Volatiles from red pepper (Capsicum spp.), In: Teranishi, R., Barrera-Benitez, H. (eds): Quality of Selected

Fruits and Vegetables of North America, ACS Symposium Series, No. 170, American Chemical Society, Washington, D.C., Chapter 12, pp. 137–146.

[59] Korany, K., Kocsis, N., Amtmann, M., Mednyanszky, Z. (2002): GC-MS investigation of aroma compounds of Hungarian red paprika (Capsicum annuum) cultivars. Journal of Food Composition and Analysis 15, 195–203.

[60] Korel, F., Bagdatlioglu, N., Balaban, M.Ö., Hisil, Y. (2002): Ground red peppers: Capsaicinoid content, Scoville scores, and discrimination by an electronic nose. J. Agric. Food chem. 50: 3257–3261.

[61] Kosuge, S., Inagaki, Y. (1959): Studies on pungent principles of red pepper. III. Determination of pungent principles. Nippon Nogei Kagaku Kaishi, 33: 470; Chem. Abstr. (1960): 54: 12404h

[62] Kozukue, N., Han, J-S., Kozukue, E., Lee, S-J., Kim, J.A., Lee, K-R., Levin, C.E., Friedman, M. (2005): Analysis of eight capsaicinoids in peppers and pepper-containing foods hy high-performance liquid chromatography and liquid chromatography-mass spectrometry. J. Agric. Food Chem. 53: 9172–9181.

[63] Krajewska, A.M., Powers, J.J. (1987): Gas chromatographic determination of capsaicinoids in green *capsicum* fruits. J. Assoc. Off. Anal. Chem. Int. 70: 926-928.

[64] Kramer, A. (1966): Parameters of quality, Food Technol. 20: 1147-1180.

[65] Krukonis, V.J. (1988): Processing with supercritical fluids. Overview and applications. In: Charpentier, B.A., Sevenants, M.R. (eds): Supercritical Fluid Extraction and Chromatography. Techniques and Applications, ACS Symposium Series 366; American Chemical Society: Washington, DC, pp. 26–43.

[66] Kulka, K. (1967): Aspects of functional groups and flavour. J. Agric. Food Chem. 15: 48–52.

[67] Kuzma, M., Molnár, Sz., Perjési, P. (2006): Development and application of a gas chromatographic method for determination of capsaicinoids, In: Abstracts of Papers, Symposium of Drug Research Committe of Hungarian Pharmaceutical Society, November 24-25, Debrecen, Hungary, p. 51

[68] Kuzma, M., Fodor, K., Boros, B., Perjési, P. (2014): Development and Validation of an HPLC-DAD Analysis for Pharmacopoeial Qualification of Industrial Capsicum Extracts. J Chromatogr Sci. *J Chromatogr Sci (2014)* doi: 10.1093/chromsci/bmu004. First published online: February 20, 2014.

[69] Lee, K.R, Suzuki, T., Kobashi, M., Hasegawa, K., Iwai, K. (1976): Quantitative micro analysis of capsaicin, dihydrocapsaicin, nordihydrocapsaicin using mass fragmentography. J. Chromatogr. 123: 119–128.

[70] Lichtenthaler, H.K., Schwender, J., Disch, A., Rohmer, M. (1997): Biosynthesis of isoprenoids in higher plant chloroplasts proceeds via mevalonate-independent pathway, FEBS Lett. 400: 271–274.

[71] Luning, P.A., Rijk, T.D., Harry, J., Wichers, H.J., Roozen, J.P., 1994a. Gas chromatography, mass spectrometry, and sniffing port analyses of volatile compounds of fresh bell peppers (Capsicum annuum) at different ripening stages. Journal of Agricultural and Food Chemistry 42, 977–983.

[72] Luning, P.A., Yuksel, D., Roozen, J.P., 1994b. Sensory attributes of bell peppers (Capsicum annuum) correlated with composition of volatile compounds. In: Maarse, H., Van der Heij, D.G. (Eds.), Proceedings of 7th Weurman Symposium. Elsevier Science Publishers, Amsterdam, pp. 241–248.

[73] Maillard, M-N, Giampaoli, P., Richard, H.M.J. (1998): Analysis of eleven capsaicinoids by reversed-phase high performance liquid chromatography. Flavour Fragrance J 12: 409–413.

[74] Manirakiza, P., Covaci, A., Shepens, P. (1999): Solid-phase extraction and gas chromatography with mass spectrometric determination of capsaicin and its analogues from chilli peppers (*Capsicum* spp.) J. Assoc. Off. Anal. Chem. Int. 82: 1399–1405.

[75] Manirakiza, P., Covaci, A., Shepens, P. (2003): Pungency principles in Capsicum – analytical determination and toxicology, In: De AK (ed): Capsicum The genus of Capsicum, Taylor and Francis, London, New York, Chapter 4

[76] McHugh, M.A., Krukonis, V.L. (1986): Supercritical fluid extraction: principles and practice; Butterworth: Stoneham, MA. pp. 13–22.

[77] Morrison, J.I. (1967): Gas chromatographic method for measuring pungency in capsicum spices, Chem. Ind. (London) 1785.

[78] Mózsik,Gy., Dömötör, A., Past, T., Vas, V., Perjési, P., Kuzma, M., Blazics, Gy., Szolcsányi, J. (2009). Capsaicinoids. From the Plant Cultivation to the Production of the Human Medical Drug. Akadémia Kiadó, Budapest.

[79] Murray, K.E., Whitfield, F.B. (1975): The occurrence of 3-alkyl-2-methoxypyrazines in raw vegetables, J. Sci. Food Agric. 26: 973–986.

[80] Niell, S., Cesio, V., Hepperle, J., Doerk, D., Kirsch, L., Kolberg, D., Scherbaum, E., Anastassiades, M., Horacio Heinzen, H. (2014): QuEChERS-Based Method for the Multiresidue Analysis of Pesticides in Beeswax by LC-MS/MS and GC×GC-TOF J. Agric. Food Chem., 62: 3675–3683.

[81] Palacio, J.J.R. (1977): Spectrophotometric determination of capsaicin, J. Assoc. Off. Anal. Chem. 60: 970–972.

[82] Pena-Alvarez, A., Ramírez-Maya, E., Alvarado-Suárez, L.A. (2009): Analysis of capsaicin and dihydrocapsaicin in peppers and pepper sauces by solid phase microextraction–gas chromatography–mass spectrometry, J. Chromatogr. A 1216: 2843–2847.

[83] Penton, Z. (1996): Flavor volatiles in fruit beverage with automated SPME. Food Testing and Analysis 2: 16–18.

[84] Peppard, T., Yang, X. (1994): Solid phase microextraction for flavour analysis. J. Agric. Food Chem. 42: 1925–1930.

[85] Perez-Parada, A., Colazzo, M., Basil, N., Dellacassa, E., Cesio, V., Heinzen, H., Fernandez-Alba, A.R. (2011): Pesticide Residues in Natural Products with Pharmaceutical Use: Occurrence, Analytical Advances and Perspectives. In: Pesticides in the Modern World - Trends in Pesticides Analysis (Stoytcheva, M., editor), InTech, 2011.

[86] Poppel, G., von Goldbochm, R.A. (1995): Epidemiologic evidence for beta-carotene and cancer prevention Am. J. Clin. Nutr. 62: S1393–S1402.

[87] Pruthi, J.S. (2003): Chemistry and quality control of *Capsicums* and *Capsicum* products, Chapter 3, In: De, A.K. (ed): Capsicum The genus of Capsicum, Taylor and Francis, London, New York pp. 25–70.

[88] Rahman, F.M.M., Buckle, K.A. (1980): Pigment changes in capsicum cultivars during maturation and ripening, J. Food Technol. 15: 241–249.

[89] Rajpoot, N.C., Govindarajan, V.S. (1981): Paper chromatographic determination of total capsaicinoids in capsicum and their oleoresins with precision, reproducibility and validation through correlation with pungency in Scoville units, J. Assoc. Off. Anal. Chem. 64: 311–318.

[90] Ravishankar, G.A, Suresh, B, Giridhar, P, Ramachandra Rao, S, Sudhakar Johnson, T (2003): Biotechnological studies on *Capsicum* for metabolite production and plant improvement. In: In: De AK (ed): Capsicum. The genus of Capsicum, Taylor and Francis, London, New York, Chapter 6, pp. 99-128.

[91] Reilly, C.A., Crouch, D.J, Yost, G.S. (2001a): Quantitative analysis of capsaicinoids in fresh pepperes, oleoresin capsicum, and pepper spray products, J. Forensic. Sci. 46: 502–509.

[92] Reilly, C.A., Crouch, D.J., Yost, G.S., Fatah, A.A. (2001b): Determination of capsaicin, dihydrocapsaicin, and nonivamide in self-defense weapons by liquid chromatography–mass spectrometry and liquid chromatography–tandem mass spectrometry., J. Chromatogr. A 912: 259-267.

[93] Reilly, C.A., Crouch, D.J., Yost, G.S., Fatah, A.A. (2002): Determination of Capsaicin, Nonivamide, and Dihydrocapsaicin in Blood and Tissue by Liquid Chromatography-Tandem Mass Spectrometry, J. Anal. Toxicol. 26: 313-319.

[94] Reineccius, G. (1994): Source book of flavors, 2nd ed., Chapmann and Hall, New York, pp. 267–273.

[95] Rodriguez-Amaya, D.B. (1997): Carotenoids and Food preparation: The retention of provitamin A carotenoids in prepared, processed, and tored foods. John Snow, Inc./ OMNI Project, 1997.

[96] Saria, A., Lembeck, F., Skofitsch, G. (1981): Determination of capsaicin in tissues and separation of capsaicin analogues by high-performance liquid chromatography, J. Chromatogr. 208: 41-46.

[97] Schweiggert, U., Carle, R., Schieber, A. (2006): Characterization of major and minor capsaicinoids and related compounds in chili pods (*Capsicum frutescens* L.) by high-performance liquid chromatography/atmospheric pressure chemical ionization mass spectrometry. Anal. Chim. Acta 557: 236–244.

[98] Scoville, W.L. (1912): Note on Capsicum, J. Amer. Pharm. Assoc. 1: 453–454.

[99] Sides, S., Robards, K., Helliwell, S. (2000): Development in extraction techniques and their application to analysis of volatiles in food. Trends in Analytical Chemistry 19 (5): 322–329.

[100] Singh, S., Jarret, R., Russo, V., Majetich, G., Shimkus, J., Bushway, R., Perkins, B. (2009): Determination of Capsinoids by HPLC-DAD in Capsicum Species, J. Agric. Food Chem. 57: 3452–3457.

[101] Simon, J.E. (1990): Essential oils and culinary herbs. In: J. Janick, J., Simon, J.E (eds): Advances in New Crops. Timber Press, Portland, OR, pp. 472–483.

[102] Spanyar, P., Blazovich, M. (1969): Thin-layer chromatography method for the determination of capsaicin, Analyst 94: 1084–1090.

[103] Spanyar, P., Kevei, E., Kiszel, M. (1957): Determination of capsaicin, Acta Chim. Acad. Sci. Hung. 11: 137–142.

[104] Spurgeon, S.L., Porter, J.W. (1983): Biosynthesis of carotenoids, In: Porter, J.W., Spurgeon, SL (eds): Biosynthesis of isoprenoid compounds, Vol. 2., Wiley, New York, pp. 1–122.

[105] Steffen, A., Pawliszyn, J., 1996. Analysis of flavor volatiles using headspace solid phase microextraction. Journal of

[106] Agricultural and Food Chemistry 44, 2187–2193.

[107] Sticher, O., Soldati, F., Joshi, R.K. (1978): High performance liquid chromatography separation and quantitative determination of capsaicin, dihydrocapsaicin, nordihydrocapsaicin and homodihydrocapsaicin in natural capsaicinoid mixtures of capsicum fruits (in German), J. Chromat. 166: 221–231.

[108] Strike, D.J., Meijerink, M.G.H., Koudelka-Hep, M. (1999): Electronic noses – A mini review, Fresenius' Anal. Chem. 364: 499–505.

[109] Suzuki, T., Iwai, K. (1984): Constituents of red pepper species: Chemistry, biochemistry, pharmacology and food science of the pungent principle of capsicum species. In: Brossi, A. (ed): The alkaloids, Academic Press Inc., New York, pp. 227–299.

[110] Suzuki, J.I., Tausing, F., Morse, R.E. (1957): Some observations on red pepper. I. A new method for the determination of pungency in red pepper. Food Technol. 11: 100-104.

[111] The United States Pharmacopoeial Convention, INC. (2005): 12601 Twinbrook Parkway, Rockwille (USP 27–NF 22)

[112] The 2006 edition of the United States Pharmacopoeia-National Formulary (*USP30–NF25)* lists *Capsicum Oleoresin* and describes its *Capsicum Oleoresin* as follows (*The USP30–NF25* Page 1611)

[113] Thomas, B.V., Schreiber, A.A., Weisskopf, C.P. (1998): Simple method for quantitation of capsaicinoids in peppers using capillary gas chromatography. J. Agric. Food Chem., 46, 2655–2663.

[114] Thompson, R.Q., Phinney, K.W., Welch, M.J., White V, E. (2005): Quantitative determination of capsaicinoids by liquid chromatography–electrospray mass spectrometry, Anal. Bioanal. Chem. 381: 1441–1451.

[115] Thresh, L.T. (1846): Isolation of capsaicin. Pharmacol. J. 6: 941

[116] Tirimanna, A.S.L. (1972): Quantitative determination of the pungent principle capsaicin of Ceylon chillies. Analyst, 97: 372–380.

[117] Todd, P.H., Bensinger, M.G., Biftu, T.J. (1975): TLC screening techniques for qualitative determination of natural and synthetic capsaicinoids. J. Chrom. Sci. 13: 577–580.

[118] Todd, P.H., Bensinger, M.G., Biftu, T.J. (1977): Determination of pungency due to capsicum by gas liquid chromatography. J. Food Sci. 42: 660–665.

[119] Zhang, Z., Pawliszyn, J. (1993): Solid phase microextraction, a solvent free alternative for sample preparation. Analytical Chemistry 65, 1843–1847.

[120] Zhang, Q., Hu, J., Sheng, L., Li, Y. (2010): Simultaneous quantification of capsaicin and dihydrocapsaicin in rat plasma using HPLC coupled with tandem mass spectrometry, J. Chromatogr. B 878: 2292–2297.

[121] Whitfield, F.B., Last, J.H. (1991). Vegetable. In: H. Maarse et al. (Eds.), Volatile Compounds in Food and Beverages. Dekker, New York, pp. 203–281

[122] Wall, M.M., Bosland, P.W. (1998): Analytical methods for color and pungency of chilies (capsicums). In Wetzel, D, Charalambous, G (eds): Instrumental Methods in Food and Beverage Analysis, Elsevier, Amsterdam, pp. 347–373.

[123] WHO guidelines for assessing quality of herbal medicines with reference to contaminats and residues. World Health Organization, 2007.

[124] Woodall, A.A., Britton, G., Jackson, M.J. (1997): Carotenoids and protection of phospholipids in solution or in liposomes against oxidation by peroxyl radicals: Relationship between carotenoid structure and protective ability. Biochim. Biophys. Acta 1336: 575–586.

[125] Woodbury, J.E. (1980): Determination of capsicum pungency by high pressure liquid chromatography and spectrofluorometric detection, J. Assoc. Off. Anal. Chem. 63: 556–558.

[126] Wu, C., Liou, S., 1986. Effect of tissue disruption on volatile constituents of bell peppers. Journal of Agricultural and

[127] Food Chemistry 34, 770–772.

Section 3

Observations with Isolated Gastric Cells Obtained from the Rat Stomach

Chapter 3

Allyl Isothiocyanate, a Pungent Ingredient of Wasabi and Mustard Oil, Impairs Gastric Paracellular Barrier in Primary Cultures from the Rat Stomach via TRPA1-Independent Pathway

Kimihito Tashima, Misako Kabashima,
Kenjiro Matsumoto, Shingo Yano,
Susan J. Hagen and Syunji Horie

Additional information is available at the end of the chapter

http://dx.doi.org/10.5772/58603

1. Introduction

Patients with peptic ulcer and functional dyspepsia avoid food intake of chilies, wasabi, and mustard oil by advised medical staffs, because the prevalent notion is that those condiments would lead to the aggravation of gastric ulcers or stomach pain. However, chilies, wasabi, and mustard oil are known to have pharmacological effects such as the ability to improve apatite and digestion traditionally. It was reported that capsaicin, a pungent ingredient of chilies, induced gastric mucosal protection, accelerated gastric healing, and regulated gastric acid secretion via capsaicin-sensitive sensory neurons from animal and human studies [1-5]. Recently, it has been shown that allyl isothiocyanate, a pungent ingredient of wasabi and mustard oil, has the protective and the aggravating effects of gastric mucosal damages in rats [6-8]. Although the underlying mechanism was investigated, it remained to be inconsistent effects of allyl isothiocyanate on gastric mucosal defense mechanisms.

Gastric mucosal defense mechanisms are essential for preventing potentially harmful elements such as acid, pepsin, and *Helicobacter pylori* (*H. pylori*), present in the gastric lumen from gaining access to the gastric mucosa. Tight junctions, which is classified as epithelial barrier in gastric mucosal defense [9], are dynamic structures located at the most apical region of cell-cell contact points. Interconnected by tight junctions, gastric epithelial cells form tight junction barrier, preventing back diffusion of acid and pepsin. Tight junction proteins are comprised of ZO-1, occludin, claudins, and junctional adhesion molecules (JAMs) [10, 11]. Occludin was the first identified transmembrane protein of tight junctions. Recently, the claudin family is supposedly composed of at least 24 members in mice and human. In the stomach, it has been reported that ZO-1, occludin, claudin-3, 4, 7, and 11 are expressed [12-14]. In addition, electrical resistance, which is an indicator for tight junction barrier, in gastric mucosa was shown the highest in the gastrointestinal tract, suggesting that tight junction barrier play critical roles in gastric mucosal defenses [11]. Indeed, it was reported that the disruption of tight junction complexes were attributed to gastric mucosal damages induced by aspirin in animal model and cell culture studies [14, 15].

1.1. Aim

The aim of the present study is (1) to develop primary cultures of gastric epithelial cells from rats that enable to investigate tight junction barrier, (2) to examine the influence of allyl isothiocyanate (AITC) on tight junction barrier using primary cultures from the rat stomachs, as compared with action of capsaicin. In this paper, it is suggested that allyl isothiocyanate breaks gastric tight junction barrier. In addition, we have established confluent primary cultures from rat stomachs for investigating tight junction barrier of gastric mucosa.

2. Materials and methods

2.1. Animals

Male Sprague-Dawley strain rats (SLC, Hamamatsu, Japan) weighing 180-220 g were used. Animals were housed under controlled environmental conditions (temperature at 24±2°C and light on 7:00 am to 7:00 pm) and fed commercial mouse chow MF (Oriental Yeast, Tokyo, Japan). Animal experiments were performed in compliance with the "Guiding Principles for the Care and Use of Laboratory Animals" approved by the Japanese Pharmacological Society and the guidelines approved by the Ethical Committee on Animal Care and Animal Experimentation of Josai International University (#12). Animals were anesthetized using sodium pentobarbital before the isolation of tissues, and euthanized by over dose of sodium pentobarbital.

2.2. Buffers for cell isolation

Medium A contained (in mM) 0.5 NaH_2PO_4, 1.0 Na_2HPO_4, 20 $NaHCO_3$, 70 NaCl, 5 KCl, 11 glucose, 50 HEPES, 2 Na_2EDTA, and 20 mg/ml BSA (fraction V). Medium B contained (in mM) 0.5 NaH_2PO_4, 1.0 Na_2HPO_4, 20 $NaHCO_3$, 70 NaCl, 5 KCl, 11 glucose, 50 HEPES, 20 mg/ml BSA (fraction V), 1.0 $CaCl_2$, and 1.5 $MgCl_2$. Medium C contained (in mM) 0.5 NaH_2PO_4, 1.0 Na_2HPO_4, 20 $NaHCO_3$, 70 NaCl, 5 KCl, 11 glucose, 50 HEPES, 1 mg/ml BSA (fraction V), 1.0 $CaCl_2$, 1.5 $MgCl_2$, and 0.5 dithiothreitol [16, 17].

2.3. Cell isolation

Cell isolation from the rat stomach was according to the methods described by Tani. et al. [16, 18] and modified by us to collect parietal cells and chief cells [19], where were located at the middle and bottom of gastric glands, from the rat stomach. In brief, three non-fasted rats were anesthetized using sodium pentobarbital. The stomach was excised, everted, and tied at both esophagus and pylorus. The everted sac was filled with 2 ml of Medium A, containing 2.5 mg/ml of protease E and placed in Medium A for 30 min (fraction 1), followed by Medium B for 120 min in a shaking water bath at 37ºC (fractions 2-4). Isolated cells from digestion fractions 4 were pelleted at 240x g in a TOMY EIX-136 centrifuge (Tokyo, Japan), re-suspended in Medium C. The cells were centrifuged at 500x g at room temperature for 10 min and then re-suspended in 1:1 mixture of Ham's F-12 and Dulbecco's minimum essential medium (DMEM/F-12), supplemented with heat-inactivated 10 % fetal bovine serum (FBS), 8 μg/ml insulin, 1 μg/ml hydrocortisone, 100 U/mL penicillin, 100 U/ mL streptomycin, and 0.25 μg/ml amphotericin B.

2.4. Primary cultured gastric epithelial cells

Isolated cells from rat stomachs were plated at density of 3.6 x 10^5 cells/cm^2 in collagen-coated Transwell filters, 35 mm-cultures dishes, and 60 mm-culture dishes. Those cells were incubated in DMEM/F12 supplemented with 10% FBS, 8 μg/ml insulin, 1 μg/ml hydrocortisone, 100 U/ mL penicillin, 100 U/ mL streptomycin, and 0.25 μg/ml amphotericin B under 5 % CO_2 in air at 37 °C by 4 days.

2.5. RGM-1 cells culture

RGM-1 cells, established by Dr. Matsui et al. [Institute of Physical and Chemical Science (RIKEN) Cell Bank and Institute of Clinical Medicine, University of Tsukuba, Tsukuba, Japan], are non-transformed gastric surface epithelial cells [20]. RGM-1 cells were cultured in DMEM/ F-12 supplemented with 10 % FBS, 100 U/mL penicillin, 100 U/mL streptomycin, and 0.25 μg/ ml amphotericin B. RGM-1 cells were plated at density of 2.8 x 10^4 cells/cm^2 in non-coated Transwell filters and incubated in 5 % CO_2 in air at 37 °C by 14-15 days.

2.6. Immunofluorescence microscopy

For histochemical identification of the isolated and 4 day-cultured cells, periodic acid-Sciff reaction (for mucus surface cells), succinic dehydrogenase activity (for parietal cells), and immunofluorescense test for pepsinogen II (for chief cells) were used [21]. Dispersed cells immediately after isolation were pelleted, re-suspended in OCT compound, and then frozen in isopentane cooled with liquid nitrogen. Frozen dispersed cells were sectioned on a cryostat (Leica, Bannockbum, IL, USA) at a thickness of 4 μm. The sections were thaw-mounted on slides glasses. Surface cells were identified by red color (neutral mucins) of the large granules when stained with periodic acid-Sciff stain [22]. Succinic dehydrogenase activity was determined by the methods of Nachlas et al [23]. The sections were incubated in the medium containing 0.2 M phosphate buffer, 0.25 M succinic acid (disodium salt), and nitro-blue tetrazolium (1 mg/ml) for 50 min at 37℃. After incubation, the sections were counterstained cell nuclei by 2 % methyl green for 15 min at 60 min. Parietal cells containing an unusual number of mitochondria among gastric epithelial cells were identified by bluish purple [24]. For immunofluorescence study of pepsinogen II for identification of chief cells, the section was incubated for 1 hr with blocking buffer containing (in mM) 150 NaCl, 10 NaH_2PO_4, 2 mg/ml of gelatin, 0.5 % fish gelatin, and 2 % BSA (globulin-free). Antibody staining was done at room temperature for 2 hr with anti-pepsinogen II antibody (BioDesign, Saco, ME). Evaluation of staining was done using a Nikon TE300 microscope (MicroVideo Instruments, Avon, MA) outfitted with an Orca charge-coupled device camera (Hamamatus Photonics) and IP Lab (Scanalytics, Fairfax, VA) image processing software. In contrast, cells grown on the 35 mm-dish were fixed for 10 min at room temperature with 4 % formaldehyde in 0.2 M phosphate buffer (pH 7.4). Fixed cells were washed with PBS, permeabilized with 0.25 % Triton X-100 containing 0.02 % saponin for 4 min at 4 °C, and then the above procedure were conducted from incubation with blocking buffer to do immunostaining and identification of each cell type. Antibody staining was done at room temperature for 2 hr with anti-cytokeratine 8/18 antibody (Novocastra, Newcastle, UK) for identification of epithelial cells and anti-vimentin antibody for fibroblasts (Novocastra, Newcastle, UK) [25, 26]. Evaluation of cell purity was done by counting the total cell number, as identified by methyl green and propidium iodide staining of nuclei, against the number of cells stained with periodic acid-Sciff, nitro blue tetrazolium, and above specific antibodies. Approximately 1,000 cells/slide were evaluated.

2.7. Electrophysiological analysis of primary cultures and RGM-1 cells

Transepithelial electrical resistance (TER) was measured in Transwell filter chambers using a "Milli-cell" ERS system (Millipore, Billerica, MA, USA). The background resistance of chambers containing medium alone was subtracted from the value of all experimental conditions. TER was evaluated 1) at 1-4 days after seeding in primary cultured epithelial cells from the rat stomach and at 4, 7, 10, 14 days after seeding in RGM-1 cells, and 2) when capsaicin, allyl isothiocyanate, cinnamaldehyde, and icilin were applied into apical compartment at every 30 min for 3 hr after apical application in 4 day-primary cultures.

2.8. Measurement of permeability in confluent primary cultures and RGM-1 cells

Mucosal (Apical or top well) to serosal (nutrient or bottom well) fluxes of mannitol were done using Transwell filters containing confluent monolayers at day 4. For these studies, 3 mM mannitol was added to the luminal solution and 3 mM D-glucose to the serosal solution. After equilibration for 30 min, 2 mCi of [^{3}H]-mannitol (15-30 Ci.mmol, NEM Life Science Products, Boston, MA) was added to the mucosal solution and the cells were returned to 37℃ in the incubator. Triplicate wells were sampled for each treatment at 1 to 3 hr after the addition of labeled mannitol. The concentration of mannitol in the serosal solution was determined by liquid scintillation as described previously in detail [26].

2.9. Fluorescence microscopy and confocal microscope for occludin, ZO-1, and claudin 4

Gastric epithelial cells grown on Transwell filters were fixed for 10 min at room temperature with 4 % formaldehyde in 0.2 M phosphate buffer (pH 7.4). Fixed cells were washed with PBS, permeabilized with 0.25 % Triton X-100 containing 0.02 % saponin for 4 min at 4 °C. Samples were then labeled with either rabbit anti-occludin antibody, rabbit anti-ZO-1 antibody, or mouse anti-claudin 4 antibody, these were followed by incubation with Gel-PBS containing with 1:200 diluted secondary FITC-conjugated goat anti-rabbit IgG or FITC-conjugated donkey anti-mouse IgG. These samples were mounted in Vectashield (Vector Labs, CA, USA). Fluorescence images were collected using an Axioskop 2 plus microscope with a plan-NEOFLUAR 40x objective. The data was analyzed using AxioVision LE Rel 4.6.3 software (Carl Zeiss Vision, Germany). Images were converted to TIFF format and composites of images were prepared using Adobe Photoshop Elements 2.0 (Adobe Co., CA, USA).

2.10. Measurement of cell viability

Cell viability was evaluated by a colorimetric assay using crystal violet [28]. In brief, primary cultured epithelial cells after apical application of pungent ingredients such as capsaicin and allyl isothiocyanate were washed with PBS to remove dead cells, fixed with methanol, air-dried, and stained with crystal violet. Stained cells were solubilized and the absorbance was measured at 590 nm using 1420 Multilabel Counter (Perkin Elmer, Shelton, CT, USA).

2.11. Reverse transcription-polymerase chain reaction

Total RNA was isolated by using an RNeasy kit (Qiagen, CA, USA) according to the manufacturer's protocol. In brief, either the confluent monolayer of primary cultured rat gastric epithelial cells, which were grown for 4 days after platting, the confluent monolayer of RGM-1 cells, or freshly isolated rat dorsal root ganglia was immediately submerged in Buffer RLT (Qiagen), which inhibited RNase activation, and was homogenized by using a Multi-beads shocker (Yasui Kikai, Osaka, Japan). Reverse transcription-polymerase chain reaction (RT-PCR) was performed by using a one-step RT-PCR Kit (Qiagen) and a thermal cycler GeneAmp PCR System 9700 (Applied Biosystems, CA, USA) for 35 cycles (TRPA1, TRPV1, and GAPDH) under the following conditions: reverse transcription at 50°C for 30 min, initial denaturation; 15 min at 95°C and then 30 sec at 94°C, followed by a 30 sec annealing step at 56°C for TRPA1, TRPV1, and GAPDH and 1 min elongation at 72°C. The primers sequences were 5′-CCC CAC TAC ATT GGG CTG CA-3′ and 5′-CCG CTG TCC AGG CAC ATC TT-3′ for rat TRPA1, 5′-TCG TCT ACC TCG TGT TCT TGT TTG-3′ and 5′-CCA GAT GTT CTT GCT CTC TTG TGC-3′ for rat TRPV1, and 5′-TCC CTC AAG ATT GTC AGC AA-3′ and 5′-AGA TCC ACA ACG GAT ACA TT-3′ for rat GAPDH. The PCR products were separated on 3% (wt/vol) agarose gel in Tris-acetate EDTA buffer, stained with ethidium bromide, and analyzed by LAS 3000 (FUJI-FILM, Tokyo, Japan). The sequence of the PCR product was analyzed using the BLAST program (NCBI).

2.12. Materials

BSA (globulin-free), crystal violet, deoxyribonuclease 1, ethidium bromide, fish gelatin, hydrocortisone, insulin, methyl green, nitro blue tetrazolium, periodic acid, protease, and icilin were from Sigma-Aldrich (MO, USA). Absolute ethanol, allyl isothiocyanate, BSA (fraction V), capsaicin, cell culture media, cinnamaldehyde, and dimethyl sulfoxide (DMSO) were from Wako Pure Chemical Industries, Inc. (Osaka, Japan). Rabbit polyclonal anti-occludin antibody, rabbit polyclonal anti-ZO-1 antibody, and monoclonal anti-claudin 4 antibody were from Zymed Laboratories (CA, USA). FITC-conjugated goat anti-rabbit IgG, FITC-conjugated donkey anti-mouse IgG, normal goat serum, and normal donkey serum were from Jackson Immune Research Laboratories (PA, USA). Serum was from GibcoBRL (CA, USA). Propidium iodide was from Molecular Probes (OR, USA). Sodium pentobarbital was from Dainippon Sumitomo Pharma Co. (Osaka, Japan). The 35 mm-and 60 mm-dish, and a collagen type I from rat tail were from Beckton Dickenson Biosciences (MA, USA). Transwell with filter (0.4 μm) was from Corning (MA, USA). Allyl isothiocyanate, capsaicin, and cinnamaldehyde were dissolved in absolute ethanol prior to dilution in cell culture medium, respectively. Icilin was dissolved in DMSO, followed by absolute ethanol prior to dilution in cell culture medium. The final concentrations of either ethanol or DMSO in the apical compartment of Transwell were less than 0.1%. The vehicles used had no pharmacological effects on the epithelial barrier in cell cultures.

2.13. Statistics

Values are presented as means±S.E.M. for three or more independent experiments.. Statistical analysis of data were done with SigmaStat software (Jandel Scientific Software, CA, USA) using a two-tailed Student's *t*-test between two groups, and multiple comparisons against a single control group were made by one-way analysis of variance (ANOVA) with Dunnett's multiple comparisons test. $P < 0.05$ was considered statistically significant.

3. Results

3.1. Identification of isolated cells from the rat gastric mucosa

Isolated cells from the rat stomach were prepared as described in methods and suspended in medium C. The identification of isolated fraction consisted of chief cells (35.6 ± 5.8 %), parietal cells (31.8 ± 2.6 %), and surface cells (10.3 ± 0.9 %) determined by fluorescent and light microscopy (Table 1). The remaining ~23 % of the cells are likely to be the non-identified immature cell, including proliferative cells and occasional endocrine cells. In addition, those isolated cells became a confluent cultures on the collagen-coating dishes by 4 days after seeding, whose cells were stained with anti-cytokeratine 8/18 antibody, a epithelial marker (data not shown), and with no staining anti-vimentin antibody, a fibroblast marker (0.11 ± 0.11 %). These results suggested that primary cultures from the rat stomach are mainly constituted of epithelial cells, including mucus surface cells, chief cells, and parietal cells, respectively.

Cell type	Values (%)	n
Chief cells	35.6±5.8	4
Parietal cells	31.8±2.6	4
Surface cells	10.3±0.9	4

Table 1. Quantification of each cell type (%) in isolated cells from the rat stomach

3.2. Tight junction barrier is formed in primary cultures from the rat stomach

When isolated gastric epithelial cells were plated, cells attached to Transwell filters by 2 days after seeding. Primary cultured epithelial cells completely covered the Transwell filters by 4 days after seeding, which were similar morphological features when cells were grown on plastic dishes (data not shown). In contrast, RGM-1 cells, which are widely used for the investigation of gastric epithelial physiology as a non-transformed gastric surface epithelial cell lines, were also attached and proliferated on Transwell filters, and formed a confluent monolayer by 4 to 5 days after seeding. Therefore, to determine whether those cultures were an appropriate model to investigate tight junction barrier, we first confirmed to form functional tight junctions. Transepithelial electrical resistance (TER) was quantified. We found that as primary cultures reached confluence at 3 to 4 days after seeding, there was a progressive increase in TER (Fig. 1A). TER at 4 days after seeding was 3069.6±582.0 Ohm.cm^2. However, RGM-1 cells did not show any increased TER, even though confluence was observed after 4 days after seeding. TER was less than about 60.0 Ohm.cm^2 throughout the experiment (Fig. 1B).

To investigate why primary cultured epithelial cells, but not RGM-1 cells, have a great high TER, we examined the localization of occludin and ZO-1 for tight junctions in the both cultures. Interestingly, it was found that the localization of occludin and ZO-1 were continuously observed at the cell-cell contact region in primary cultures from the rat stomach (Fig. 2A and B). In RGM-1 cells, occludin was no expressed at the tight junction region, although ZO-1 was only continuously expressed at the cell-cell contact point (Fig. 2C and D). It is suggested that primary cultures from the rat stomach, but not RGM-1 cells, form functional tight junction barrier.

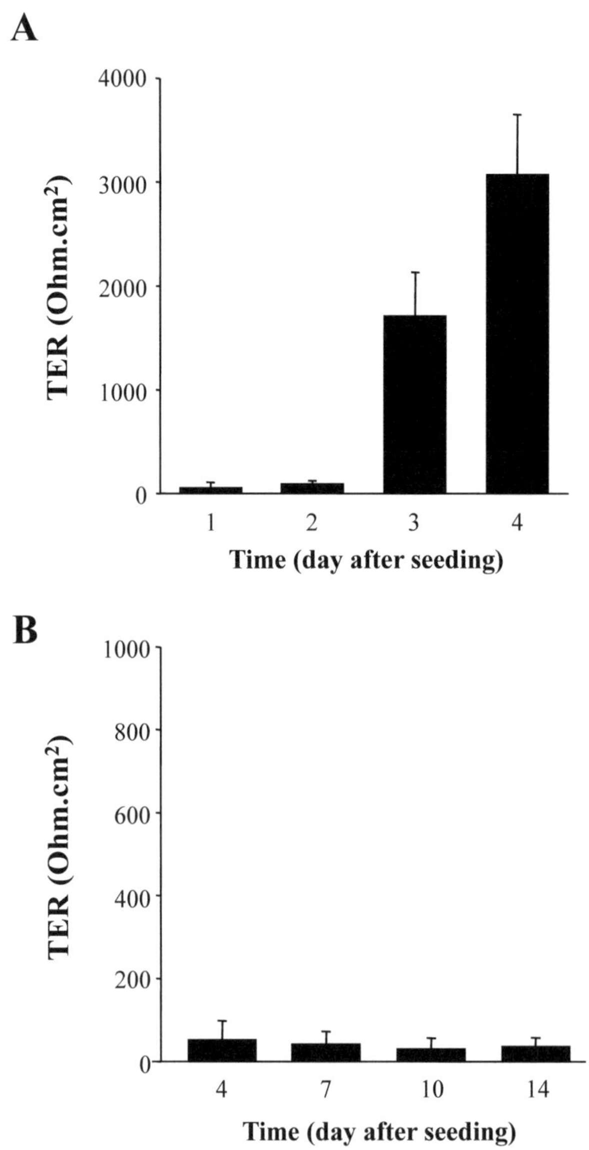

Figure 1. Progressive increased TER in primary cultures from the rat stomach, but not RGM-1 cells. Isolated cells from the rat stomach and RGM-1 cells were grown on Transwell filters. TER was measured from 1 to 4 days after seeding of primary cultures (A) and at 4, 7, 10, 14 days after seeding of RGM-1 cells (B). Data represent means±S.E.M. from 4 independent experiments. Note that primary cultures from the rat stomach produced a great high TER after 3 to 4 days after seeding, when they formed a confluent monolayer.

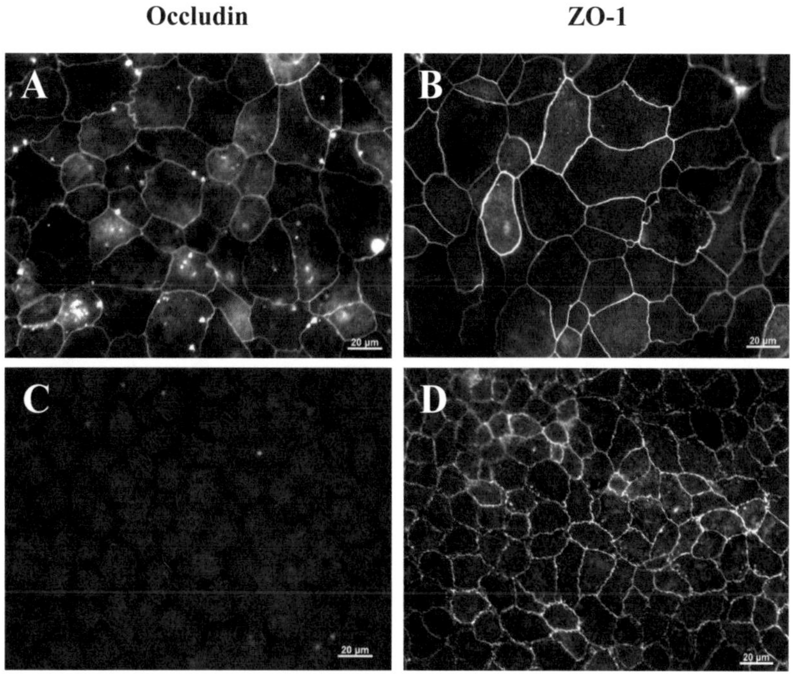

Figure 2. Immunolocalization of occludin and ZO-1 in primary cultures from the rat stomach and RGM-1 cells. The expression is anti-occludin staining (A, C) and anti-ZO-1 staining (B, D) for tight junction. Primary cultures were grown to confluent by 4 days after seeding (A, B), and RGM-1 cells were grown confluent enough by 14 days after seeding on Transwell filters (C, D). Those cells were fixed directly on the filter, incubated with each specific antibody, and evaluated by a fluorescence microscope. Note that the localization of the both occludin and ZO-1 was observed at the entire region of cell-cell contact in primary cultures from the rat stomach, yet occludin, but not ZO-1, did not localize at the cell-cell contact region in RGM-1 cells. Bar (A, B, C, D)=20 µm.

3.3. Allyl isothiocyanate alters tight junction barrier in primary cultures from rat stomachs

To determine the effects of pungent ingredients such as allyl isothiocyanate and capsaicin on tight junction barrier, we next examined TER and the mannitol flux using confluent cultures at 4 days after seeding. Allyl isothiocyanate and capsaicin are applied into the apical side (luminal or top compartment), because the apical side of gastric epithelial cells would be exposed to those pungent ingredients when people intake condiments such as wasabi, mustard oil, chili etc. It was found that 100 µM of allyl isothiocyanate induced a progressive decreased in TER in a time-dependent manner as compared with control (Fig. 3A). TER loss was apparent within 1 hr and fell by about 60 % following 3 hr of application. However, the lower concentration of allyl isothiocyanate (1 and 10 µM) did not affect TER. In contrast, capsaicin failed to affect TER in primary cultures from the rat stomach, even at high concentration (300 µM) of capsaicin (Fig.3C). Permeability was inversely correlated to TER, where cells applied with 100 µM of allyl isothiocyanate produced most permeable cultures among all groups (Fig. 4A and B). Permeability is no change when the lower concentration of allyl isothiocyanate (10 µM) and 300 µM of capsaicin were applied.

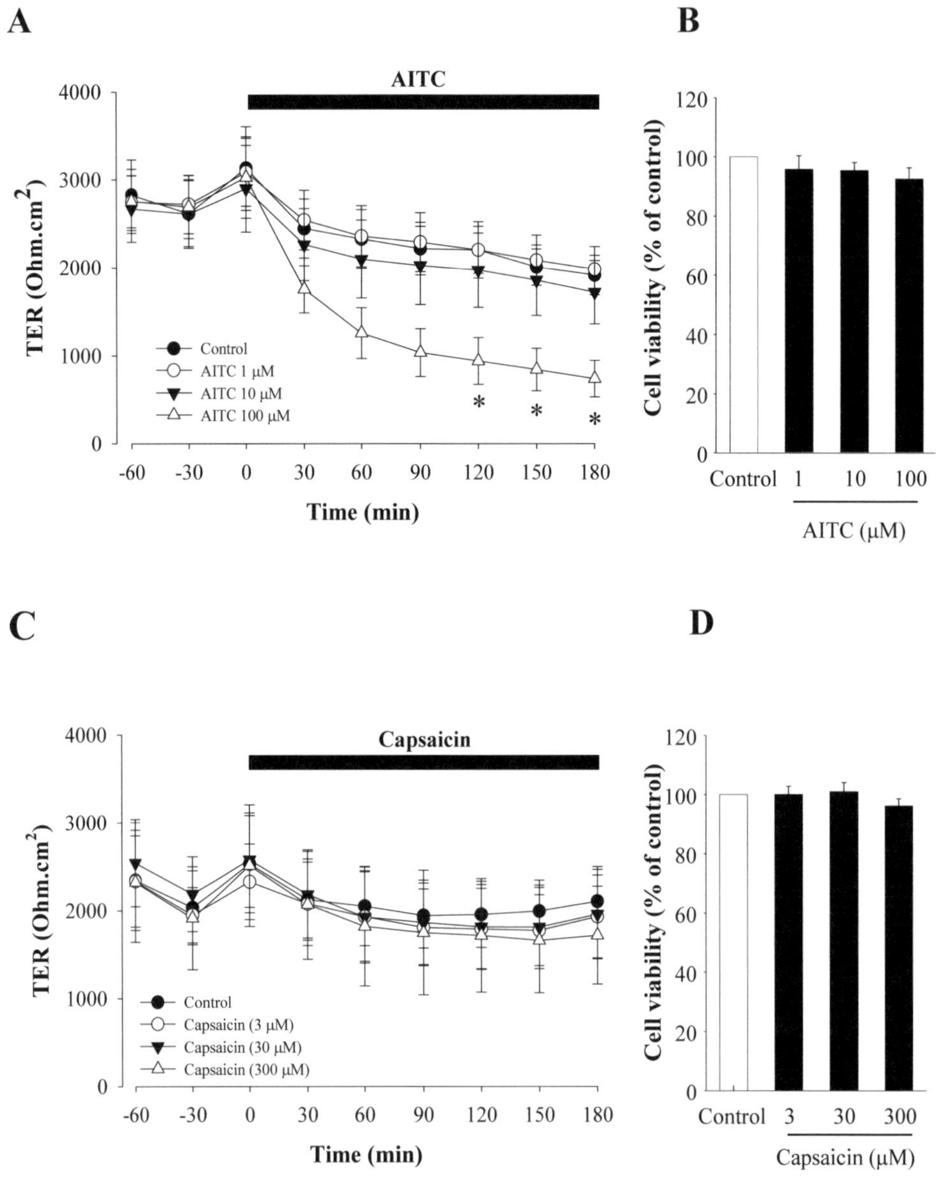

Figure 3. Effect of allyl isothicyanate and capsaicin on TER and cell viability in primary cultures from the rat stomach. Transwell-grown primary cultures from the rat stomach were incubated for 3 hr with allyl-isothiocyanate (A, B) and capsaicin (C, D) each at the indicated concentrations in the apical side. Data for the time-course analysis of TER (A, C) and cell vability (B, D) represent means ± S.E.M. from 3~6 independent experiments. *P<0.05 by ANOVA with Dunnett's multiple comparisons test compared with control. Note that the high dose (100 μM) of allyl-isothiocyanate in the apical side produced a significant decrease in TER in primary cultures from the rat stomach with no affecting cell viability, although the lower dose of allyl-isothiocyanate (1 and 10 μM) did not any alter in TER and cell viability. In addition, notice that capsaicin did not affect TER and cell viability in primary cultures.

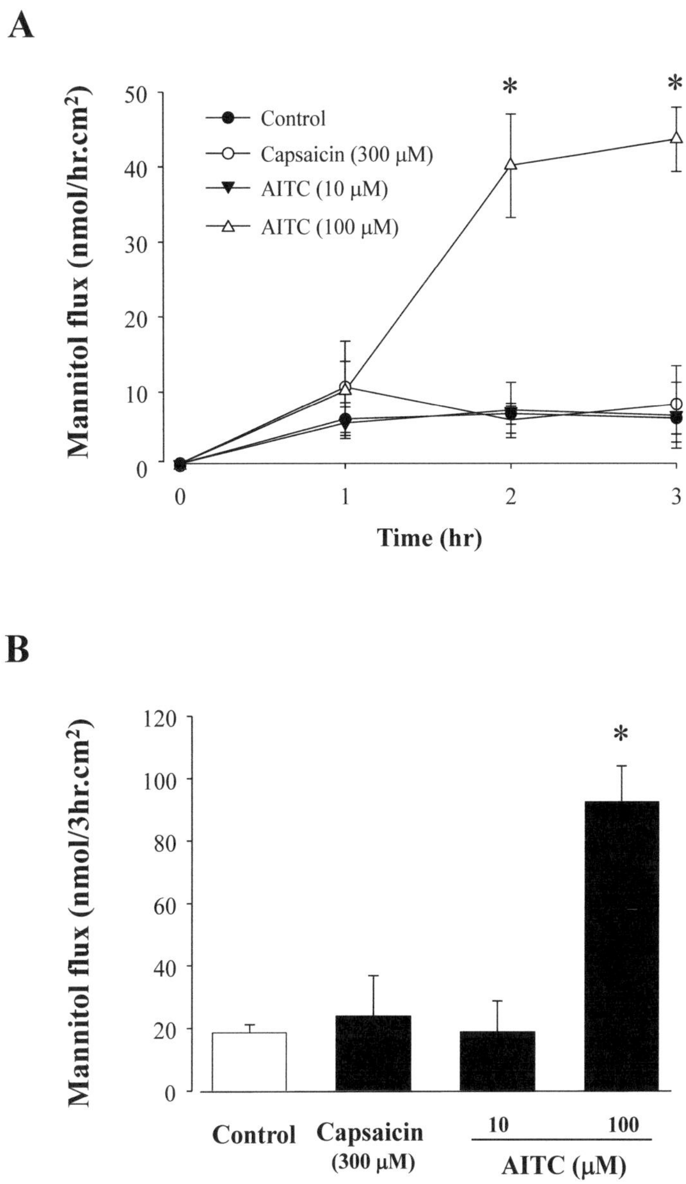

Figure 4. Effect of capsaicin and allyl isothiocyanate on [^{3}H]-mannitol flux in primary cultures from the rat stomach. Isolated cells from the rat stomach were grown to confluence at 4 days after seeding on Transwell filters. The permeability of [^{3}H]-mannitol (MW=182.17) was measured as the flux from the apical to basolateral chambers each hour for 3 hours. *A*: data indicate the [^{3}H]-mannitol flux and presented as means ± S.E.M. of values determines every 1 hr after apical application of capsaicin and allyl isothiocyanate from 3 independent experiments. *$P<0.05$ by ANOVA with Dunnett's multiple comparisons test compared with control. *B*: data show total [^{3}H]-mannitol flux for 3 hr after apical application of capsaicin and allyl isothiocyanate from 3 independent experiments. *$P<0.05$ by ANOVA with Dunnett's multiple comparisons test compared with control. Note that primary cultures from the rat stomach show a low permeability in nature, however the apical application of high concentration of AITC (100 μM), but not low concentration of AITC (10 μM) and capsaicin, produced a high permeable monolayer in primary cultures from the rat stomach.

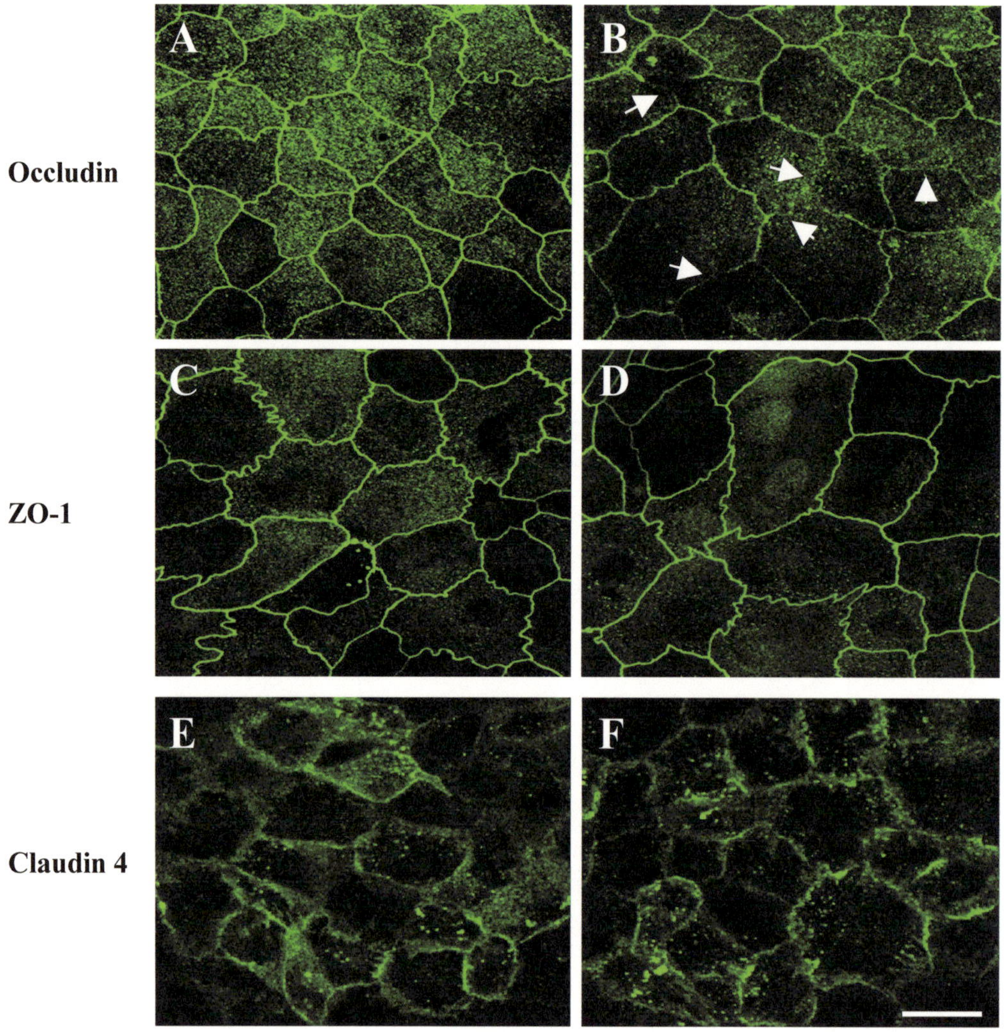

Figure 5. Discontinuous expression of occludin in response to high concentration of allyl isothiocyanate (AITC) in primary cultured epithelial cells from the rat stomach. The green label is anti-occludin antibody (A, B), anti-ZO-1 antibody (C, D), or, anti-claudin 4 antibody (E,F) staining for tight junction. AITC (100 μM) or control (containing 0.1% ethanol) was added for 3 hr in the apical side of transwell-grown primary cultures. Cells were fixed directly on the transwell filter, followed by incubation with anti-occludin antibody, anti-ZO-1 antibody, or, anti-claudin 4 antibody, and evaluated by fluorescence microscope. Note that the continuous expression of occludin, ZO-1, and, claudin 4 at the cell-cell contact region in primary cultures were observed in control, yet the application of AITC (100 mM) induced the discontinuous expression of occludin, but not ZO-1 and claudin 4, at the cell-cell contact region (arrows). Bar=20 mm.

To confirm the loss of tight junction barrier in response to allyl isothiocyanate, we assessed localization of ZO-1, occludin, and claudin 4 for tight junctions in primary cultures by immunocytochemistry. Those proteins are well-characterized tight junction components in the stomach and has been reported that dislocation of tight junction proteins lead to the pathogenesis of gastrointestinal tract such as *H. pylori*-induced gastritis [29]. When vehicle was applied for 3hr, ZO-1, occludin, and claudin 4 were located to the cellular margins (Fig. 5A, C, and E). In contrast, the distribution of occludin was aberrant with discontinuous expression of the cell-cell contact point, when 100 μM of allyl isothiocyanate was applied for 3 hr (Fig. 5B). However, the distribution of ZO-1 and claudin 4 applied by allyl isothiocyanate was found no deference as compared with vehicle-treated groups (Fig. 5D and F).

To determine that the decreased TER and the mannitol flux were not due to allyl isothiocyanate-induced alterations in cell viability, we measured the cell viability of primary cultures at the end of each experiment. Fig. 3B and D demonstrate that primary cultures with allyl isothicianate or capsaicin did not significantly alter cell viability, suggesting that in this system, TER loss following application of allyl isothiocyanate is likely due to modulation of tight junction barrier.

3.4. Allyl isothiocyanate-induced disruption of tight junction barrier is produced via TRPA1-independent pathway

Recently, allyl isothiocyanate is known as an activator of transient receptor potential A1 (TRPA1), which is considered to be a chemosensor in several sensory tissues including gastrointestinal tract [30]. Additionally, it has been well known that TRPA1 is co-expressed with TRPV1, which is ion channel targeted by capsaicin, on neuronal cells such as dorsal root ganglia and trigeminal ganglia. Therefore, to investigate the possibility that loss of tight junction barrier in response to allyl isothiocyanate was attributed to TRPA1 in primary cultures from rat stomachs, we examined (1) the mRNA expression of TRPA1 and TRPV1, and (2) the effect of cinnamaldehyde and icilin, other TRPA1 channel activators, on TER in primary cultures from rat stomachs. We found that not only TRPV1 mRNA (predicted size: 347 bp) but also TRPA1 mRNA (predicted size: 487 bp) were expressed in the primary cultures from rat stomachs (Fig. 6A). By contrast, TRPV1 mRNA was only expressed in RGM-1 cells (Fig. 6B), which is agreement with previous reports [31, 32]. In positive controls samples from the rat dorsal root ganglia, TRPA1 and TRPV1 mRNA were also observed (data not shown). The mRNA expression levels of glyceraldehyde-3-phosphate-dehydroxgenase were unchanged among all tested samples so that the mRNA expression analysis by using RT-PCR was done appropriately, suggesting that TRPA1 and TRPV1 are periphery expressed at mRNA levels in native gastric epithelial cells in rats. Therefore, we investigate the effect of cinnamaldehyde and icilin, the other TRPA1 activators, on TER. When apical application of neither cinnamaldehyde (3-300 μM) nor icilin (1-100 μM) for 3 hr induced decrease in TER (Fig. 7A, C) and cell viability (Fig. 7B, D) in primary cultures from rat stomachs. In addition, TER reduction in response to100 μM of allyl isothiocyanate was not inhibited in the presence of 10 μM of ruthenium red, which is a nonselective TRP channel inhibitor (data not shown) [33]. These results suggested that allyl isothiocyanate breaks tight junction barrier in primary cultures not via the pathway of TRPA1 channels activation.

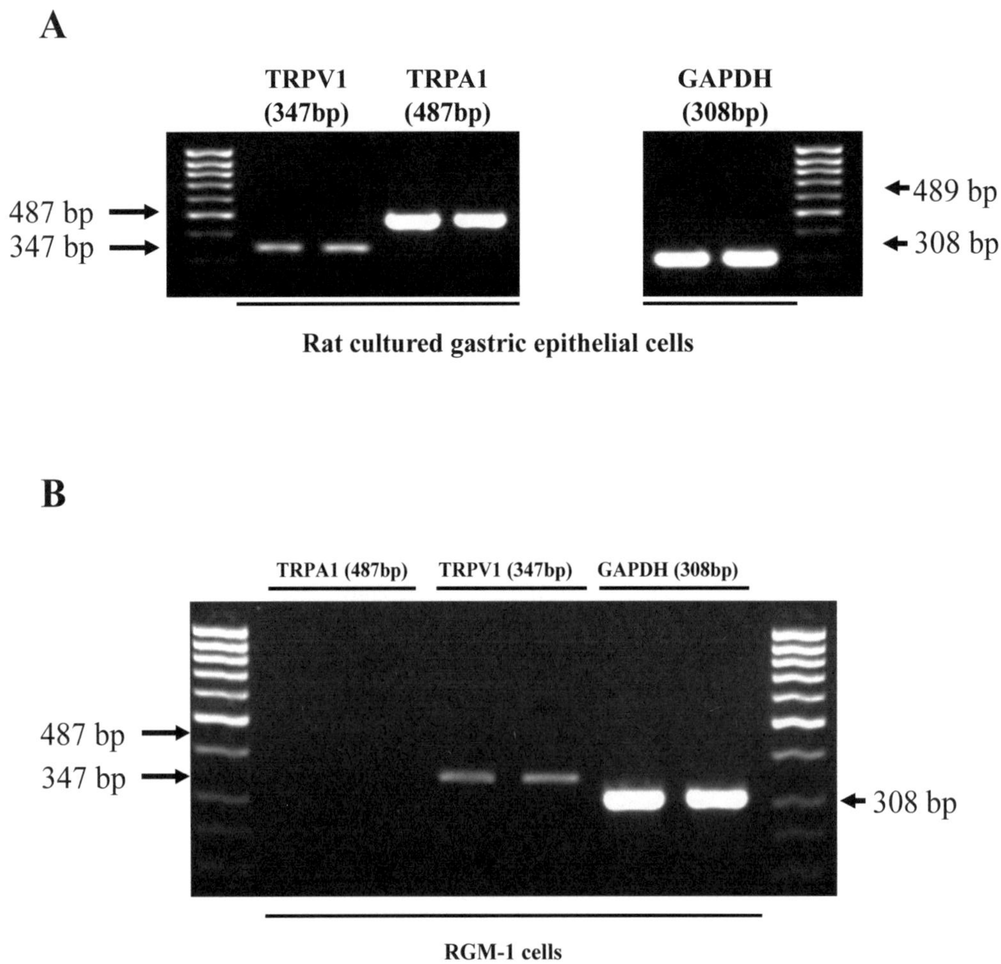

Figure 6. Expression of TRPV1, TRPA1, and, TRPM8 mRNA in primary cultures from the rat stomach, and the expression of TRPV1 and TRPA1 mRNA in RGM-1 cells by RT-PCR. Total RNA was isolated from rat dorsal root ganglia, primary cultures from the rat stomach, and RGM-1 cells. Data showed the mRNA expression of TRPV1 and TRPA1 in primary cultures from the rat stomach (A), and in RGM-1 cells (B). The mRNA levels were analyzed by PCR (35 cycles) using primers for TRPA1, TRPV1, and GAPDH. Rat DRG was used as positive control samples for TRPA1, TRPV1, and TRPM8 mRNA. Predicted sizes of PCR products are TRPA1 (487 bp), TRPV1 (347 bp), and GAPDH (308 bp), respectively. M: marker. GAPDH was the control for assay efficiency.

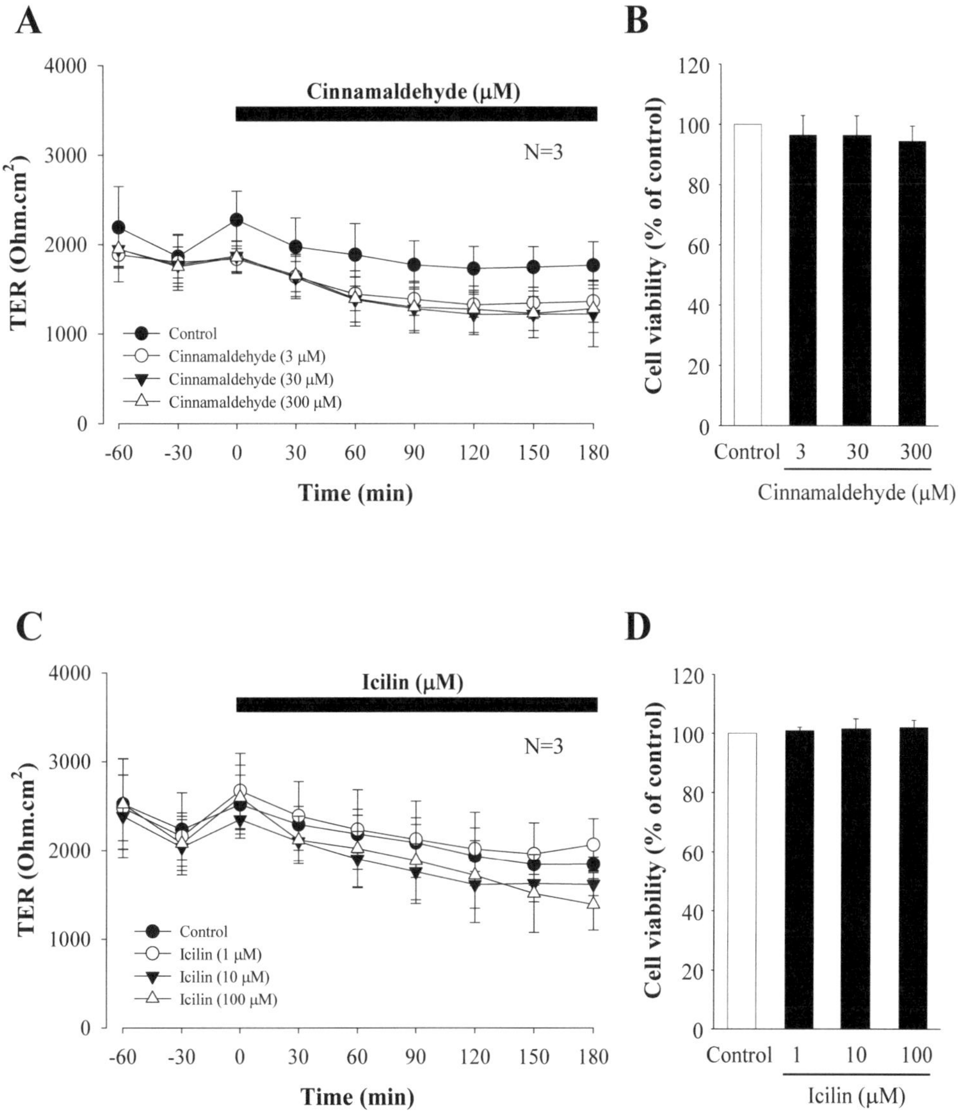

Figure 7. Effect of cinnamaldehyde and icilin, the other TRPA1 antagonist, on TER and cell viability in primary cultures from the rat stomach on AITC-induced TER reduction and cell viability in primary cultures from the rat stomach. Trans-well-grown primary cultures from the rat stomach were incubated for 3 hr with cinnamaldehyde (A, B) and icilin (C, D) each at the indicated concentrations in the apical side. Data for the time-course analysis (A, C) and cell viability (B, D) represent means ± S.E.M. from 3 independent experiments. Note that the application of cinnamaldehyde and icilin, which are TRPA1 agonists, did not affect TER and cell viability.

4. Discussion

Previous investigations into mechanism by which noxious substances, including acid, *H. pylori,* non-steroidal anti-inflammatory drugs (NSAIDs), and dietary nitrate, disrupts the tight junctions barrier have been limited by the lack of testable gastric epithelial cells models that form functional tight junction barrier. The present study has utilized a biologically relevant in vitro model of the influence of condiments such as wasabi, mustard oil, and chilies on gastric epithelial cell to demonstrate that exposure of allyl isothiocyanate, a pungent ingredient of wasabi and mustard oil, induced a progressive loss of TER which is followed by disruption of occludin at the levels of the tight junctions, but not capsaicin which is a pungent ingredient of chilies. Our results have also identified TRPA1, which is activated by allyl isothiocyanate and are expressed in native rat gastric epithelia cells, is not involved in tight junction barrier dysfunction.

4.1. Confluent primary cultures with a great high TER

Isolated cells from the rat stomach, which are consisted of not only surface cells but also parietal cells, chief cells, and non-identified immature cells, were grown a confluent monolayer with a great high TER (>2000 Ohm.cm^2), whose cultures are also identified as epithelial cells. In previous reports, TER in gastric mucosa was shown the highest in the gastrointestinal tract (>2000 Ohm.cm^2) to prevent mucosal damages from exposure of luminal acid and pepsin [11], suggesting that tight junction barrier plays critical roles in gastric mucosal defenses as epithelial barriers. Although MDCK cells, T-84 cells, AGS cells, and MNK 28 cells [34] are frequently used to study aspect tight junction barrier, those cells are not of gastric origin or gastric adenocarcinoma cells so that those experimental data might not faithfully replicate the physiology of gastric epithelial cells. In addition, RGM-1 cells as a non-transformed cell line established from the rat stomach is a very useful cell culture models for investigation of gastric epithelial physiology [20, 28]. However, we found that RGM-1 cells is not able to form tight junction barrier with a high TER, although our results revealed that occludin expression was not located at cell-cell contact region in RGM-1 cells, whereas ZO-1 expression was continuously located at tight junctions regions. It has been reported that occludin-/-mice produced histological abnormalites in the gastric epithelium, which were complete loss of parietal and mucus cell hyperplasia, suggesting that occludin is involved in not only epithelial barrier formation but also epithelial differentiation in the stomach [35, 36]. It has been shown that the expression of tight junction proteins are at the cell-cell contact points which is identified as mature epithelial or endothelial cells in physiological condition, whereas down regulation of tight junction proteins is associated with survival and metastatic potential in human gastric cancer [37]. Shimokawa et al. [38] reported that RGM-1 cells had no secretory granules and the abundance of polyribosomes by using electron microscopic analysis, suggesting that RGM-1 cells are undifferentiated and proliferating mucous progenitor cells, not mature and differentiated mucous neck cells. In agreement with those previous reports, the lock of occludin expression at tight junction regions in RGM-1 cells is due to characterize as immature gastric epithelial cell line such as proliferating mucus progenitor cells. So that primary cultures from the rat stomach was mimicked to the gastric epithelium, which is stand against noxious substances such as gastric acid and pepsin.

4.2. Allyl isothiocyanate, but not capsaicin, breaks tight junction barrier, which is independent on TRPA1

We next explored the alteration of tight junction barrier in response to allyl isothiocyanate and capsaicin in primary cultures from the rat stomach. That is because the digestive properties of capsaicin and allyl isothiocyanate were attributed to enhancement of digestive functions such as acid secretion [5], motility [39, 40], and mucosal blood flow [41, 42]. However, little is known those pungent ingredients of condiments affect gastric epithelial barrier. Although some reports showed that very high concentration of capsaicin (5 mM) in luminal side decreased in TER in the human intestinal epithelial cell line HCT-8 [43], there is no report about allyl isothiocyanate. In the present studies, it was observed the luminal application of capsaicin (300 μM) did not have any changes in tight junction barrier, whereas the luminal application of allyl isothiocyanate at high concentration (100 μM) induced the decreased tight junction barrier in primacy cultures from the rat stomach. Yet, the low concentration of allyl isothiocyanate (<10 μM) did not provide any alteration of tight junction barrier in primary cultures. Indeed, the localization of tight junction proteins including occludin, ZO-1, and claudin 4 were continuously expressed at the cell-cell region in control group. However, the discontinuous expression of occludin, but not ZO-1 and claudin 4, was observed in the group treated with high concentration of allyl isothiocyanate in primary cultures, suggesting that dislocation of occludin provide the loss of tight junction barrier in response to allyl isothiocyanate.

It has been reported that TRPA1 is expressed primarily in small diameter, nociceptive neurons, where its activation likely contributes to a variety of sensory processes, including thermal nociception and inflammatory hyperalgesia [44]. TRPA1 is an excitatory ion channels targeted by irritant compounds derived from plants including wasabi, mustard, and cinnamon [45]. TRPA1 expression has been demonstrated in gastrointestinal tract [40, 46], especially it was showed that TRPA1 protein expression in gastric sensory neurons in rat using immunohistochemistry [47]. Although little was known about the expression of TRPA1 in non-neuronal cells, Nozawa et al. [48] and Kono et al. [49] recently reported that TRPA1 was expressed in serotonin-containing enterochromaffin cells in the rat small intestine and rat intestinal epithelial cells. These findings let us speculate that gastric epithelial cells express TRPA1 functionally. Interestingly, in the present study, TRPA1 mRNA was also found to be clearly expressed in primary cultures from the rat stomach which are epithelial cells identified with the anti-cytokeratine 8/18 antibody, although there was no observation of the expression of TRPA1 mRNA in RGM-1 cells. These data indicated that TRPA1 was located on not only gastric sensory neuron but also native gastric epithelial cells. Therefore, we asked if the loss of tight junction barrier in response to allyl isothiocyanate was mediated by TRPA1 in primary cultures. It was analyzed by using the other TRPA1 activator cinnamaldehyde and icilin [50], so that it was observed those TRPA1 activator did not provide the loss of tight junction barrier at all. Additionally, it was also observed allyl isothiocyanate-induced tight junction's alteration was not dose-dependently, and was not inhibited by the pretreatment of a non-selective TRP blocker ruthenium red (data not shown), suggesting that the loss of tight junctions in response to allyl isothiocyanate was not mediated by TRPA1 in primary cultures of the rat stomach.

5. Conclusion

In conclusion, it is suggested that allyl-isothiocyanate breaks gastric tight junction barrier via TRPA1-independent pathways. In addition, we have established a unique technique to form the confluent primary cultures from rat stomachs with a great high TER.

Terminology

TJ: tight junction

RGM-1 cells: rat gastric epithelial cell line

TER: Transepithelial electrical resistance

TRPV1: transient receptor potential vanilloid type 1

TRPA1: transient receptor potential ankyrin 1

ZO-1: zonula occludens-1

S.E.M: standard error of mean

Acknowledgements

The authors thank Dr. Hirofumi Matsui for providing RGM-1 cells and Miwa Yoshida for effort in analysis of tight junction barrier in RGM-1 cells for this work. This work was supported by a JSPS KAKENHI Grant Number 18790127 and by a grant from the Hamaguchi Fundation for the advancement of biochemistry.

Present address of M. Kabashima: Pharmaceutical department, Red Cross Fukuoka Hospital, 3-1-1 Ookusu, Minami-ku, Fukuoka, 815-8555, Japan. Present address of K. Matsumoto: Department of Pharmacology and Experimental Therapeutics, Divison of Pathological Sciences, Kyoto Pharmaceutical University, 5 Nakauchi Misasagi Yamashina-ku, Kyoto 607-8414, Japan. Present address of S. Yano: Faculty of Pharmaceutical Sciences, Teikyo Heisei University, 4-21-2 Nakano Nakano-ku, Tokyo 164-8530, Japan.

http://dx.doi.org/10.5772/58603

Author details

Kimihito Tashima[1*], Misako Kabashima[2], Kenjiro Matsumoto[3], Shingo Yano[2], Susan J. Hagen[4] and Syunji Horie[4]

*Address all correspondence to: ktashima@jiu.ac.jp

1 Lab. of Pharmacology, Faculty of Pharmaceutical Science, Josai International University, Togane, Japan

2 Lab. of Molecular Pharmacology and Pharmacotherapeutics, Graduate School of Pharmaceutical Sciences, Chiba University, Chiba, Japan

3 Lab. of Pharmacology, Faculty of Pharmaceutical Science, Josai International University, Togane, Japan

4 Dept. of Surgery, Beth Israel Deaconess Medical Center, Boston, Massachusetts, USA

The authors have no competing interests.

References

[1] Holzer P: Neural gastroenterology and motility; Neural regulation of gastrointestinal blood flow. In: Johnson LR (ed.) Physiology of the Gastrointestinal Tract. Fourth Edition, Academic Press; 2006. P 817-839

[2] Kang JY, Teng CH, Wee A, Chen FC: Effect of capsaicin and chilli on ethanol induced gastric mucosal injury in the rat. Gut. 1995; 36: 664-669

[3] Takeuchi K, Ueshima K, Ohuchi T, Okabe S: The role of capsaicin-sensitive sensory neurons in healing of HCl-induced gastric mucosal lesions in rats. Gastroenterology. 1994; 106:1524-1532

[4] Mózsik G, Debreceni A, Abdel-Salam OM, Szabó I, Figler M, Ludány A, Juricskay I, Szolcsányi J: Small doses of apsaicin given intragastrically inhibit gastric basal acid secretion in healthy human subjects. J Physiol Paris 1999; 93: 433-436

[5] Okumi H, Tashima K, Matsumoto K, Namiki T, Terasawa K, Horie S: Dietary agonists of TRPV1 inhibit gastric acid ecretion in mice. Planta Med. 2012; 78: 1801-1806

[6] Matsuda H, Ochi M, Nagatomo A et al: Effect of allyl isothiocyanate from horseradish on several experimental gastric esions in rats. Eur J Pharmacol 2007; 571: 172-181

[7] zumi N, Hayashi S, Sugihara T, Kato S, Takeuchi K: Biphasic effect of Japanese horseradish and mustard on gastric ulcerogenic responses in rats. Gastroenterology 2008; 134 (Suppl 1): A240 (abstract).

[8] Tashima K, Raimura M, Matsumoto K, Chino A, Namiki T, Terasawa K, Horie S: Effect of allyl isothiocyanate, a pungent ingredient of wasabi and mustard oil, on gastric mucosal blood flow and ulcerogenesis in rats: comparison with apsaicin. Gastroenterology 2010; 138: (Suppl 1): S-721 (abstract)

[9] Laine L, Takeuchi K, Tarnawski A: Gastric mucosal defense and cytoprotection: bench to bedside. Gastroenterology 2008; 135: 41-60

[10] Tsukita S, Furuse M, Itoh M: Multifunctional Strands in tight junctions. Nat Rev Mol Cell Biol 2001; 2: 285-293

[11] Ma TY, Anderson JM: Tight junction and the intestinal barrier. In: Johnson LR (ed.) Physiology of the Gastrointestinal Tract. Fourth Edition, Academic Press; 2006. P 1559-1594

[12] Oshima T, Miwa H, Joh T: Aspirin induces gastric epithelial barrier dysfunction by activating p38 MAPK via claudin-7. Am J Physiol Cell Physiol. 2008; 295: C800-806

[13] Kimura Y, Shiozaki H, Hirao M, Maeno Y, Doki Y, Inoue M, Monden T, Ando-Akatsuka Y, Furuse M, Tsukita S, Monden M: Expression of occludin, tight-junction-associated protein, in human digestive tract. Am J Pathol. 1997; 151:45-54

[14] Rahner C, Mitic LL, Anderson JM: Heterogeneity in expression and subcellular localization of claudins 2, 3, 4, and 5 in he rat liver, pancreas, and gut. Gastroenterology. 2001;120: 411-422

[15] Meyer RA, McGinley D, Posalaky Z: Effects of aspirin on tight junction structure of the canine gastric mucosa. Gastroenterology 1986; 91: 351-359

[16] Tani S, Tanaka T.: Direct inhibition of pepsinogen secretion from rat gastric chief cells by somatostatin. Chem Pharm Bull (Tokyo). 1990; 38: 2246-2248

[17] Hadjiagapiou C, Schmidt L, Dudeja PK, Layden TJ, Ramaswamy K: Mechanism(s) of butyrate transport in Caco-2 cells: ole of monocarboxylate transporter 1. Am J Physiol Gastrointest Liver Physiol. 2000; 279: G775-780

[18] Tani S, Tanaka T, Kudo Y, Takahagi M: Pepsinogen secretion from cultured rat gastric mucosal cells. Chem Pharm Bull Tokyo). 1989; 37: 2188-2190

[19] Tashima K, Zhang S, Ragasa R, Nakamura E, Seo JH, Muvaffak A, Hagen SJ: Hepatocyte growth factor regulates the development of highly pure cultured chief cells from rat stomach by stimulating chief cell proliferation in vitro. Am J Physiol Gastrointest Liver Physiol. 2009;296: G319-329

[20] Kobayashi I, Kawano S, Tsuji S, Matsui H, Nakama A, Sawaoka H, Masuda E, Takei Y, Nagano K, Fusamoto H, Ohno T, Fukutomi H, Kamada T: RGM1, a cell line de-

rived from normal gastric mucosa of rat. In Vitro Cell Dev Biol Anim. 1996; 32: 259-261

[21] Schwenk M, Thiedemann KU, Giebel J: Diversity of cell-cell interactions formed by gastric parietal cells in culture: morphological study on guinea pig cells. J Submicrosc Cytol Pathol. 1993; 25: 333-340

[22] Matsumoto A, Asada S, Saitoh O, Tei H, Okumura Y, Hirata I, Ohshiba S: A study on gastric ulcers induced by long-term asting in rats. Scand J Gastroenterol (Suppl) 1989; 162: 75-78

[23] Nachlas MM, Tsou KC, DE Souza E, Cheng CS, Seligman AM: Cytochemical demonstration of succinic dehydrogenase by the use of a new p-nitrophenyl substituted ditetrazole. J Histochem Cytochem. 1957; 5: 420-436

[24] to S. Functional Gastric Morphology. In: Johnson LR. (ed.) Physiology of the Gastrointestinal Tract. Second Edition, Raven Press; 1987. P817-851.

[25] Brembeck FH, Moffett J, Wang TC, Rustgi AK: The keratin 19 promoter is potent for cell-specific targeting of genes in ransgenic mice. Gastroenterology. 2001; 120: 1720-1728

[26] Basque JR, Chailler P, Perreault N, Beaulieu JF, Ménard D: A new primary culture system representative of the human gastric epithelium. Exp Cell Res. 1999; 253: 493-502

[27] Abdul-Ghaffar Al-Shaibani TA, Hagen SJ: Regulation of acid secretion and paracellular permeability by F-actin in the bullfrog, Rana catesbeiana. Am J Physiol Gastrointest Liver Physiol. 2002; 282: G519-526

[28] Nakamura E, Hagen SJ: Role of glutamine and arginase in protection against ammonia-induced cell death in gastric pithelial cells. Am J Physiol Gastrointest Liver Physiol. 2002; 283: G1264-1275

[29] Wroblewski LE, Shen L, Ogden S, Romero-Gallo J, Lapierre LA, Israel DA, Turner JR, Peek RM Jr. Helicobacter pylori dysregulation of gastric epithelial tight junctions by urease-mediated myosin II activation. Gastroenterology. 2009; 136: 236-246

[30] Kaji I, Yasuoka Y, Karaki S, Kuwahara A: Activation of TRPA1 by luminal stimuli induces EP4-mediated anion secretion in human and rat colon. Am J Physiol Gastrointest Liver Physiol. 2012; 302: G690-701

[31] Kato S, Aihara E, Nakamura A, Xin H, Matsui H, Kohama K, Takeuchi K: Expression of vanilloid receptors in rat gastric pithelial cells: role in cellular protection. Biochem Pharmacol. 2003; 66:1115-1121

[32] Hayashi S, Nakamura E, Kubo Y, Takahashi N, Yamaguchi A, Matsui H, Hagen SJ, Takeuchi K: Impairment by allyl sothiocyanate of gastric epithelial wound repair through inhibition of ion transporters. Physiol Pharmacol. 2008; 59: 691-706

[33] Hashimoto K, Oshima T, Tomita T, Kim Y, Matsumoto T, Joh T, Miwa H: Oxidative stress induces gastric epithelial permeability through claudin-3. Biochem Biophys Res Commun. 2008; 376: 154-157

[34] Saitou M, Furuse M, Sasaki H, Schulzke JD, Fromm M, Takano H, Noda T, Tsukita S. Complex phenotype of mice acking occludin, a component of tight junction strands. Mol Biol Cell. 2000;11: 4131-4142

[35] Schulzke JD, Gitter AH, Mankertz J, Spiegel S, Seidler U, Amasheh S, Saitou M, Tsukita S, Fromm M: Epithelial transport and barrier function in occludin-deficient mice. Biochim Biophys Acta. 2005; 1669: 34-42

[36] Ohtani S, Terashima M, Satoh J, Soeta N, Saze Z, Kashimura S, Ohsuka F, Hoshino Y, Kogure M, Gotoh M: Expression of tight-junction-associated proteins in human gastric cancer: downregulation of claudin-4 correlates with tumor aggressiveness and survival. Gastric Cancer. 2009; 12: 43-51

[37] Shimokawa O, Matsui H, Nagano Y, Kaneko T, Shibahara T, Nakahara A, Hyodo I, Yanaka A, Majima HJ, Nakamura Y, Matsuzaki Y: Neoplastic transformation and induction of H+,K+-adenosine triphosphatase by N-methyl-N'-nitro-N-nitrosoguanidine in the gastric epithelial RGM-1 cell line. In Vitro Cell Dev Biol Anim. 2008; 44: 26-30

[38] McNamara CR, Mandel-Brehm J, Bautista DM, Siemens J, Deranian KL, Zhao M, Hayward NJ, Chong JA, Julius D, Moran MM, Fanger CM: TRPA1 mediates formalin-induced pain. Proc Natl Acad Sci U S A. 2007; 104: 13525-13530

[39] Matsumoto K, Kurosawa E, Terui H, Hosoya T, Tashima K, Murayama T, Priestley JV, Horie S: Localization of TRPV1 nd contractile effect of capsaicin in mouse large intestine: high abundance and sensitivity in rectum and distal colon. Am Physiol Gastrointest Liver Physiol. 2009; 297: G348-360

[40] Penuelas A, Tashima K, Tsuchiya S, Matsumoto K, Nakamura T, Horie S, Yano S: Contractile effect of TRPA1 receptor gonists in the isolated mouse intestine. Eur J Pharmacol. 2007; 576:143-150

[41] Raimura M, Tashima K, Matsumoto K, Tobe S, Chino A, Namiki T, Terasawa K, Horie S: Neuronal nitric oxide ynthase-derived nitric oxide is involved in gastric mucosal hyperemic response to capsaicin in rats. Pharmacology. 2013; 92: 60-70

[42] Tashima K, Yoshikubo M, Raimura M, Ozone K, Okumi H, Matsumoto K, Chino A, Namiki T, Horie S: Allyl sothiocyanate, a dietary activator of TRPA1, increases gastric mucosal blood flow through TRPV1-expressing and non-xpressing sensory nerves in rats. Gastroenterology 2011; 140 (Suppl 1): S471 (abstract)

[43] ensen-Jarolim E, Gajdzik L, Haberl I, Kraft D, Scheiner O, Graf J: Hot spices influence permeability of human intestinal pithelial monolayers. J Nutr. 1998; 128: 577-581

[44] Trevisani M, Siemens J, Materazzi S, Bautista DM, Nassini R, Campi B, Imamachi N, Andrè E, Patacchini R, Cottrell GS, Gatti R, Basbaum AI, Bunnett NW, Julius D, Gep-

petti P. 4-Hydroxynonenal, an endogenous aldehyde, causes pain nd neurogenic inflammation through activation of the irritant receptor TRPA1. Proc Natl Acad Sci U S A. 2007; 104: 13519-13524

[45] Bautista DM, Movahed P, Hinman A, Axelsson HE, Sterner O, Högestätt ED, Julius D, Jordt SE, Zygmunt PM: Pungent products from garlic activate the sensory ion channel TRPA1. Proc Natl Acad Sci U S A. 2005; 102: 12248-11252

[46] Poole DP, Pelayo JC, Cattaruzza F, Kuo YM, Gai G, Chiu JV, Bron R, Furness JB, Grady EF, Bunnett NW: TRPA1 gonists delay gastric emptying in rats through serotonergic pathways. Gastroenterology. 2011; 141: 565-575

[47] Kondo T, Obata K, Miyoshi K, Sakurai J, Tanaka J, Miwa H, Noguchi K: Transient receptor potential A1 mediates gastric distention-induced visceral pain in rats. Gut. 2009; 58:1342-1352

[48] Nozawa K, Kawabata-Shoda E, Doihara H, Kojima R, Okada H, Mochizuki S, Sano Y, Inamura K, Matsushime H, Koizumi T, Yokoyama T, Ito H: TRPA1 regulates gastrointestinal motility through serotonin release from nterochromaffin cells. Proc Natl Acad Sci U S A. 2009; 106: 3408-3413

[49] Kono T, Kaneko A, Omiya Y, Ohbuchi K, Ohno N, Yamamoto M: Epithelial transient receptor potential ankyrin 1 TRPA1)-dependent adrenomedullin upregulates blood flow in rat small intestine. Am J Physiol Gastrointest Liver Physiol. 2013; 304: G428-436

[50] Bandell M, Story GM, Hwang SW, Viswanath V, Eid SR, Petrus MJ, Earley TJ, Patapoutian A: Noxious cold ion channel TRPA1 is activated by pungent compounds and bradykinin. Neuron. 2004; 41: 849-857

Section 4

Observations with Capsaicin(oids) in the Gastrointestinal Tract of Animals

Chapter 4

Cooperative Effects of Neuronal Nitric Oxide Synthase and Endothelial Nitric Oxide Synthase on Gastric Hyperemic Response to Intragastric Capsaicin

Syunji Horie, Masaki Raimura, Kenjiro Matsumoto,
Takao Namiki, Katsutoshi Terasawa,
John V. Priestley and Kimihito Tashima

Additional information is available at the end of the chapter

http://dx.doi.org/10.5772/58557

1. Introduction

1.1. Capsaicin-sensitive afferent nerves

Capsaicin-sensitive afferent nerves play an important role in maintaining the integrity of the gastric mucosa. Stimulation of these nerves by capsaicin has been demonstrated to protect gastric mucosa from a variety of noxious stimuli through increased gastric mucosal blood flow (GMBF) [1, 2]. The binding site of capsaicin has been cloned, and named transient receptor potential vanilloid type 1 (TRPV1), a nonselective cation channel [3]. It is reported that capsaicin stimulates these afferent nerves through activation of TRPV1, resulting in gastric mucosal protection [4] and gastric hyperemic response [5], which are mediated by both calcitonin gene-related peptide (CGRP) and nitric oxide (NO) [6, 7]. Indeed, it has been shown that gastric mucosal vasodilation induced by intragastric application of capsaicin was reduced by the inhibitor of NO synthase (NOS), N^G-nitro-L-arginine methyl ester (L-NAME) [8].

1.2. Nitric oxide synthase

NO has been reported to affect gastric mucosal blood flow [9]. In mammals, three isoforms of NOS encoded by different genes have been identified [10]. The constitutively expressed isoforms include neuronal NOS (nNOS) present in the neuron and endothelial NOS (eNOS) present in the endothelium lining the vasculature. Inducible NOS (iNOS) requires a stimulus (cytokines and lipopolysaccharides) for expression in specific cell types such as macrophages, neutrophils, and epithelial cells. Therefore, eNOS-derived NO is assumed to contribute to the gastric hyperemic response to capsaicin although the gastric mucosa has been shown to contain not only eNOS [11, 12] but also nNOS [11] and iNOS [13].

Interestingly, Chen et al. [14] speculated that NO comes from not only endothelium but also nitroxidergic nerves in the submucosa in gastric vasodilation response to capsaicin. However, it has not been studied which NOS isoforms contribute to gastric hyperemic responses to capsaicin thus far.

1.3. Aim

In the present report, we examined to determine the roles of NOS isoforms on gastric hyperemic response to capsaicin in urethane-anesthetized rats by using pharmacological tools, including N^5-[imino (propylamino) methyl]-L-ornithine, (NPLA; a selective nNOS inhibitor), N^5-(l-iminoethyl)-L-ornithine (L-NIO; a selective eNOS inhibitor), and 1400W (a selective iNOS inhibitor). In addition, we investigated the localization relationship of nNOS and TRPV1-expressing nerves in rat stomachs by using immunohistochemical analysis.

2. Material and methods

2.1. Animals

Male Sprague–Dawley strain rats (SLC, Hamamatsu, Japan) weighing 180–220 g were used. Animals were housed under controlled environmental conditions (temperature, 24 ± 2°C and lights on 7:00 am to 7:00 pm) and fed commercial rat chow MF (Oriental Yeast, Tokyo, Japan). The animals were kept in individual cages with raised mesh bottoms to prevent coprophagy, and they were deprived of food but allowed free access to tap water for 18 h before the experiments. Animal experiments were performed according to the "Guiding Principles for the Care and Use of Laboratory Animals" approved by the Japanese Pharmacological Society and the guidelines approved by the Ethical Committee on Animal Care and Animal Experimentation of Josai International University (#52). The number of animals used was kept to the minimum necessary for meaningful interpretation of the data.

2.2. Preparations and drugs used

Atenolol, capsaicin, CMC, dimethyl sulfoxide (DMSO), *dl*-isoproterenol, and urethane (ethyl carbamate) were obtained from Wako Pure Chemical Industries (Osaka, Japan). L-arginine, L-NAME, and omeprazole were from Sigma-Aldrich (St. Louis, MO, USA). NPLA and L-NIO came from Tocris Cookson (Ellisville, MO, USA). N-(4-t-Butylphenyl)-4-(3-chlopyridin-2-yl) tetrahydropyrazine-1(2H)-carboxamide (BCTC) was purchased from BIOMOL (Plymouth Meeting, PA, USA). Capsaicin was dissolved in Tween 80-ethanol solution (10% ethanol, 10% Tween 80, and 80% saline) for s.c. injection or suspended in 0.5% CMC for mucosal application. Omeprazole was suspended in 0.5% CMC for i.p. injection. BCTC was dissolved in DMSO prior to dilution in saline, and the final concentration of DMSO was less than 1.0%. Other drugs were dissolved in saline with no organic solvent or detergent. Each drug was prepared immediately before use and was given in a volume of 0.5 ml/100 g of body wt. in the case of i.p. and s.c. administration or in a volume of 0.1 ml/100 g of body wt. in case of i.v. administration. Control animals received the vehicle alone.

2.3. Gastric mucosal blood flow

The measurement of gastric blood flow was carried out as described previously [15]. The animals were anesthetized with urethane (1.25 g/kg, i.p.). The stomach was exposed through a midline incision, delivered onto the abdominal surface by gentle traction on the spleen, and pylorus was ligated. The lucite chamber was used for maintaining ex vivo conditions of gastric mucosa. The lucite chamber, known as the ex vivo chamber, consists of two parts: one part is a lucite base and the other is plastic rim which has two holes on the side wall. Two holes are cannulated for perfusing the mucosa with saline (154 mmol/l NaCl, 37°C) at a flow rate of 1 ml/min. The lucite base was lowered over the animals, and the stomach was drawn though the center hole with the forceps applied only to the forestomach. The stomach was then opened along the greater curvature from the middle part of the forestomach to the area where the epiploic artery is terminated, and the edges were pinned out by gently stretching the glandular mucosa. The plastic rim was then applied and tightened down on the mucosa. Under these conditions, the exposed area was exclusively the glandular mucosa, mostly consisting of corpus region. The chamber was set at the level of the abdominal wall so that the external wall of the stomach remained inside the abdominal cavity. The body temperature was maintained at a temperature similar to that of the rectum at around 37°C by using a small animal warmer and thermometer (Bio Research Center, Model BWT-100, Nagoya, Japan). Gastric mucosal blood flow was measured by laser-Doppler flowmetry (Advance, Model ALF-21N, Tokyo, Japan) and by a non-touching probe (1 mm in diameter) on the surface of the corpus mucosa. After gastric mucosal blood flow was well stabilized, the perfusion was discontinued, the luminal solution was removed, and then the mucosa was exposed to 2 ml of capsaicin for 10 min. After application, the mucosa was rinsed with saline, another 2 ml of saline was instilled, and the perfusion resumed. Changes in the gastric mucosal blood flow were continuously monitored and recorded for 2-h test periods by using the PowerLab system (Model ML845; AD Instruments, Bella Vista, NSW, Australia).

2.4. Experimental procedures

A TRPV1 antagonist *N*-(4-*t*-butylphenyl)-4-(3-chlopyridin-2-yl) tetrahydropyrazine-1(2H)-carboxamide (BCTC) (0.8 mmol/L, i.g.) [16], a non-selective NOS inhibitor N^G-nitro-L-arginine methyl ester (L-NAME; 5 and 10 mg/kg, i.v.), a nNOS selective inhibitor NPLA (0.02 and 0.2 mg/kg, i.v.), an eNOS selective inhibitor L-NIO (3 and 10 mg/kg, i.v.), and an iNOS selective inhibitor 1400W (3 and 10 mg/kg, i.v.) were administered 20 min before exposing the stomach to 2 ml of capsaicin for 10 min. In one group, L-arginine (300 mg/kg, i.v.) was administered twice 40 min and 60 min before the application of capsaicin.

2.5. Chemical deafferentation

Chemical deafferentation was performed two weeks before the experiment by successive injections of capsaicin subcutaneously once daily for 3 d (20, 30, and 50 mg/kg) [17]. All capsaicin injections were performed under ether anesthesia, and the rats were pretreated with the beta-adrenergic receptor agonist isoproterenol (0.01 mg/kg, i.m.) and the selective beta 1-adrenergic antagonist atenolol (0.01 mg/kg, i.m.) to counteract the respiratory impairment associated with capsaicin injection. To check for the effectiveness of the treatment, a drop of a 0.1 mg/ml solution of capsaicin in 0.5% carboxymethyl cellulose solution (CMC) was instilled into one eye of each rat, and the protective wiping movements were counted [18].

2.6. Immunohistochemical study

The immunohistochemical procedures were performed as described previously [4]. The corpora of rat stomachs were fixed by immersion in fresh 4% paraformaldehyde in 0.1 mol/l phosphate buffer (pH 7.4) for 2 h at 4°C, and washed three times with phosphate-buffered saline (PBS). They were cryoprotected overnight in 0.1 mol/l phosphate buffer containing 20% sucrose. The tissues were frozen in OCT mounting medium (Sakura Finetek Europe, Zoeterwoude, The Netherlands), and sectioned on a cryostat (Leica, Hemel Hempstead, UK) at a thickness of 60 μm. The tissue sections were thaw-mounted onto Superfrost Plus slides (BDH Laboratory Supplies, Poole, UK). Prior to staining, the slide-mounted sections were incubated in PBS containing 0.3% hydrogen peroxide for 30 min to quench endogenous peroxidase activity and washed with PBS. The sections were successively incubated in 10% normal donkey serum containing 0.2% Triton X-100, 0.1% sodium azide in PBS for 1 h, and polyclonal anti-TRPV1 antibody (1:15000) for 40 h at room temperature. TRPV1 immunoreactivity was detected using a polyclonal antiserum raised in rabbit against the carboxy terminus of rat TRPV1 provided by Dr. David Julius. After washes in PBS, the sections were incubated with biotinylated donkey anti-rabbit immounoglobulin G (1:400; Jackson Immunoresearch Laboratories, West Grove, PA, USA) for 90 min at room temperature. After further washes, the sections were incubated in stretavidin biotin-peroxidase complex (1:5 in PBS; Vectastain Elite ABC kit, Vector Laboratories, Peterborough, UK) for 1 h at room temperature followed by fluorescein tyramide (1:75; TSA kit, PerkinElmer Life Sciences, Boston, MA, USA). In control experiments, the TRPV1 antibody was omitted from the staining procedures to verify the specificity of the staining. No immunolabeling was observed in these controls.

Double staining of the section with TRPV1 antiserum combined with protein gene product 9.5 (PGP 9.5) and nNOS antisera was also performed. TRPV1 staining was carried out first using the TSA procedure with FITC, following by PGP 9.5 or nNOS staining using indirect labeling procedure as described below. The sections were incubated for 40 h at room temperature in the PGP 9.5 or nNOS primary antibody solution, and then washed three times for 10 min each in PBS. To visualize the labeling, sections were then incubated for 4 h with the corresponding secondary antibody linked to tetramethyl rhodamine isothiocyanate (TRITC, 1:400; Jackson Immunoresearch Laboratories). Antisera were diluted in PBS containing 0.2% Triton X-100 and 0.1% sodium azide. Two sets of controls were processed for this double labeling. First, the primary antibodies in the first and second stainings were omitted from the staining procedures.

No immunolabeling was observed in this control. Second, only the primary antibody in the second staining was omitted from the staining procedures. In this control, FITC labeling of TRPV1 fibers was seen, but TRITC labeling was not.

2.7. Microscopy

Sections were viewed on either a Leica epifluorescence microscope using Y3 (TRITC) and L4 (FITC) filter blocks, or on a upright Zeiss confocal laser scanning microscope system (LSM510) and ×20, ×40 Plan Neofluar objectives. On the latter system, single tracking mode was used for single FITC labeling. Sections were scanned in multitracking mode (to avoid channel cross talk) when double labeling was done with FITC (488 nm) and TRITC (543 nm). Each image was produced by projecting all the slices of the stack onto one plane. Final plates were prepared using Adobe Photoshop.

2.8. Statistics

The data are presented as the means ± S.E.M. from 3–7 rats per group. The statistical significance of differences between two groups was assessed using Student's *t*-test. Multiple comparisons against a single control group were made by a one-way analysis of variance ANOVA with Bonferroni correction. The level of significance was set at 0.05. Sigma Stat 3.1 software (Jandel Scientific Software, San Rafael, CA, USA) procedure was applied for statistical analysis.

3. Results

3.1. Effects of intragastric capsaicin on gastric mucosal blood flow

Intragastric capsaicin (0.33, 1, and 3.3 mmol/l) induced gastric hyperemic responses in a concentration-dependent manner: a significant effect was observed at concentrations greater than 1 mmol/l (Fig. 1B). The response of gastric mucosal blood flow to capsaicin (0.33, 1, and 3.3 mmol/l) during intragastric application for 10 min was 121.5 ± 2.6%, 146.4 ± 8.9%, and 178.6 ± 12.9%, respectively. Interestingly, gastric mucosal blood flow in response to 3.3 mmol/l capsaicin remained significantly high despite the removal of capsaicin from the chamber (Fig. 1A). At 20 and 50 minutes after removal of capsaicin, gastric mucosal blood flow showed a persistent increase (about ~120–130%) as compared to pre-application values (Fig. 1C). Mucosal application of the control solution (0.5% CMC) did not increase gastric mucosal blood flow. Since the effect of capsaicin on gastric mucosal blood flow reached the maximum values during the application and remained significantly elevated after removal of capsaicin at 3.3 mmol/l, this concentration was used in the following experiments for examining the effects of various agents on the gastric mucosal blood flow in response to capsaicin.

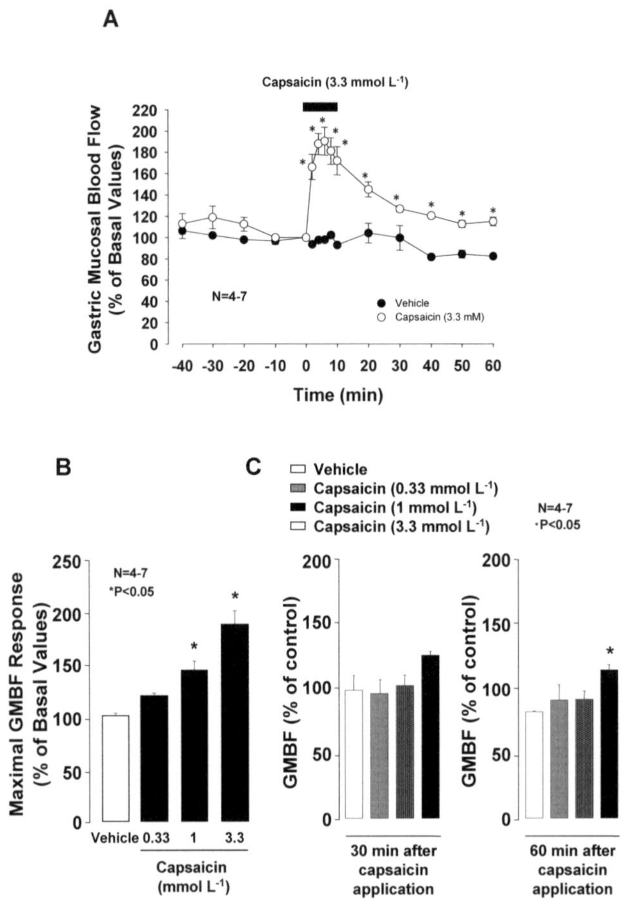

Figure 1. Effect of mucosal application of capsaicin on gastric mucosal blood flow (GMBF) in the ex vivo stomach of anesthetized rats. Figure A shows the time course of analysis for GMBF in response to capsaicin (3.3 mmol/l) in anesthetized rats. Capsaicin was topically applied to the mucosa for 10 min from time 0, and the stomach was perfused with saline before and after the application. The data are expressed as a % increase of baseline values and represent the means ± S.E. of values obtained every 2 or 10 min from 4 to 7 rats. * indicates statistically significant difference at P<0.05 compared to the group treated with control (0.5% CMC). Figure B shows the maximum GMBF response during capsaicin (0.33–3.3 mmol/l) application, and figure C shows the GMBF response at 20 and 50 min after removal of capsaicin (0.33–3.3 mmol/l). The data are expressed as a % increase of baseline values, and represent the means ± S.E. from 4 to 7 rats. * indicates statistically significant difference at P<0.05 compared to the group treated with control (0.5% CMC). Note that GMBF in response to capsaicin (3.3 mmol/l) was significantly increased during application, and remained moderately elevated even after removal of capsaicin from the chamber.

The increased gastric mucosal blood flow in animals in response to capsaicin (3.3 mmol/l) was totally abolished in the animals when the mucosa was exposed to a TRPV1 antagonist BCTC (0.8 mmol/l) (Fig. 2). The maximum response of gastric mucosal blood flow induced by 3.3 mmol/l capsaicin in the presence of BCTC was 102.4 ± 6.1% throughout the experiment. A similar phenomenon was observed in the animals following chemical deafferentation by consecutive injections of capsaicin (neurotoxic dose: total 100 mg/kg, s.c.) at two weeks before the experiment (Fig. 2). In those animals, the gastric mucosal blood flow remained unchanged during and after exposure of the mucosa to capsaicin (3.3 mmol/l), the maximum response was 103.1 ± 4.2%. It was found that intragastric capsaicin produced a significant and persistent increase in gastric mucosal blood flow via activation of TRPV1 expressed in capsaicin-sensitive sensory nerves in anesthetized rats.

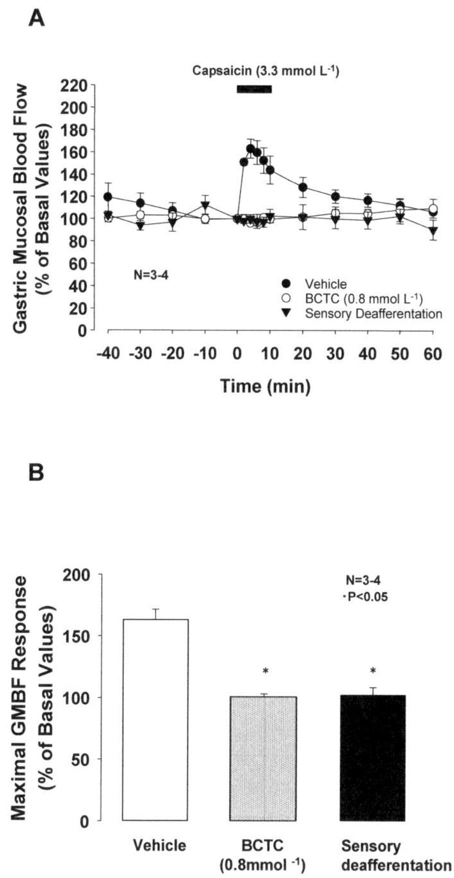

Figure 2. Effects of BCTC, a TRPV1 antagonist, and sensory deafferentation on gastric mucosal blood flow (GMBF) induced by mucosal application of capsaicin in the ex vivo stomach of anesthetized rats. Figure A shows the time course of analysis for GMBF response to capsaicin (3.3 mmol/l) in anesthetized rats treated with BCTC or sensory deafferentation. Capsaicin was topically applied to the mucosa for 10 min and the stomach was perfused with saline before and after the application. BCTC (0.8 mmol/l) was applied to the chamber for 30 min, starting at 20 min before the capsaicin application. Chemical deafferentation (capsaicin pretreatment) was performed 2 weeks before the experiment by consecutive injections of capsaicin s.c. once daily for 3 days (total dose: 100 mg/kg). The data are expressed as a % increase of baseline values and represent the mean ± S.E. of values obtained every 2 or 10 min from 3 to 4 rats. * indicates statistically significant difference at P<0.05 compared to the group treated with vehicle. Figure B shows a maximum response of GMBF induced by mucosal application of capsaicin (3.3 mmol/l). The data are expressed as a % increase of baseline values and represent the mean ± S.E. from 3 to 4 rats. * indicates statistically significant difference at P<0.05 compared to the group treated with vehicle. Note that increased GMBF in response to capsaicin was completely abolished by BCTC and sensory deafferentation.

3.2. Effects of L-NAME, a non-selective NOS inhibitor, and combined treatment with L-arginine on gastric mucosal blood flow in response to capsaicin

Gastric mucosal blood flow was temporarily increased after the injection of L-NAME was injected but immediately returned to the baseline value (Fig. 3A). The increase in gastric mucosal blood flow in response to capsaicin (3.3 mmol/l) seen in control rats apparently attenuated by L-NAME in a dose-dependent manner. The maximum response of gastric mucosal blood flow in response to capsaicin in animals treated with L-NAME (5 and 10 mg/kg) was 138.8 ± 11.6% and 125.6 ± 11.6%, respectively (Fig.3B). The administration of 300 mg/kg L-arginine, a substrate for NOS, twice reversed the inhibitory effects of L-NAME (10 mg/kg) on gastric hyperemic response both during and after removal of capsaicin (Fig. 3). Thus, gastric hyperemia in response to capsaicin was attributable to both NO-dependent hyperemia during the application, followed by NO-dependent hyperemia alone after removal of capsaicin in anesthetized rats.

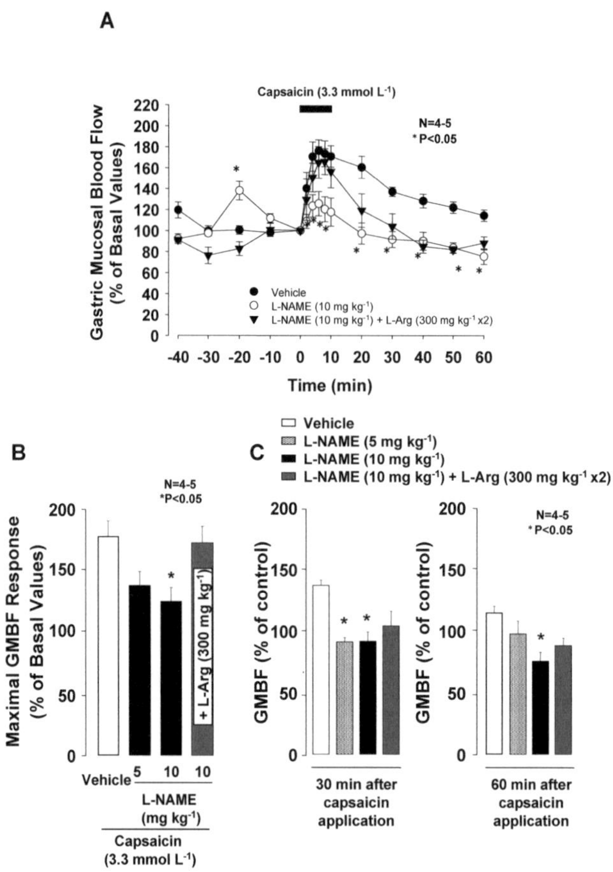

Figure 3. Effects of L-NAME, a non-selective NOS inhibitor, and combined treatment with L-arginine (300 mg/kg, x2) on gastric mucosal blood flow (GMBF) induced by mucosal application of capsaicin in the ex vivo stomach of anesthetized rats. Figure A shows the time course of analysis for GMBF response to capsaicin (3.3 mmol/l) in anesthetized rats

pretreated with L-NAMA and L-arginine. Capsaicin (3.3 mmol/l) was topically applied to the mucosa for 10 min and the stomach was perfused with saline before and after the application. L-NAME (5 and 10 mg/kg) was given via intravenous injection 20 min before capsaicin application. L-NAME by itself showed the temporary increase of GMBF when was injected, but immediately returned to baseline value. L-arginine (300 mg/kg) was given via intravenous injection 40 and 60 min before capsaicin application. The data are expressed as a % increase of baseline values and represent the means ± S.E. of values obtained every 2 or 10 min from 4 to 5 rats. * indicates statistically significant difference at P<0.05 compared to the group treated with vehicle (saline). Figure B shows the maximum response of GMBF during capsaicin (3.3 mmol/l) application in animals with L-NAME (5 and 10 mg/kg) or L-NAME (10 mg/kg) plus L-arginine (300 mg/kg, x2). Figure C shows a response of GMBF at 20 and 50 min after removal of capsaicin (3.3 mmol/l) with L-NAME (5 and 10 mg/kg) or L-NAME (10 mg/kg) plus L-arginine (300 mg/kg, x2). The data are expressed as a % increase of baseline values and represent the mean ± S.E. from 4 to 5 rats. * indicates statistically significant difference at P<0.05 compared to the group treated with vehicle (saline). Note that increased GMBF during and after removal of capsaicin was significantly inhibited by L-NAME (10 mg/kg), whose response was reversed by pretreatment with L-arginine (300 mg/kg, x2).

3.3. Effect of NPLA, a selective nNOS inhibitor, on gastric mucosal blood flow in response to capsaicin

The roles of different isoforms of NOS in the gastric hyperemia induced by capsaicin were investigated by using selective NOS inhibitors including a nNOS inhibitor NPLA, an eNOS inhibitor L-NIO, and an iNOS inhibitor 1400W. Administration of the nNOS-specific inhibitor NPLA alone did not significantly affect gastric mucosal blood flow (Fig. 4A). Interestingly, the increase in gastric mucosal blood flow in response to capsaicin (3.3 mmol/l) during the application, but not after removal, was apparently decreased by 0.2 mg/kg NPLA. The maximum responses of gastric mucosal blood flow during capsaicin application in animals treated with NPLA (0.02 and 0.2 mg/kg) were 182.1 ± 26.6% and 141.9 ± 8.9%, respectively (Fig. 4B). In contrast, the persistent increase in gastric mucosal blood flow after removal of capsaicin was not affected by NPLA (0.2 mg/kg), with the responses being 138.3 ± 17.3% and 126.5 ± 15.1%, respectively (Fig. 4C).

3.4. Effect of L-NIO, a selective eNOS inhibitor, on gastric mucosal blood flow in response to capsaicin

Administration of the selective eNOS inhibitor L-NIO (10 mg/kg) by itself temporarily increased gastric mucosal blood flow, but the gastric mucosal blood flow immediately returned to the baseline value (Fig. 5A). The gastric hyperemic response after treatment with capsaicin during the application was not significantly affected by L-NIO (3 and 10 mg/kg), and the maximum responses being 158.7 ± 8.4% and 160.0 ± 9.6%, respectively (Fig. 5B). However, the persistent increase in gastric mucosal blood flow after removal of capsaicin was obviously attenuated by L-NIO (10 mg/kg) (Fig. 5A, C). In treatment with L-NIO (10 mg/kg), the gastric mucosal blood flow responses at 20 and 50 min after removal of capsaicin were 96.2 ± 7.2% and 89.5 ± 6.2%, respectively.

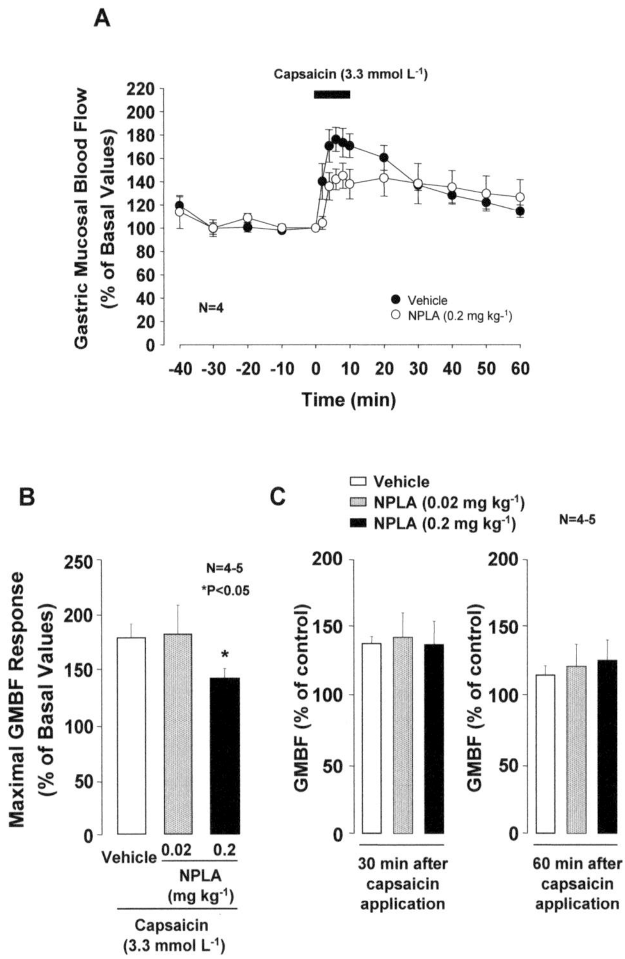

Figure 4. Effect of NPLA, a selective neuronal NOS inhibitor, on gastric mucosal blood flow (GMBF) induced by capsaicin in the ex vivo stomach of anesthetized rats. Figure A shows the time course of the effect of NPLA (0.2 mg/kg) on GMBF response to capsaicin (3.3 mmol/l) in anesthetized rats. Capsaicin (3.3 mmol/l) was topically applied to the mucosa for 10 min and the stomach was perfused with saline before and after the application. NPLA (0.2 mg/kg) was given via intravenous injection 20 min before capsaicin application. The data are expressed as a % increase of baseline values and represent the means ± S.E. of values obtained every 2 or 10 min from 4 rats. * indicates statistically significant difference at $P<0.05$ compared to the group treated with vehicle (saline). Figure B shows the maximum response of GMBF response during capsaicin (3.3 mmol/l) application in animals with NPLA (0.02 and 0.2 mg/kg). Figure C shows a response of GMBF at 20 and 50 min after removal of capsaicin (3.3 mmol/l) with NPLA (0.02 and 0.2 mg/kg). The data are expressed as a % increase of baseline values and represent the means ± SE from 4 to 5 rats. * indicates statistically significant difference at $P<0.05$ compared to the group treated with vehicle (saline). Note that increased GMBF during capsaicin application was inhibited by NPLA, yet persistent increase in GMBF after removal of capsaicin was not affected by NPLA.

http://dx.doi.org/10.5772/58557

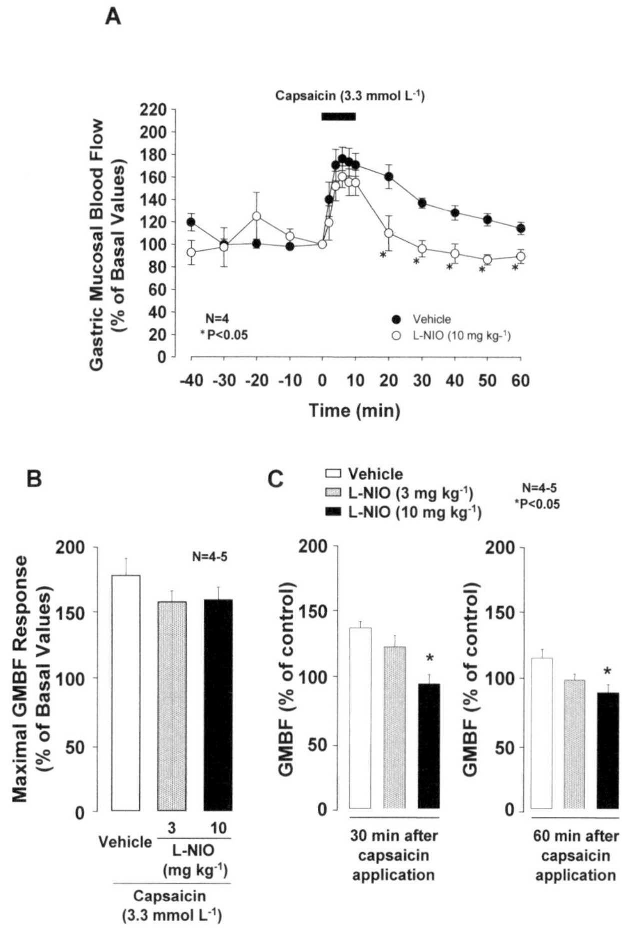

Figure 5. Effect of L-NIO, a selective endothelial NOS inhibitor, on gastric mucosal blood flow (GMBF) induced by capsaicin in the ex vivo stomach of anesthetized rats. Figure A shows the time course of analysis for the effect of L-NIO (10 mg/kg) on GMBF response to capsaicin (3.3 mmol/l) in anesthetized rats. Capsaicin (3.3 mmol/l) was applied topically to the mucosa for 10 min and the stomach was perfused with saline before and after the application. L-NIO (10 mg/kg) was injected intravenously 20 min before capsaicin application. L-NIO by itself induced a temporary increase of GMBF when injected, but it immediately returned to baseline value. The data are expressed as a % increase of baseline values and represent the means ± S.E. of values obtained every 2 or 10 min from 4 rats. * indicates statistically significant difference at $P<0.05$ compared to the group treated with vehicle (saline). Figure B shows the maximum response of GMBF response during capsaicin (3.3 mmol/l) application in animals with L-NIO (3 and 10 mg/kg). Figure C shows the response of GMBF at 20 and 50 min after removal of capsaicin (3.3 mmol/l) with L-NIO (3 and 10 mg/kg). The data are expressed as a % increase of baseline values and represent the means ± S.E. from 4–5 rats. * indicates statistically significant difference at $P<0.05$ compared to the group treated with the vehicle (saline). Note that L-NIO significantly inhibited persistent increase of GMBF after removal of capsaicin, although GMBF response during capsaicin application was not affected by L-NIO.

3.5. Effect of 1400W, a selective iNOS inhibitor, on gastric mucosal blood flow in response to capsaicin

Gastric mucosal blood flow remained unchanged by the administration of an iNOS selective inhibitor 1400W (10 mg/kg) (Fig. 6). In addition, the increased gastric mucosal blood flow I response to capsaicin was not also affected by 1400W (3 and 10 mg/kg) (Fig. 6).

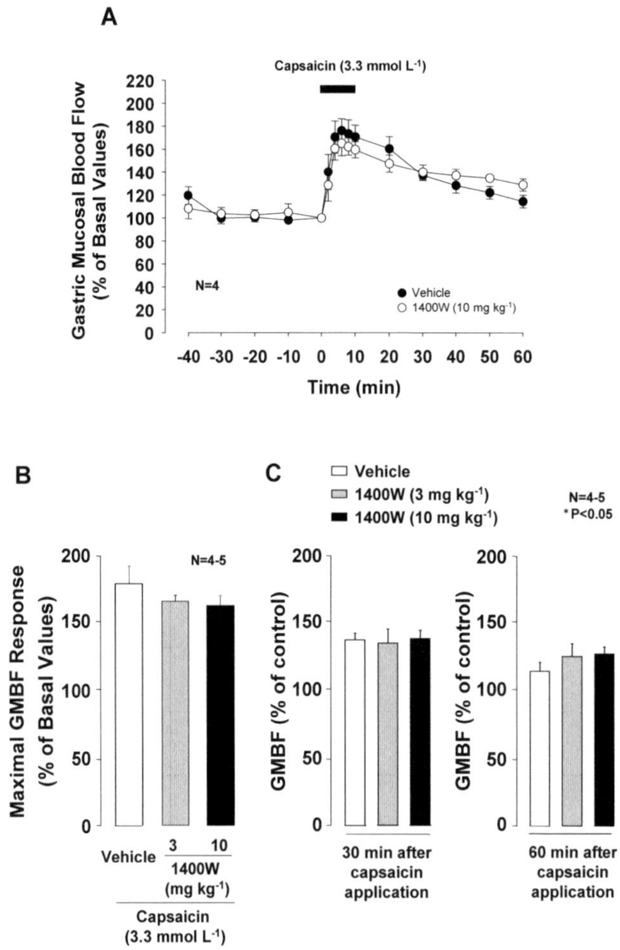

Figure 6. Effect of 1400W, a selective inducible NOS inhibitor, on gastric mucosal blood flow (GMBF) induced by capsaicin in the ex vivo stomach of anesthetized rats. Figure A shows the time course of analysis for the effect of 1400W (10 mg/kg) on GMBF response to capsaicin (3.3 mmol/l) in anesthetized rats. Capsaicin (3.3 mmol/l) was topically applied to the mucosa for 10 min and the stomach was perfused with saline before and after the application. 1400W (3 and 10 mg/kg) was given via intravenous injection 20 min before capsaicin application. The data are expressed as a % increase of baseline values and represent the means ± S.E. of values obtained every 2 or 10 min from 4 rats. Figure B shows the maximum response of GMBF response during capsaicin (3.3 mmol/l) application in animals treated with 1400W (3 and 10 mg/kg). Figure C shows the responses of GMBF (3.3 mmol/l) at 20 and 50 min after removal of capsaicin. The data are expressed as a % increase of baseline values and represent the mean ± S.E. from 4 to 5 rats. Note that increased GMBF in response to capsaicin was not affected by 1400W.

http://dx.doi.org/10.5772/58557

3.6. TRPV1-immunoreactivity in corpus and antrum of stomach

Extensive TRPV1-immunoreactivity was detected in fundus, corpus and antrum of the stomach [4, 19]. Immunoreactivity was present in all layers of the corpus and in all cases appeared axon-like in nature (Fig. 7A). This identification was confirmed by double labeling with the pan axonal marker PGP 9.5, which confirmed that all TRPV1 immunoreactive structures were also PGP 9.5 immunoreactive (Figure 7C). However, not all PGP 9.5-immunoreactive fibers were TRPV1-immunoreactive, reflecting the fact that only a subpopulation of neural elements in the stomach expresses TRPV1. TRPV1 immunoreactivity was also not seen in the PGP 9.5 immunoreactive cell bodies of the myenteric plexus or submucosal plexus. In control experiments, TRPV1-immunoreactivity was not observed in any corpus sections processed without the primary antibody. Similar observation was obtained in all layers of antrum of the stomach [4].

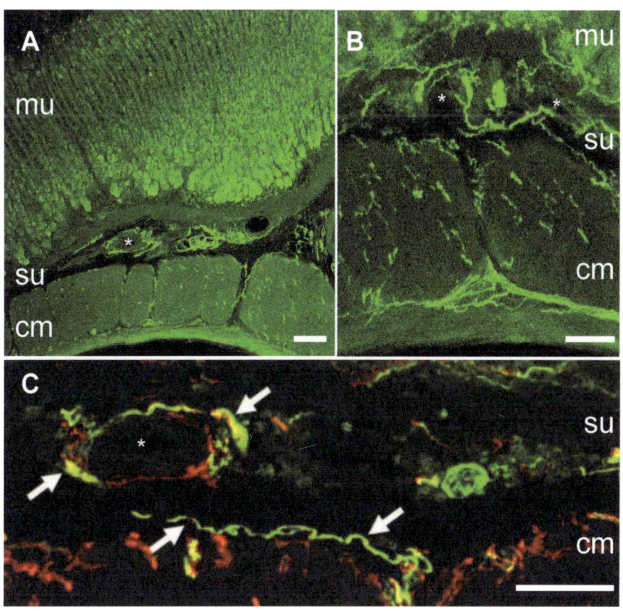

Figure 7. Distribution of TRPV1-immunoreactivity in corpus of rat stomach. mu: mucosa; su: submucosa; cm: circular muscle. (A) A low magnification image showing that TRPV1-immunoractivity is present in all layers of corpus. Asterisk indicates a blood vessel. (B) A high magnification image showing that TRPV1-immunoractivity is present in submucosal and muscular layers of corpus. TRPV1-immunoreactive fibers are observed associated with small blood vessels (asterisk) or along and in the lamina muscularis mucosae. Numerous TRPV1-immunoreactive fibers are found around blood vessels (asterisks) in the submucosal layer. TRPV1-immunoreactive axons are sparse in longitudinal smooth muscle but isolated varicose fibers are present. Fibers are abundant in circular muscle layer where they run parallel to muscle fibers. A large number of nerve fibers are seen in circular smooth muscle layer and in the myenteric nerve plexus. (C) Co-localization of TRPV1-positive neurons with protein gene product 9.5 (PGP 9.5) in corpus submucosa. Rat stomach sections were dual-labelled with TRPV1 in green and PGP 9.5 in red. Merged image is shown in (C). Arrows indicate the co-localization of TRPV1 immunoreactivity with PGP 9.5 immunoreactivity. All TRPV1 immunoreactive structures are PGP 9.5 immunoreactive. Note that in circular smooth muscle, the TRPV1 immunoreactive axons represent a relatively small population of the total population of PGP 9.5 immunoreactive axons. Scale bars are 100 μm in (A) and 50 μm in (B), (C).

The TRPV1-immunoreactive varicose fibers were present in the mucosa along gastric glands of corpus and antrum, although Ward et al. (2003) did not observe TRPV1 immunoreactive fibers that penetrate the mucosa [20]. A few TRPV1-immunoreactive varicose nerve fibers were observed in the lamina propria, mainly in association with small vessels or along the muscularis mucosae of antrum and corpus [4, 19]. Numerous TRPV1-immunoreactive axons were also found around arterioles in the submucosal layer. A dense TRPV1-innervation of the submucosal blood vessels was seen running along the major arterioles (Fig. 7B). Occasionally fibers formed baskets around the vessels [4].

3.7. Coexistence of TRPV1 and nNOS

Many TRPV1 axons were also observed to be immunoreactive for nNOS (Figure 8). A few axons of this type were present in the mucosa and smooth muscle layers but were particularly abundant in the vicinity of blood vessels in the submucosa [21]. Numerous TRPV1-immunoreactive axons were found around arterioles in the mucosal and submucosal layer.

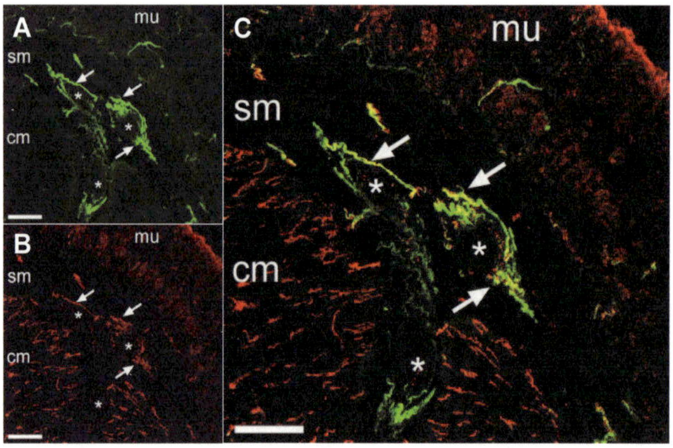

Figure 8. Confocal images showing co-localization of TRPV1-and neuronal NOS-immnuoreactivities in corpus submucosa and muscle. Labeling for TRPV1 (A: green) and neuronal NOS (B: red) is shown separately, and merged in (C). Double immunolabeling for TRPV1 and neuronal NOS demonstrated co-localization in many but not all axons. This photo shows abundant TRPV1 axons containing neuronal NOS in the submucosa, with a high density of immounoreactive axons around blood vessels (asterisk). mu: mucosa; sm: submucosa; cm: circular muscle. Scale bars is 100 μm.

4. Discussion

This report showed that intragastric application of capsaicin facilitates an initial increase in gastric mucosal blood flow by NO mainly derived from nNOS after stimulating capsaicin-sensitive sensory nerves, and also the persistent increase in gastric mucosal blood flow after removal of capsaicin is attributed to eNOS/NO in the rat stomach.

Topical application of capsaicin causes dilatation of the submucosal and mucosal arterioles in the rat stomach [22, 23], but it has not been fully elucidated how capsaicin really activates primary afferent vasodilator neurons in the stomach. Primary afferent neurons express TRPV 1 channels, which mediates the gastrointestinal vasodilator effect of capsaicin. By the use of the TRPV1 blocker BCTC, it was found that this TRPV1 channels appear to participate in the capsaicin-induced hyperemia in the rat stomach [21]. Nerve-selective ablation of capsaicin-sensitive afferent neurons has revealed that the mucosal hyperemic response to local capsaicin administration in the rat stomach is mediated by primary afferent vasodilator neurons that originate in the dorsal root ganglia. It was inferred that the capsaicin-induced increase of blood flow is relayed entirely by a peripheral reflex circuit via the TRPV1 activation. The gastric hyperemic response to capsaicin results from an axon reflex between mucosal and submucosal collaterals of afferent neurons [24]. Evidence for an axon reflex-type innervation has been found in submucosal arterioles of the guinea pig ileum in which focal application of capsaicin evokes vasodilatation that spreads beyond the application site [25].

It is known that NO, the endothelium-derived vasodilator, plays an important role in the regulation of the resting gastric mucosal microcirculation [26, 27]. Indeed, an increase in both systemic arterial blood pressure and gastric mucosal blood flow was observed under physiological conditions in rats after a bolus administration of L-NAME.

The gastric mucosal blood flow responses to capsaicin were markedly inhibited by a non-selective NOS inhibitor L-NAME, which indicated that NO is mainly involved in those hyperemic responses. However, L-NAME did not completely inhibit the increases in gastric mucosal blood flow as much as BCTC. This result suggests that gastric mucosal hyperemia in response to capsaicin is attributable not only to NO but also to other mediators including CGRP and prostaglandins (PGs). Several studies have shown that endogenous PGs, contributes to gastric hyperemic responses to capsaicin by sensitizing TRPV1-expressing afferent nerves, which was revealed by the treatment of indomethacin (5 mg/kg, s.c.) and the animals lacking IP receptors [28]. In addition, Chen et al. reported the interaction of NO and CGRP in gastric vasodilation through sensory nerves [14]. Our results can be explained on the basis of the previous findings that BCTC functionally antagonizes the action of capsaicin at the peripheral terminals of sensory nerves and inhibits the release of some transmitters such as CGRP and NO from capsaicin-sensitive afferent nerves. Further, the submucosal application of CGRP induced dose-dependent dilation of gastric submucosal arterioles, which was significantly decreased by L-NAME [23]. However, the dilation induced by submucosal CGRP was decreased to a much lesser degree by inhibition of NO synthesis than that induced with intragastric capsaicin [14]. This indicates that NO released by CGRP is not the only source of submucosal NO in capsaicin-induced vasodilation, and there may be other source of submucosal NO, such as from nitroxidergic nerves that has not been determined thus far [29]. The existence of capsaicin-sensitive nitroxidergic nerves is hypothesized by some reports, but it was not proved [6].

NO is synthesized from L-arginine by NOS in various cells. NOS is present not only in vascular endothelial cells (eNOS) but also in perivascular nerves (nNOS) [10, 30]. It is well known that NO is a vasodilator that increases gastric mucosal blood flow, and this gas mediator is important in the modulation of gastric mucosal integrity through interaction with sensory nerves [6]. The increase in gastric mucosal blood flow responses to capsaicin is mitigated by

N^G-monomethyl L-arginine, and the gastroprotection induced by capsaicin is also decreased by the NOS inhibitor [8, 31]. Previous studies have shown that gastric hyperemia caused by acid back-diffusion or exogenous CGRP is mediated partly by NO, but which NOS isoform is involved in those hyperemic responses has not been investigated in any of the studies thus far. In addition, the source of NO involved in the actions of capsaicin was not identified [29]. That is because highly selective inhibitors for NOS isoforms had not been developed at that time. We investigated which NOS isoform mediates the increased gastric mucosal blood flow in response to capsaicin by using newly developed NOS inhibitors.

In this study, NPLA and L-NIO were adopted as selective nNOS and eNOS inhibitors, respectively. It was reported that the potency of inhibition for nNOS by NPLA is 3158 times that for iNOS and 149-fold that for eNOS, whose selectivity for nNOS/iNOS and nNOS/eNOS are ratio of the inverse of IC_{50} values [32, 33]. L-NIO and 1400W were also reported to be as selective inhibitors for eNOS and iNOS, respectively [34, 35].

Intravenous injection of L-NIO alone of L-NAME alone produced a temporary increase in gastric mucosal blood flow, although intravenous injection of NPLA did not affect the gastric mucosal blood flow. Therefore, eNOS-derived NO homeostatically regulates gastric mucosal blood flow under physiological conditions. In the increased gastric mucosal blood flow in responses to capsaicin, NPLA significantly decreased the maximum response of gastric mucosal blood flow during the application of capsaicin, but NPLA did not affect the increase in gastric mucosal blood flow after removal of capsaicin. In contrast, L-NIO significantly decreased gastric mucosal blood flow responses after removal of capsaicin, but did not affect the maximum response of gastric mucosal blood flow induced by capsaicin during the application. These results suggested that nNOS/NO, which may be released from TRPV1-expressing nerves stimulated by capsaicin, plays an important role in gastric hyperemia during the luminal application of capsaicin (as in the early phase). eNOS/NO plays a role in regulating gastric mucosal blood flow responses after removal of capsaicin (as in the late phase). On the other hand, intravenous injection of 1400W did not affect the baseline value of gastric mucosal blood flow as well as the increase in gastric mucosal blood flow in response to capsaicin.

Our results were consistent with those reported previously that eNOS was expressed mostly in the vasculature throughout the gastric mucosa in rats, but the expression of iNOS was hardly observed in the gastric mucosa of normal rats by using immunohistochemical analysis [11, 12]. These findings support our hypothesis that eNOS/NO plays a role in the resting state responses of gastric mucosal blood flow in the late phase, while iNOS/NO plays no role in the increased GMBF in response to capsaicin.

In our immunohistochemical studies, TRPV1 immunoreactivity was detected in mucosal and submucosal layers of the corpus of the rat stomach. Many TRPV1 nerve fibers contain nNOS, but not all axons do. In addition, numerous TRPV1-immunoreactive axons were also found around arterioles in the submucosal layer. These data led us to speculate that the capsaicin-induced increase in gastric mucosal blood flow could be attributed to the time-dependent interaction of both nNOS/NO and eNOS/NO. Namely, it is suggested that capsaicin stimulates TRPV1 nerves and releases CGRP and NO from the sensory nerve endings. The NO is immediately provided by nNOS and dilates the blood vessels in the early phase. On the other hand, NO derived from eNOS, but not nNOS, maintains the persistent dilation of the blood vessels after capsaicin application in rat stomachs (in the late phase) (Fig. 9).

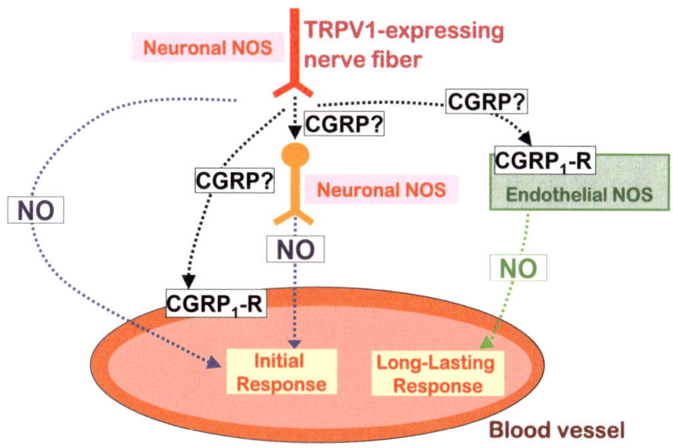

Figure 9. Putative mechanism underlying increase of gastric mucosal blood flow due to activation of TRPV1 channels. Capsaicin increases blood flow in the rat stomach by a peripheral axon reflex-like circuit. Capsaicin excites primary afferent neurons that originate in the dorsal root ganglia and that arborize into several branches that innervate mucosa and submucosal arterioles. The reflex hyperemia is mediated by calcitonin gene-related peptide (CGRP) and nitric oxide (NO) that form most likely in the endothelium. The involvement of NO derived from nNOS in hyperemia is newly clarified. The primary afferent neurons release NO/nNOS to dilate blood vessels.

Stimulation of sensory nerves leads to gastric hyperemic response, which is mediated partly by NO formation, but it is not clear whether the NO is derived solely from endothelial cells or is also released directly by extrinsic and/or intrinsic nerves [6, 14]. We have reported that abundant TRPV1 axons containing nNOS in the submucosa with a high density of immunoreactive axons around blood vessels [21]. Therefore, our study suggests that capsaicin is likely to induce vasodilatation by inducing NO release from TRPV1-expressing sensory fibers.

5. Conclusion

The mucosal application of capsaicin increased gastric mucosal blood flow by releasing NO derived from nNOS after stimulating capsaicin-sensitive sensory nerves. The contribution of nNOS-derived NO in gastric hyperemic responses to the activation of TRPV1 by capsaicin has been reported using not only pharmacological but also immunohistochemical techniques. We also demonstrated the interaction between nNOS/NO and eNOS/NO on the increased gastric mucosal blood flow by capsaicin in time-dependently, whose hyperemic responses were composed of the both nNOS/NO in the early phase and eNOS/NO in the late phase.

Terminology

1400W: a selective inducible NOS inhibitor

ANOVA: analysis of variance

BCTC: *N*-(4-*t*-butylphenyl)-4-(3-chloropyridin-2-yl)tetrahydropyrazine-1(2H)-carboxamide: a TRPV1 antagonist

CGRP: calcitonin gene-related peptide

GMBF: gastric mucosal blood flow

iNOS: inducible NO synthase

eNOS: endothelial NO synthase

L-NIO: N^5-(l-iminoethyl)-L-ornithine: a selective endothelial NOS inhibitor

nNOS: neuronal NO synthase

NO: nitric oxide

NPLA: N^5-[imino (propylamino) methyl]-L-ornithine: a selective nNOS inhibitor

TRPV1: transient receptor potential vanilloid type 1

S.E.M.: standard error of mean

Acknowledgements

This work was supported by Grants-in-Aid for Scientific Research from the Ministry of Education, Culture, Sports and Technology, Japan.

Author details

Syunji Horie[1*], Masaki Raimura[2], Kenjiro Matsumoto[1], Takao Namiki[2], Katsutoshi Terasawa[3], John V. Priestley[4] and Kimihito Tashima[1]

*Address all correspondence to: shorie@jiu.ac.jp

1 Laboratory of Pharmacology, Faculty of Pharmaceutical Sciences, Josai International University, Togane, Japan

2 Department of Frontier Japanese-Oriental (Kampo) Medicine, Graduate School of Medicine, Chiba University, Chiba, Japan

3 Department of Kampo Medicine, Chiba Central Medical Center, Chiba, Japan

4 Neuroscience Centre, St. Bartholomew's and the Royal London School of Medicine and Dentistry, Queen Mary University of London, London, United Kingdom

Kimihito Tashima, Laboratory of Pharmacology, Faculty of Pharmaceutical Sciences, Josai International University, Togane, Japan

The authors have no competing interests.

References

[1] Lippe IT, Pabst MA, Holzer P: Intragastric capsaicin enhances rat gastric acid elimination and mucosal blood flow by afferent nerve stimulation. Br J Pharmacol 1989; 96: 91–100

[2] Matsumoto J, Takeuchi K, Okabe S: Characterization of gastric mucosal blood flow response induced by intragastric capsaicin in rats. Jpn J Pharmacol 1991; 57: 205–213

[3] Caterina MJ, Schumacher MA, Tominaga M, Rosen TA, Levine JD, Julius D: The capsaicin receptor: a heat-activated ion channel in the pain pathway. Nature 1997; 389: 816–824

[4] Horie S, Yamamoto H, Michael GJ Uchida M, Belai A, Watanabe K, Priestley JV, Murayama T: Protective role of vanilloid receptor type 1 in HCl-induced gastric mucosal lesions in rats. Scand J Gastroenterol 2004; 39: 303–312

[5] Tashima K, Nakashima M, Kagawa S, Kato S, Takeuchi K: Gastric hyperemic response induced by acid back-diffusion in rat stomachs following barrier disruption-relation to vanilloid type-1 receptors. Med Sci Monit 2002; 8: BR157–BR163

[6] Holzer P: Neural emergency system in the stomach. Gastroenterology 1998; 114: 823–839

[7] Lambrecht N, Burchert M, Respondek M, Müller KM, Peskar BM: Role of calcitonin gene-related peptide and nitric oxide in the gastroprotective effect of capsaicin in the rat. Gastroenterology 1993; 104: 1371-1380

[8] Whittle BJ, Lopez BJ, Moncada S: Nitric oxide mediates rat mucosal vasodilation induced by intragastric capsaicin. Eur J Pharmacol 1992; 218: 339–341

[9] Wallace JL, Miller MJ: Nitric oxide in mucosal defense: a little goes a long way. Gastroenterology 2000; 119: 512–520

[10] Knowles RG, Moncada S: Nitric oxide synthases in mammals. Biochem J 1994 298: 249–258

[11] Price KJ, Hanson PJ, Whittle BJ: Localization of constitutive isoforms of nitric oxide synthase in the gastric glandular mucosa of the rat. Cell Tissue Res 1996; 285: 157–163

[12] Kato S, Kawahara R, Yasuda M, Amagase K, Takeuchi K: Aggravation of cold–restraint stress–induced gastric lesions in adjuvant arthritic rats: pathogenic role of inducible and endothelial nitric oxide. J Pharmacol Sci 2009; 111: 244–252

[13] Phillipson M, Henriksnäs J, Holstad M, Sandler S, Holm L: Inducible nitric oxide synthase is involved in acid-induced gastric hyperemia in rats and mice. Am J Physiol 2003; 285: G154-G162

[14] Chen RY, Guth PH: Interaction of endogenous nitric oxide and CGRP in sensory neuron-induced gastric vasodilation. Am J Physiol 1995; 268: G791-G796

[15] Takeuchi K, Ishihara Y, Okada M, Niida H, Okabe S: A continuous monitoring of mucosal integrity and secretory activity in rat stomach: a preparation using a lucite chamber. Jpn J Pharmacol 1989; 49: 235–244

[16] Pomonis JD, Harrison JE, Mark L, Bristol DR, Valenzano KJ, Walker K: N-(4-Tertiary-butylphenyl)-4-(3-cholorphyridin-2-yl)tetrahydropyrazine-1(2H)-carbox-amide (BCTC), a novel, orally effective vanilloid receptor 1 antagonist with analgesic properties: II. in vivo characterization in rat models of inflammatory and neuropathic pain. J Pharmacol Exp Ther 2003; 306: 387–393

[17] Esplugues JV, Ramos EG, Gil L, Esplugues J: Influence of capsaicin-sensitive afferent neurons on the acid secretory responses of the stomach in vivo. Br J Pharmacol 1990; 100: 491–496

[18] Yonei Y, Holzer P, Guth PH: Laparotomy-induced gastric protection against ethanol injury is mediated by capsaicin-sensitive sensory neurons. Gastroenterology 1990; 99: 3–9

[19] Horie S, Michael GJ, Priestley JV: Co-localization of TRPV1-expressing nerve fibers with calcitonin-gene-related peptide and substance P in fundus of rat stomach. Inflammopharmacology 2005;13(1-3):127-37.

[20] Ward SM, Bayguinov J, Won KJ, Grundy D, Berthoud HR: Distribution of the vanilloid receptor (VR1) in the gastrointestinal tract. J Comp Neurol. 2003; 465(1): 121-135

[21] Raimura M, Tashima K, Matsumoto K, Tobe S, Chino A, Namiki T, Terasawa K, Horie S: Neuronal nitric oxide synthase-derived nitric oxide is involved in gastric mucosal hyperemic response to capsaicin in rats. Pharmacology 2013; 92(1-2):60-70.

[22] Saeki T, Ohno T, Boku K, Saigenji K, Katori M, Majima M: Mechanism of prevention by capsaicin of ethanol-induced gastric mucosal injury--a study in the rat using intravital microscopy. Aliment Pharmacol Ther 2000; Suppl 1: 135–144

[23] Chen RY, Li DS, Guth PH: Role of calcitonin gene-related peptide in capsaicin-induced gastric submucosal arteriolar dilation. Am J Physiol 1992; 262: H1350-H1355

[24] Holzer P, Livingston EH, Guth PH: Sensory neurons signal for an increase in rat gastric mucosal blood flow in the face of pending acid injury. Gastroenterology 1991; 101:416-423.

[25] Vanner S, Bolton M: Neural circuitry of capsaicin-sensitive afferents innervating submucosal arterioles in guinea pig ileum. Am J Physiol 1996;270:G948-G955

[26] Pique JM, Whittle BJ, Esplugues JV: The vasodilator role of endogenous nitric oxide in the rat gastric microcirculation. Eur J Pharmacol 1989; 174:293–296

[27] Tepperman BL, Whittle BJ: Endogenous nitric oxide and sensory neuropeptides interact in the modulation of the rat gastric microcirculation. Br J Pharmacol 1992; 105:171–175

[28] Takeuchi K, Kato S, Takeeda M, Ogawa Y, Nakashima M, Matsumoto M: Facilitation by endogenous prostaglandins of capsaicin-induced gastric protection in rodents through EP2 and IP receptors. J Pharmacol Exp Ther 2003; 304: 1055–1062

[29] Holzer P: Neural regulation of gastrointestinal blood flow. In: Johnson LR (ed.) Physiology of the Gastrointestinal Tract, Fourth Eddition, Academic Press; 2006. p817-839.

[30] Moncada S, Palmer RMJ, Higgs A: Nitric oxide: physiology, pathophysiology, and pharmacology. Pharmacol Rev 1991; 43: 109-142

[31] Whittle BJ, Lopez BJ, Moncada S: Regulation of gastric mucosal integrity by endogenous nitric oxide: interactions with prostaglandins and sensory neuropeptides in the rat. Br J Pharmacol 1990; 99: 607–611

[32] Cooper GR, Mialkowski K, Wolff DJ: Cellular and enzymatic studies of Nω-propyl-L-ariginine and S-Ethyl-N-[4-trifluoromethyl phenyl]isothiourea as reversible, slowly dissociating inhibitors selective for the neuronal nitric oxide synthase isoforms. Arch Biochem Biophys 2000; 375: 183–194

[33] Zhang HQ, Fast W, Marletta MA, Martasek P, Silverman RB: Potent and selective inhibition of neuronal nitric oxide synthase by N omega-propyl-L-arginine. J Med Chem 1997; 40:3869-3870

[34] Wolff DJ, Lubeskie A, Gauld DS, Neulander MJ: Inactivation of nitric oxide synthases and cellular nitric oxide formation by N^6-iminoethyl-L-lysine and N^5-iminoetyl-L-irnithine. Eur J Pharmacol 1998; 350: 325–334

[35] László F, Whittle BJ: Actions of isoform-selective and non-selective nitric oxide synthase inhibitors on endotoxin-induced vascular leakage in rat colon. Eur J Pharmacol 1997; 334:99-102

Chapter 5

Modulation of Capsaicin-Induced Gastric Protection by Endogenous Prostaglandins through EP2/IP Receptors

Koji Takeuchi

Additional information is available at the end of the chapter

http://dx.doi.org/10.5772/58337

1. Introduction

Gastric mucosal integrity is maintained by multiple factors, including both paracrine and neuronal factors [1-4]. The former includes prostaglandins (PGs) [1] and nitric oxide (NO) [2], while capsaicin-sensitive afferent neurons play a central role in neuronal protection in the stomach [3]. Previous studies demonstrated that capsaicin, a selective stimulator of these afferent neurons, protected the gastric mucosa against various ulcerogenic stimuli such as nectrotizing agents [3]. The protective effects of capsaicin were shown to be mediated by these afferent neurons because they were completely attenuated by the chemical ablation of these neurons following a pretreatment with a large dose of capsaicin [3, 5]. The binding site of capsaicin has been cloned and named the transient receptor potential vaniloid type 1 receptor (TRPV1), a nonselective cationic channel [6]. Capsaicin is assumed to stimulate these afferent neurons by activating TRPV1, which results in the liberation of the neurotransmitter, calcitonin gene-related peptide (CGRP) and gastric protection.

Several studies, including our own, have showed that the protective effects of capsaicin were mitigated by the prior administration of indomethacin, which indicated the involvement of endogenous PGs in this action [6-9]. Endogenous PGs were previously shown to sensitize sensory neurons to nociceptive stimuli [10, 11]. Therefore, endogenous PGs are assumed to play a supportive role in the mechanism underlying capsaicin-induced gastric protection, possibly by sensitizing these afferent neurons, because capsaicin-induced gastric cytoprotection was shown to be attenuated by indomethacin.

On the other hand, recent pharmacological studies have classified PGE_2 receptors into four specific G protein-coupled subtypes, EP1 to EP4 [12]. The distribution of these receptors is considered to explain the multiple effects of PGE_2 in various tissues including the gastrointestinal tract. Mice lacking various receptors for prostanoids have been established [13, 14], and the roles of specific PG receptors in the various biological actions of PGs have been demonstrated using these "knockout mice" [15]. We performed a series of experiments to identify the EP receptor subtypes mediating the gastrointestinal protection afforded by PGE_2 using various models in both rats and EP receptor knockout mice, and found that PGE_2, administered exogenously or generated endogenously, provided gastric protection against HCl/ethanol mediated by EP1 receptors [16, 17]. However, the relationship between the EP receptor subtype and facilitation of capsaicin-induced gastric protection by PGs remains unknown.

We here investigated the role of endogenous PGs in the gastric protective action of capsaicin against HCl/ethanol-induced damage in rats, mainly in relation to PGE_2 and EP receptors. Furthermore, because an animal model lacking various receptors for prostanoids is now available [13, 15, 18], we also evaluated the protective activity of capsaicin in knockout mice lacking EP1 or EP3 receptors and also in some cases IP receptors. In addition, we also examined the gastric hyperemic response to capsaicin in these knockout mice in order to provide functional evidence for the modulatory role of PGs in capsaicin-induced protective effects.

2. Methods

ANIMALS: Male Sprague-Dawley rats (200-220 g) and C57BL/6 mice (25-30 g) were used. Mice lacking the EP1, EP3, or IP receptors were generated as described previously [13, 15, 19, 20]. In brief, the mouse genes encoding the EP1, EP3, and IP receptors were individually disrupted, and chimaeric mice were generated. These animals were then back crossed with C57BL/6 mice, and the resulting heterozygous litter mates [EP1 (+/-), EP3 (+/-) or IP (+/-),] were bred to produce homozygous EP1 (-/-), EP3 (-/-), or IP (-/-) mice. Homozygous mice were born at the predicted Mendelian frequency, grew normally, lived longer than 1 year and were fertile. The distribution of the EP1, EP3, and IP receptor genes was verified by northern blot hybridization, which failed to detect messenger RNAs encoding the respective receptors in EP1 (-/-), EP3 (-/-), and IP (-/-) mice. These knockout mice were deprived of food, but allowed free access to tap water for 18 hr before the experiments. All studies were performed using 4~8 animals per group.

INDUCTION OF GASTRIC LESIONS: Rats were administered 1 ml of HCl/ethanol (60% in 150 mM HCl) p.o. through esophageal intubation, and killed 1 hr later under deep ether anesthesia. The stomachs were removed, inflated by injecting 10 ml of 1% formalin for 10 min to fix the tissue walls, and opened along the greater curvature. The area (mm^2) of hemorrhagic lesions that developed in the stomach was measured under a dissecting microscope with a square grid (x10). Capsaicin (1-10 mg/kg) was given p.o. 30 min before the administration of HCl/ethanol. PGE_2 (0.3 mg/kg) was given i.v. 10 min prior to the HCl/ethanol treatment. In some cases, indomethacin (5 mg/kg) or ONO-AE-829 (5 and 10 mg/kg), the EP1 receptor antagonist [20], was given s.c. 30 min before the administration of PGE_2 or capsaicin. In

http://dx.doi.org/10.5772/58337

addition, the protective effects of PGE_2 and capsaicin on HCl/ethanol were also examined in rats with the chemical ablation of capsaicin-sensitive sensory neurons. Chemical deafferentation was induced by s.c. injections of capsaicin once a day for three consecutive days (total dose: 100 mg/kg) 2 weeks before the experiment [5]. All capsaicin injections were performed under ether anesthesia, and rats were pretreated with terbutaline (0.1 mg/kg, i.m.) and aminophylline (10 mg/kg, i.m.) to counteract the respiratory impairment associated with capsaicin injections. The effectiveness of the treatment was tested by examining protective wiping movements of the eye. In a separate experiment, we examined the rescue effect of various subtype-specific EP agonists on the protective effects of capsaicin in indomethacin-treated rats. Animals were first administered indomethacin (5 mg/kg) s.c., followed by capsaicin p.o. 30 min later, and were then given HCl/ethanol p.o. 30 min following the capsaicin treatment. Butaprost (an EP2 agonist: 3 mg/kg), ONO-NT-012 (an EP3 agonist: 3 mg/kg) or 11-deoxy PGE_1 (an EP3/EP4 agonist: 1 mg/kg) was administered i.v. 10 min before the capsaicin treatment. Animals were killed 1 hr after the administration of HCl/ethanol. In another experiment, wild-type mice and EP1, EP3, or IP receptor knockout mice were administered HCl/ethanol p.o. in a volume of 0.3 ml, and killed 1 hr later [16]. The stomach was then removed and treated with formalin, and the mucosa was examined for hemorrhagic lesions under a dissecting microscope, as described previously. Capsaicin (10 mg/kg) was given p.o. to half of the animals in each group 30 min before the administration of HCl/ethanol. In addition, indomethacin (5 mg/kg) or ONO-AE-829 (10 mg/kg) was given s.c. 30 min before the administration of capsaicin in wild-type mice.

MEASUREMENT OF GASTRIC MUCOSAL BLOOD FLOW (GMBF): GMBF was measured in both wild type mice and EP1-, EP3-, or IP-receptor knockout mice according to methods described in our previous study [21, 22]. Under urethane anesthesia, the abdomen was opened through a midline incision, and the stomach exposed, mounted on an *ex-vivo* chamber (the exposed area; 0.7 mm^2), and superfused at a rate of 0.5 ml/min. Gastric mucosal blood flow was measured by a laser Doppler flowmeter (ALF-21, Advance, Tokyo, Japan) and by placing a probe gently on the surface of the corpus mucosa using a balance (Medical Agent, Kyoto, Japan). Changes in mucosal blood flow were monitored on a recorder (U-228, Tokai-irika, Tokyo, Japan). After mucosal blood flow had stabilized, the solution in the chamber was withdrawn, and the mucosa was then exposed to 0.2 ml of cicaprost, a PGI_2 analogue (5 μg/ml), or capsaicin (1 mg/ml) for 10 min. After the application of these agents, the mucosa was rinsed with saline, another 0.2 ml of saline was instilled, and perfusion was resumed. Indomethacin (5 mg/kg) was given s.c. to some of wild type mice 30 min before the application of capsaicin.

MEASUREMENT OF MUCOSAL PGE_2 AND 6-keto PGF_1< LEVELS: PGE_2 levels in the rat gastric mucosa and those of 6-keto $PGF_1\alpha$ in the mouse stomach were measured 30 min after the p.o. administration of capsaicin (10 mg/kg). Some of the rats used were pretreated with caspsaicin for sensory deafferentation. In some cases, indomethacin (5 mg/kg) was administered s.c. 30 min before the capsaicin treatment. Under ether anesthesia, the stomachs were quickly removed, opened along the greater curvature, and rinsed with ice-cold saline. To separate the mucosal layer, the corpus mucosa was placed between two glass slides, squeezed with a rubber band, and placed in hexane-frozen Dry Ice and acetone. These glasses were separated, and the mucosa was collected, weighed, and put in a tube containing 100% ethanol plus 0.1 M indomethacin [17, 23]. The samples were then homogenized, and centrifuged for 10 min at 12000 g at 4°C. The supernatant of each sample was used to determine PGE_2 and 6-keto $PGF_1\alpha$ levels by EIA using PGE_2-and 6-keto PGF_1<-kits, respectively (Cayman Chemical Co., Ann Arbor, MI).

PREPARATION OF DRUGS: The drugs used in the present study were capsaicin (Nakarai Tesque, Kyoto, Japan), prostaglandin E_2 (PGE_2), 11-deoxy prostaglandin E_1 (11-deoxy PGE_1) (Funakoshi, Tokyo, Japan), ONO-AE-829, butaprost, and ONO-NT-012 (Ono, Osaka, Japan), terbutaline (Fujisawa, Osaka, Japan), aminophylline (Eisai, Tokyo, Japan), and indomethacin (Sigma Chemicals, St. Louis, Mo). Capsaicin was dissolved in Tween 80-ethanol solution (10% ethanol, 10% Tween 80, 80% saline, w/w) for s.c. injections, while indomethacin was suspended in saline with a drop of Tween 80 (Wako, Osaka, Japan). ONO-AE-829 was dissolved in saline. PGE_2 and other EP receptor ligands were first dissolved in absolute ethanol and then diluted with saline to the desired concentration. Each agent was prepared immediately before use and given in a volume of 0.5 ml per 100 g body weight (rat) or 0.1 ml per 10 g body weight (mouse) for its p.o. and s.c. administration, respectively, and given i.v. in a volume of 0.1 ml per 100 g body weight (rat). Control animals received saline instead of the active agent.

STATISTICS: Data are presented as the mean±SE for 4~8 animals per group. Statistical analyses were performed using a two-tailed Dunnett's multiple comparison test, and values of $P<0.05$ were regarded as significant.

3. Results

3.1. Effect of capsaicin on HCl/ethanol-induced gastric lesions in rats

The oral administration of HCl/ethanol (60% in 150 mM HCl) produced multiple lesions in the glandular mucosa, along the long axis of the rat stomach. These lesions were dose-dependently prevented in animals pretreated with capsaicin (1-10 mg/kg) p.o. before the challenge with HCl/ethanol, and a significant effect was obtained at doses over 3 mg/kg, with the inhibition at 10 mg/kg being 81.6% (Figure 1A). The protective effects of capsaicin (10 mg/kg) were completely attenuated by the chemical ablation of sensory neurons as well as prior administration of indomethacin (5 mg/kg), but not by ONO-AE-829 (10 mg/kg)(Figure 1B). The severity of HCl/ethanol-induced gastric lesions was also significantly reduced by the prior i.v. administration of PGE_2 (0.03 mg/kg), with the inhibition being 82.1% (Figure 2). The protective effects of PGE_2 were significantly mitigated by the pretreatment with the EP1 antagonist, ONO-AE-829 (10 mg/kg), but not by chemical deafferentation. The degree of protection afforded by PGE_2 in the presence of ONO-AE-829 at 10 mg/kg was 19.8%, which was significantly less than that observed in vehicle-treated normal rats.

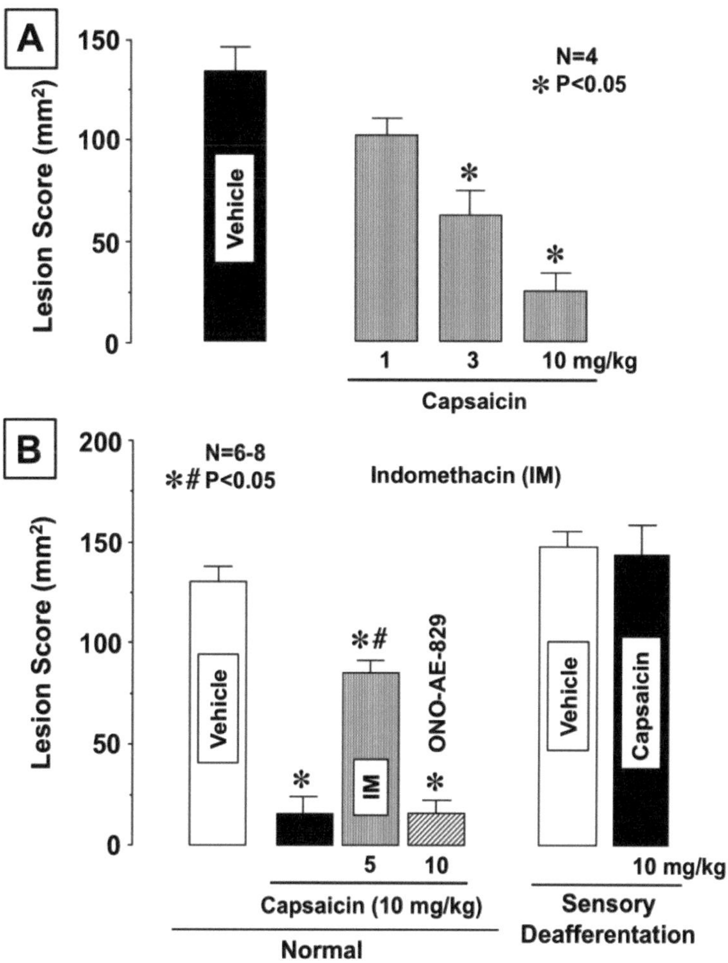

Figure 1. Dose-response relationship for the protective effects of capsaicin against HCl/ethanol-induced gastric lesions in rats (A), and the effects of indomethacin (5 mg/kg), ONO-AE-829 (10 mg/kg), or sensory deafferentation on the mucosal protective effects of capsaicin (B). Animals were administered 1 ml of HCl/ethanol (60% in 150 mM HCl), and killed 1 hr later. Capsaicin (1-10 mg/kg) was administered p.o. 30 min before HCl/ethanol. Indomethacin (5 mg/kg) or ONO-AE-829 (10 mg/kg) was given s.c. 30 min before capsaicin. Sensory deafferentation was achieved with 3 consecutive s.c. injections of capsaicin (total 100 mg/kg) 2 weeks before the experiment. Data are presented as means±SE from 4-8 rats. Significantly different at P<0.05: *from the control; # from the vehicle.

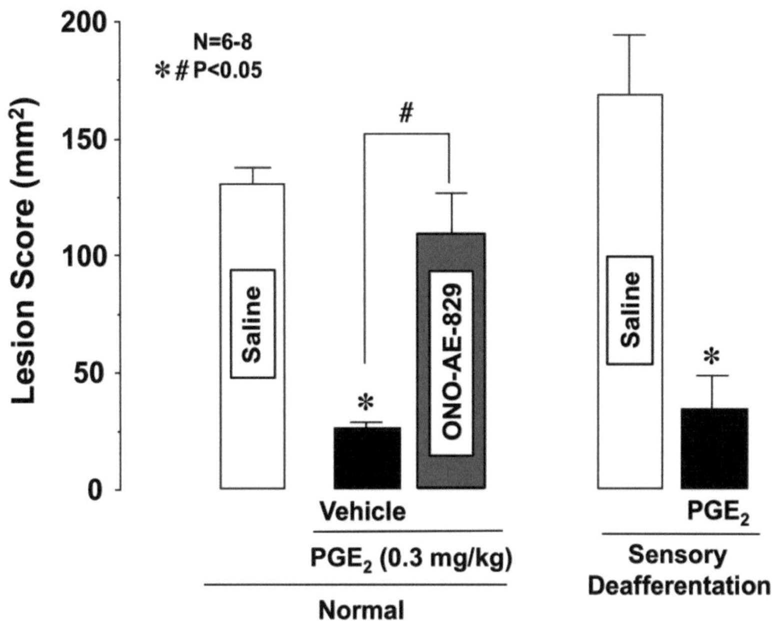

Figure 2. Effects of ONO-AE-829 or sensory deafferentation on the protective action of PGE_2 against HCl/ethanol in the rat stomach. Animals were administered 1 ml of HCl/ethanol (60% in 150 mM HCl), and killed 1 hr later. PGE_2 (0.3 mg/kg) was given i.v. 10 min before HCl/ethanol. ONO-AE-829 (10 mg/kg) was administered s.c. 30 min before PGE_2. Sensory deafferentation was induced with 3 consecutive s.c. injections of capsaicin (total 100 mg/kg) 2 weeks before the experiment. Data are presented as means±SE from 6-8 rats. Significantly different at $P<0.05$: *from the control; # from the vehicle.

The oral administration of capsaicin (10 mg/kg) did not affect the mucosal PGE_2 content when measured 0.5 hr after its administration (not shown). The prior administration of indomethacin (5 mg/kg, s.c.) markedly reduced PGE_2 levels in the presence of capsaicin. As in normal rats, capsaicin did not significantly affect mucosal PGE_2 levels in sensory deafferented animals.

3.2. Reversal of capsaicin-induced protection by EP agonists in indomehtacin-pretreated rats

To investigate the roles of PGE_2 and EP receptors in capsaicin-induced gastric protection, we examined the rescue effects of various subtype-specific EP agonists on capsaicin in the presence of indomethacin. The oral administration of capsaicin (10 mg/kg) markedly protected against HCl/ethanol-induced gastric lesions (Figure 3A). This effect of capsaicin was significantly mitigated by the prior administration of indomethacin (5 mg/kg), and the degree of inhibition was reduced to 29.7%. When these animals were given various EP agonists i.v. 20 min after indomethacin, the protective effects of capsaicin were again observed in rats pretreated with butaprost (an EP2 agonist). Neither ONO-NT-012 (an EP3 agonist) nor 11-deoxy PGE_1 (an EP3/EP4 agonist) rescued the effects of capsaicin against HCl/ethanol in the presence of indomethacin. None of the EP agonists (i.v.) used, including butaprost, significantly protected against HCl/ethanol by themselves (Figure 3B).

http://dx.doi.org/10.5772/58337

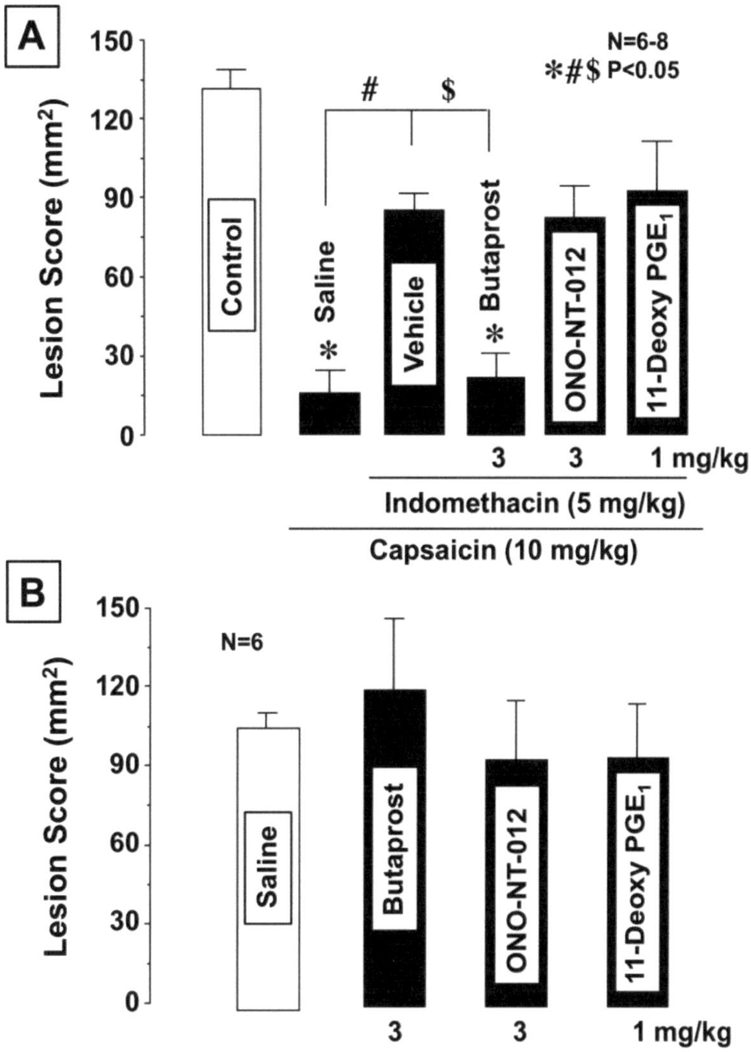

Figure 3. A: Effects of various EP agonists on the mucosal protective action of capsaicin against HCl/ethanol-induced gastric lesions in the rat stomach in the presence of indomethacin. Animals were given 1 ml of HCl/ethanol (60% in 150 mM HCl) and killed 1 hr later. Capsaicin (10 mg/kg) was administered p.o. 30 min before HCl/ethanol. Indomethacin (5mg/kg) was given s.c. 30 min before capsaicin. Various EP agonists were given i.v. 10 min before capsaicin. Data are presented as means±SE from 6-8 rats. Significantly different at $P<0.05$: *from the control; # from the saline; $ from vehicle. **B:** Effects of various EP agonists on HCl/ethanol-induced gastric lesions in the rat stomach. Various EP agonists were given i.v. 10 min before HCl/ethanol. Data are presented as means±SE from 6 rats.

3.3. Gastric cytoprotection against HCl/ethanol by capsaicin in mice

To further investigate the relationship between capsaicin-induced gastric protection and EP receptor subtype, we examined the protective effects of capsaicin against HCl/ethanol in both wild-type and knockout mice lacking EP1 or EP3 receptors. In addition, since other study reported a role for PGI_2 in the release of CGRP in the stomach following capsaicin stimulation [19], the protective effect of capsaicin was also examined in IP receptor knockout mice. The intragastric administration of HCl/ethanol (0.3 ml) also caused hemorrhagic lesions in the mouse stomach (Figure 4). HCl/ethanol led to the development of gastric lesions in EP1, EP3, and IP receptor knockout mice, similar to wild-type mice, and the severity of these lesions was similar among these groups. The severity of these lesions in wild-type mice was also reduced by the prior p.o. administration of capsaicin (10 mg/kg). This agent significantly reduced the severity of these lesions in animals lacking either EP1 or EP3 receptors. However, capsaicin failed to protect the stomach against HCl/ethanol in IP receptor knockout mice, and the lesion score in these animals was not significantly different from that observed in IP receptor knockout animals without the capsaicin pretreatment.

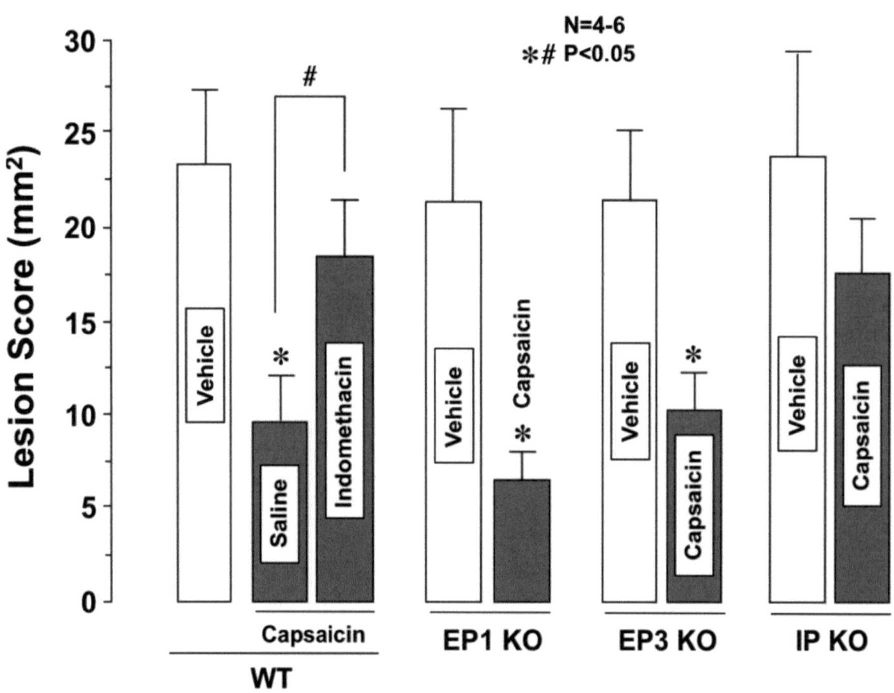

Figure 4. Effects of capsaicin on HCl/ethanol-induced gastric lesions in wild-type and knockout mice lacking EP1, EP3 or IP receptors. Animals were administered 0.3 ml of HCl/ethanol (60% ethanol in 150 mM HCl) p.o. and killed 1 hr later. Capsaicin (10 mg/kg) was given p.o. 30 min before HCl/ethanol. In wild-type mice, indomethacin (5 mg/kg) was given s.c. 30 min before administration of capsaicin. Data are presented as means±SE from 4-6 mice. Significantly different at $P<0.05$; *from the vehicle in the corresponding group; # from saline.

The oral administration of capsaicin (10 mg/kg) did not significantly affect 6-keto $PGF_1\alpha$ levels, which was similar to the effects observed on PGE_2 content in the rat stomach (not shown). Indomethacin (5 mg/kg) markedly decreased 6-keto $PGF_1\alpha$ levels in the presence of capsaicin. Similarly, capsaicin had no effect on 6-keto $PGF_1\alpha$ levels in IP receptor knockout mice.

3.4. Effect of capsaicin on gastric mucosal blood flow in mice

Under urethane anesthesia, the chambered stomachs of both wild type mice and those lacking EP1, EP3, or IP receptors showed a relatively constant GMBF during a 2-hr test period. The mucosal application of capsaicin (1 mg/ml) for 10 min caused a marked increase in GMBF in wild type mice, and this effect was significantly attenuated by the prior administration of indomethacin (5 mg/ml) (Figure 5). A significant increase in GMBF by capsaicin was also observed in both EP1 and EP3 receptor knockout mice. However, the gastric hyperemic response to capsaicin was almost completely absent in animals lacking IP receptors, and GMBF values were significantly lower than those in control wild type mice, at most of the time points measured after the application of capsaicin.

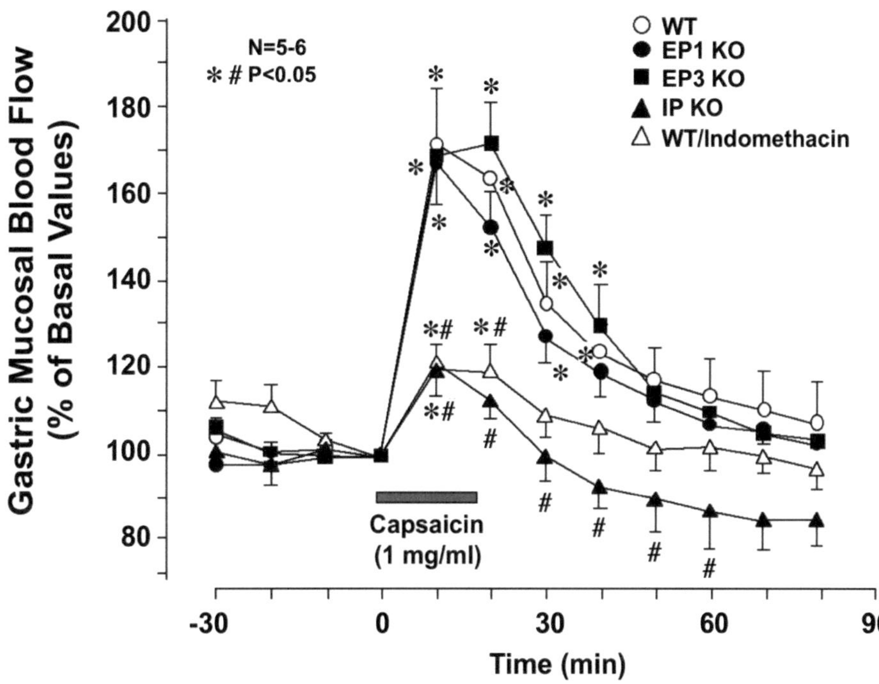

Figure 5. Effects of capsaicin on GMBF in wild type mice and knockout mice lacking EP1, EP3 or IP receptors under urethane anesthetized conditions. Capsaicin was applied to the chamber at a concentration of 1 mg/ml for 10 min (100 μl), and GMBF was measured before and after its application. Indomethacin was administered s.c. at a dose of 5 mg/kg 30 min before capsaicin in wild-type mice. Data are expressed as an increase in GMBF (a % of basal values) and presented as means±SE of values determined every 10 min from 5-6 mice per group. Significantly different at $P<0.05$: *from the corresponding basal values (time 0) in the corresponding group: # from wild type mice.

4. Commentary

PGs, either endogenous or exogenous derivatives, have been shown to act on multiple receptors [12]. Capsaicin affords gastric protection by stimulating afferent C-fibers [3], and this action is partly dependent on endogenous PGs [5, 8, 9, 24]. We previously examined the relationship between EP receptor subtypes and gastric protection against HCl/ethanol in rats using various EP agonists and found that the gastroprotective action afforded by endogenous or exogenous PGs was mediated by EP1 receptors [16, 17]. However, the EP receptor subtypes or other prostanoid receptors responsible for this phenomenon has yet to be established. The present study was conducted to determine the prostanoid receptor(s) involved in capsaicin-induced gastric protection.

First, we confirmed that PGE_2 prevented the development of HCl/ethanol-induced gastric lesions, and this action was attenuated by the EP1 antagonist, ONO-AE-829 [16]. This result was also verified in EP receptor knockout mice, with this protection being completely absent in mice lacking EP1 receptors [16, 17]. These results strongly suggest that the protective effects of exogenous PGE_2 in the stomach were mainly mediated by the activation of EP1 receptors. On the other hand, endogenous PGs play a role in the gastric cytoprotection induced by the oral administration of capsaicin [5, 8, 9]. As shown in this study, the protective effects of capsaicin against HCl/ethanol were dose-dependent, and were attenuated by the chemical ablation of capsaicin-sensitive sensory neurons. The protective effects of capsaicin were also significantly mitigated by the prior administration of indomethacin, which indicated the involvement of endogenous PGs in these effects. However, in contrast to the adaptive cytoprotection induced by a mild irritant [17], the effects of capsaicin were not affected by the selective EP1 antagonist, ONO-AE-829. This was confirmed by the stimulatory effects of capsaicin on gastric HCO_3^- secretion which were attenuated by indomethacin and capsazepine, but not ONO-8711 (an EP1 antagonist) [25]. Furthermore, neither the stimulation of sensory neurons by capsaicin nor sensory deafferentation affected mucosal PGE_2 levels in the stomach. Many studies have shown that mild irritants increased the production of PGE_2 in the stomach [14, 17]. These findings suggest that although endogenous PGs are involved in the gastric cytoprotection induced by both mild irritants and capsaicin, the mode of action appears to be different in these two cases. The stimulation of afferent neurons by capsaicin was assumed to increase the production of PGs in the stomach, but exerted protective effects in the stomach, that were partly dependent on endogenous PGs.

In the present study, we administered various EP agonists to indomethacin-treated animals, to determine whether the inhibitory effect of indomethacin on capsaicin-induced gastric protection was reversed by exogenous PGE_2, and if so, which EP receptor subtype was responsible for this action. The protective effects of capsaicin were significantly restored, even in the presence of indomethacin, by the prior administration of butaprost, the EP2 agonist, but not by the EP3 or EP4 agonist. In addition, the protective effects of capsaicin were significantly enhanced in the presence of butaprost, which strongly suggested a supportive role for EP2 receptors in capsaicin-induced gastric protection. These results are supported by the findings of Haupt et al [26], who reported the involvement of the EP2 receptor in the potentiation of afferent neuronal discharges by PGE_2 in the rat jejunum. Jenkins et al [27] also demonstrated that the activation of DP, EP, and IP receptors could each cause the release of CGRP from trigeminal neurons, and that the predominant EP receptor subtype involved may be the EP2 receptor. In the present study, neither of these EP agonists, including butaprost, offered any protection against HCl/ethanol-induced gastric damage by themselves. Furthermore, capsaicin-induced gastric protection was not affected by the EP1 antagonist, which excluded the involvement of EP1 receptors in the facilitation of this action by endogenous PGs. The significant level of protection afforded by capsaicin was also observed in knockout mice lacking EP1 and EP3 receptors, which confirmed that capsaicin-induced gastric protection did not involve EP1 or EP3 receptors. We could not confirm the involvement of EP2 receptors in this action because EP2 knockout mice were not available in our laboratory.

In contrast, we demonstrated that capsaicin failed to exhibit a cytoprotective effect against HCl/ethanol-induced gastric lesions in IP-receptor knockout mice. We previously showed that 20 mM taurocholate, as a mild irritant, protected the stomach against HCl/ethanol even in IP receptor knockout mice, which was similar to that observed in wild-type mice. These results suggested the absence of the involvement of PGI_2 in the mechanism responsible for adapative cytoprotection [17]. We also reported that the adaptive cytoprotection induced by taurocholate was attenuated by ONO-AE-829, the EP1 antagonist, as well as indomethacin, and was not observed in EP1 receptor knockout mice [17]. The present results obtained in knockout mice suggest that IP receptors are also involved in the protective effects of capsaicin in the stomach, in addition to EP2 receptors. The exact mechanism by which endogenous PGs contributes to the protective action of capsaicin is currently unknown. Previous studies have suggested that endogenous PGs may sensitize sensory neurons to nociceptive stimuli [10, 11]. Boku et al. [19] reported the lack of CGRP release in response to mild injuries in the stomachs of IP-receptor knockout mice. Oishi et al. [10] demonstrated, using IP-receptor knockout mice, that PGI_2 was a major nociceptive mediator in the acetic acid-induced writhing reaction. Since capsaicin-induced gastric cytoprotection was attenuated by indomethacin and was absent in IP-receptor knockout mice, endogenous PGI_2 may play a supportive role in the mechanism responsible for capsaicin-induced gastric cytoprotection, possibly by sensitizing sensory neurons [17, 28]. However, capsaicin did not have any effect on either PGE_2 production in the rat stomach or PGI_2 production in the mouse stomach. Thus, PGs generated constitutively may maintain the sensitivity of these neurons to the capsaicin stimulation.

Intragastric capsaicin has been shown to increase GMBF in the rat stomach, and this effect was attenuated by sensory deafferentation following a capsaicin pretreatment [9, 14, 29]. Although gastric hyperemia is not the exclusive mechanism responsible for gastric cytoprotection induced by PGE_2 or the stimulation of capsaicin-sensitive afferent neurons [16, 30], GMBF is considered to be a factor in capsaicin-induced gastric protection under certain experimental conditions [7, 29]. We previously reported that the gastric hyperemic response to capsaicin was also significantly mitigated by indomethacin, which suggested the involvement of endogenous PGs in this response [14]. In the present study, we confirmed that intragastric capsaicin markedly increased GMBF in wild type mice in an indomethacin-sensitive manner. This effect was also observed in EP1 or EP3 receptor knockout mice, but was completely absent in animals lacking IP receptors, similar to the gastroprotective effects of capsaicin. These results may provide functional evidence for the modulatory role of IP receptors in the facilitation of gastric protection mediated by capsaicin-sensitive afferent neurons by endogenous PGs.

The results of the present study suggest that capsaicin exhibits gastric cytoprotective effects as well as gastric hyperemic response, essentially by stimulating sensory neurons, and this partly depended on endogenous PG levels. The facilitative effects of endogenous PGs were mediated by EP2 and IP receptors, which may have sensitized the sensory neurons to capsaicin, even though capsaicin increased the production of PGI_2 but not PGE_2 in the gastric mucosa. However, whether endogenous PGs modulated the effects of capsaicin by interacting with TRPV1 remains unknown; however, capsaicin previously exhibited gastric protective effects by activating TRPV1 [31]. Endogenous phosphatidyl-inositol-4, 5-bisphosphate (PtdIns(4, 5) P_2) was shown to inhibit TRPV1, and this was alleviated by agents that activated phospholipase C [32, 33]. Therefore, PGs may sensitize these afferent neurons to capsaicin through EP2/IP receptors by somehow releasing TRPV1 from PtdIns(4, 5)P_2-mediated inhibition.

5. Summary

Capsaicin provided gastric cytoprotection essentially through the stimulation of sensory neurons, and this partly depended on endogenous PGs. PGs facilitated the protective effects of capsaicin, and this response was mediated by EP2 and IP receptors, possibly by sensitizing the sensory neurons to capsaicin, even though capsaicin increased the production of PGI_2 but not PGE_2 in the gastric mucosa (Figure 6). Although endogenous PGs are also known to be involved in the adaptive cytoprotection induced by mild irritants, this is different from that of capsaicin and is mediated by the activation of EP1 receptors with a concomitant increase in the production of mucosal PGE_2.

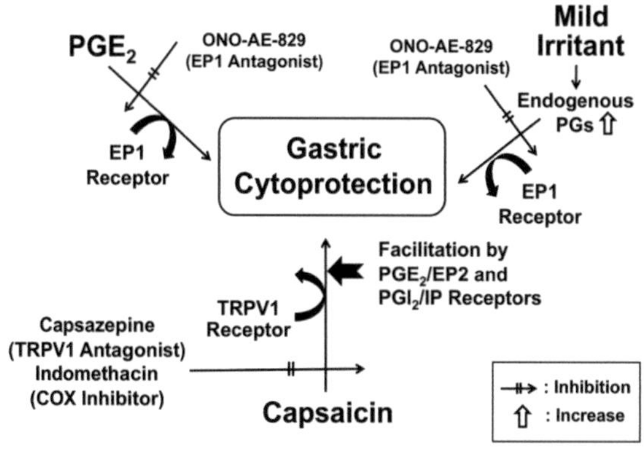

Figure 6. Mechanisms underlying the gastric cytoprotection induced by PGE_2, mild irritants, and capsaicin. Exogenous PGE_2 provides direct gastric cytoprotection, and this was mediated by the activation of EP1 receptors and completely blocked by the EP1 antagonist, ONO-AE-829. A mild irritant increased endogenous PGE_2 production in the stomach and exhibited adaptive gastric cytoprotection. This action was prevented by indomethacin as well as the EP1 antagonist. On the other hand, capsaicin exhibited gastric cytoprotective effects, essentially mediated by capsaicin-sensitive afferent neurons via the activation of TRPV1 receptors, and this effect was completely attenuated by the TRPV1 antagonist, capsazepine. Although capsaicin increased the production of PGI_2 but not PGE_2 in the gastric mucosa, this protective effect was facilitated by endogenous PGs through PGE_2/EP2 and PGI_2/IP receptors.

http://dx.doi.org/10.5772/58337

Acknowledgements

The authors are greatly indebted to Professor Shu Narumiya, Kyoto University Faculty of Medicine, for kindly supplying EP1, EP3, and IP receptor-knockout mice and Ono Pharmaceutical Company for supplying various EP agonists and antagonists. We also thank the students at the Department of Pharmacology and Experimental Therapeutics, Kyoto Pharmaceutical University, Kyoto, Japan, for their technical collaboration.

Author details

Koji Takeuchi[1,2*]

Address all correspondence to: takeuchi@mb.kyoto-phu.ac.jp

1 Department of Pharmacology & Experimental Therapeutics, Kyoto Pharmaceutical University, Yamashina, Kyoto, Japan

2 General Incorporated Association, Kyoto Research Center for Gastrointestinal, Diseases, Karasuma-Oike, Kyoto, Japan

The author declares no conflict of interest.

References

[1] Robert A, Nezamis JE, Lancaster C, Davis JP, Field SO, Hanchar AJ. Mild irritants prevent gastric necrosis through "adaptive cytoprotection" mediated by prostaglandins. Am J Physiol 1983; 245: G113-21.

[2] Whittle BJR, Lopez-Belmote J, Moncada S. Regulation of gastric mucosal integrity by endogenous nitric oxide: Interaction with prostaglandins and sensory neuropeptides in the rat. Br J Pharmacol 1990; 99: 607-11.

[3] Holzer P, Sametz W. Gastric mucosal protection against ulcerogenic factors in the rat mediated by capsaicin-sensitive afferent neurons. Gastroenterology 1986; 91: 975-81.

[4] Holzer P. Neural emergency system in the stomach. Gastroenterology 1998; 114: 823-39.

[5] Takeuchi K, Niida H, Matsumoto J, Ueshima K, Okabe S. Gastric motility changes in capsaicin-induced cytoprotection in the rat stomach. Jpn J Pharmacol 1991; 55: 147-55.

[6] Caterina MJ, Schumacher MA, Tominaga M, Rosen T, Levine JD, Lulius D. The capsaicin receptor: a heat-activated ion channel in the pain pathway. Nature 1997; 389: 316-24.

[7] Takeuchi K, Ohuchi T, Narita M, Okabe S. Capsaicin-sensitve sensory nerves in recovery of gastric mucosal integrity after damage by sodium taurocholate in rats. Jpn J Pharmacol 1993; 63: 479-85.

[8] Uchida M, Yano S, Watanabe K. The role of capsaicin-sensitive afferent nerves in protective effect of capsaicin against absolute ethanol-induced gastric lesions in rats. Jpn J Pharmacol 1991; 55: 279-82.

[9] Brzozowski T, Drozdowicz D, Szlachcic A, Pytko-Polonczyk J, Majka J, Konturek SJ. Role of nitric oxide and prostaglandins in gastroprotection induced by capsaicin and papaverine. Digestion 1993; 54: 24-31.

[10] Ohishi S, Ueno A, Matsumoto H, Murata T, Ushikubi F, Narumiya S. Evidence for involvement of prostaglandin I_2 as a major nociceptive mediator in acetic acid-induced writhing reaction: a study using IP-receptor disrupted mice. Adv Exp Med Biol 1999; 469: 265-8.

[11] Ueno A, Naraba H, Ikeda Y, Ushikubi F, Murata T, Narumiya S, Ohishi S. Intrinsic prostacyclin contributes to exudation induced by bradykinin or carrageenin: a study on the paw edema induced in IP-receptor-deficient mice. Life Sci 2000; 66: PL155-60.

[12] Coleman RA, Smith WL, Narumiya S. Classification of prostanoid receptors: Properties, distribution, and structure of the receptors and their subtypes. Pharmacol Rev 1994; 46: 205-29.

[13] Sugimoto Y, Namba T, Honda A, Hayashi Y, Negishi M, Ichikawa A, Narumiya S. Cloning and expression of a cDNA for mouse prostaglandin E receptor EP3 subtype. J Biol Chem 1992; 267: 6463-6.

[14] Matsumoto J, Takeuchi K, Ueshima K, Okabe S. Role of capsaicin-sensitive afferent neurons in mucosal blood flow response of rat stomach induced by mild irritants. Dig Dis Sci 1992; 37: 1336-44.

[15] Ushikubi F, Segi E, Sugimoto Y, Murata T, Matsuoka T, Kobayashi T, Hizaki H, Tuboi K, Katsuyama M, Ichikawa A, Tanaka T, Yoshida N and Narumiya S. Impaired febrile response in mice lacking the prostaglandin E receptor subtype 3. Nature 1998; 395: 281-4

[16] Araki H, Yagi K, Suzuki K, Furukawa O, Takeuchi K. Roles of prostaglandin E receptor subtypes in cytoprotective action of prostaglandin E_2 in rat stomachs. Alimental Pharmacol Ther 2000; 14 (Suppl 1): 18-25.

[17] Takeuchi K, Araki H, Umeda M, Komoike Y, Suzuki K. Adaptive gastric cytoprotection is mediated by prostaglandin EP1 receptors: A study using rats and knockout mice. J Pharmacol Exp Ther 2001; 297: 1160-5.

[18] Oida H, Namba T, Sugimoto Y, Ushikubi F, Ohishi H, Ichikawa A, Narumiya S. In situhybridization studies of prostacyclin receptor mRNA expression in various mouse organs. Br J Pharmacol 1995; 116: 2828-37.

[19] Boku K, Ohno T, Saeki T, Hayashi H, Hayashi I, Katori M, Murata T, Narumiya S, Saigenji K, Majima M. Adaptive cytoprotection mediated by prostaglandin I_2 is attributable to sensitization of CRGP-containing sensory nerves. Gastroenterology 2001; 120: 134-43.

[20] Watabe A, Sugimoto Y, Honda A, Irie A, Namba T, Negishi M, Ito S, Narumiya S, Ichikawa A. Cloning and expression of cDNA for a mouse EP1 subtype of prostaglandin E receptor. J Biol Chem 1993; 27: 20175-8.

[21] Takeuchi K, Komoike Y, Takeeda M, Ukawa H. Gastric mucosal ulcerogenic responses following barrier disruption in knockout mice lacking prostaglandin EP1 receptors. Aliment Pharmacol Ther 2002; 16: 74-82.

[22] Futaki N, Takahashi S, Yokoyama M, Arai I, Higuchi S, Otomo S. NS-398, a new antiinflammatory agent, selectively inhibits prostaglandin G/H synthase/ cyclooxygenase (COX-2) activity in vitro. Prostaglandins 1994; 47: 55-9

[23] Holzer P, Livingston EH, Saria A, Guth PH. Sensory neurons mediate protective vasodilatation in rat gastric mucosa. Am J Physiol 1991; 260: G363-70.

[24] Takeuchi K, Matsumoto J, Ueshima K, Okabe S. Role of capsaicin-sensitive afferent neurons in alkaline secretory response to luminal acid in the rat duodenum. Gastroenterology 1991; 101: 954-61.

[25] Aihara E, Hayashi M, Sasaki Y, Kobata A, Takeuchi K. Mechanisms underlying capsaicin-stimulated HCO_3^-secretion in the stomach: Comparison with mucosal acidification. J Pharmacol Exp Ther 2005; 315: 423-32.

[26] Haupt W, Jiang W, Kreis ME, Grundy D. Prostaglandin EP receptor subtypes have distinctive effects on jejunal afferent sensitivity in the rat. Gastroenterology 2000; 119: 1580-9.

[27] Jenkins DW, Feniuk W, Humphrey PPA. Characterization of the prostanoid receptor types involved in mediating calcitonin gene-related peptide release from cultured rat trigeminal neurons. Br J Pharmacol 2001; 134: 1296-302.

[28] Fukushima K, Aoi Y, Kato S, Takeuchi K. Gastroprotective action of lafutidine mediated by capsaicin-sensitive afferent neurons without interaction with TRPV1 and involvement of endogenous prostaglandins. World J Gastroenterol 2006; 12: 3031-37.

[29] Takeuchi K, Kato S, Ogawa Y, Kanatsu K, Umeda M. Role of endogenous prostacyclin in gastric ulcerogenic and healing responses: A study using IP-receptor knockout mice. J Physiol Paris 2001; 95: 75-80.

[30] Stroff T, Plate S, Ebrahim JS, Ehrlich KH, Respondek M, Peskar BM. Tachykinin-induced increase in gastric mucosal resistance: role of primary afferent neurons, CGRP, and NO. Am J Physiol 1996; 271: G1017-27.

[31] Yamamoto H, Horie S, Uchida M, Tsuchiya S, Murayama T, Watanabe K. Effects of vanilloid receptor agonists and antagonists on gastric antral ulcers in rats. Eur J Pharmacol 2001; 432: 203-10.

[32] Premkumar LS, Ahern GP. Induction of vanilloid receptor channel activity by protein kinase C. Nature 2000; 408: 985-90.

[33] Chuang HH, Prescott ED, Kong H, Shields S, Jordt SE, Basbaum AI, Chao MV, Julius D. Bradykinin and nerve growth factor release the capsaicin receptor from PtdIns(4, 5)P2-mediated inhibition. Nature 2001; 411: 957-62.

Chapter 6

Mechanism of Capsaicin-Stimulated Gastric HCO^{3-} Secretion – Comparison with Mucosal Acidification

Koji Takeuchi and Eitaro Aihara

Additional information is available at the end of the chapter

http://dx.doi.org/10.5772/58336

1. Introduction

The gastric mucosa is maintained in an intact state by multiple protective mechanisms including humoral and neuronal factors, in spite of its exposure to acid and other chemical hazards [1]. Capsaicin-sensitive afferent neurons play a central role in neuronal mechanisms taking place in the stomach [2]. These afferent neurons have been shown to regulate various gastric functions such as secretion, mucosal blood flow (GMBF), and motility, and modulate the mucosal integrity of the stomach [2-5]. Vanilloid type 1 receptor (VR1), a nonselective cationic channel, has recently been cloned as the binding site of capsaicin [6], and more recently, has been identified as a member of the transient receptor potential (TRP) family of ion channels [7]. Although the TRP family is activated by a diverse range of stimuli, including the depletion of intracellular Ca^{2+}stores [6], the VR1 receptor remains the only channel activated by vanilloids such as capsaicin and is now known as TRPV1 [8]. Capsaicin stimulates these afferent neurons via TRPV1, resulting in the release of calcitonin gene-related peptide (CGRP), the predominant neurotransmitter of spinal afferents in the rat stomach, and thus, exerts a gastroprotective action [9]. CGRP has been shown to induce endothelial cells to release nitric oxide (NO), and this molecule is known to strongly mediate the action of CGRP [2]. Other studies have also demonstrated that activation of the bradykinin B2 receptor caused the opening of TRPV1 and modified the action of capsaicin [10, 11].

The secretion of HCO_3^- from surface epithelial cells is a protective mechanism in the stomach, with HCO_3^- working in collaboration with mucus gel, which adheres to the surface of mucosa [1]. We previously reported that capsaicin increased duodenal HCO_3^- secretion mediated by endogenous prostaglandins (PGs) and NO as well as capsaicin-sensitive afferent neurons [12, 13]. We also demonstrated that PGE_2 stimulated HCO_3^- secretion through EP1 receptors in the stomach and EP3/EP4 receptors in the duodenum [14, 15], while the action of capsaicin in the duodenum required the presence of prostacyclin (PGI_2) IP receptors [16]. However, few studies have examined the mechanisms involved in gastric HCO_3^- secretion in response to capsaicin.

We here described the regulatory mechanism underlying capsaicin-induced gastric HCO_3^- secretion, in relation to sensory neurons, TRPV1, PGs, NO, and bradykinin B2 receptors, and compared it to that of the acid-induced response. In addition, because we found that responses to capsaicin and acid in the duodenum differed concerning PGI_2/IP dependency [16], we also examined these responses in the stomach using mice lacking EP1, EP3 or IP receptors.

2. Methods

ANIMALS: Male SD rats (220-260 g, Nippon Charles River, Shizuoka, Japan) and male C57BL/6 mice (25-30 g) were used. Mice lacking the EP1, EP3, or IP receptors were generated as described previously [17, 18]. These rats and knockout mice were deprived of food, but allowed free access to tap water for 18 hr before the experiments. Studies were performed under urethane anesthesia (1.25 g/kg, i.p.) using 4~8 animals per group.

DETERMINATION OF GASTRIC HCO_3^- SECRETION: The secretion of HCO_3^- was measured in the chambered stomach as described previously [5]. The abdomen was incised and the stomach was exposed, mounted on a chamber (exposed area, rat: 3.1 cm^2, mouse: 0.7 cm^2), and superfused with saline that was gassed with 100% O_2 and kept in a reservoir. The secretion of HCO_3^- was measured at pH 7.0 using a pH-stat method (Hiranuma Comtite-8, Mito, Japan) and by adding 2 mM HCl to the reservoir. Acid secretion was completely inhibited by omeprazole given i.p. at a dose of 60 mg/kg to unmask HCO_3^- in the stomach. After basal HCO_3^- secretion had stabilized, animals were subjected to the following treatment. Capsaicin (0.03~0.3 mg/ml) or NOR-3 (a NO donor: 3 mg/ml) was topically applied to the chamber for 10 min, while PGE_2 (1 mg/kg) or bradykinin (30 μg/kg) was given i.v. as a single injection. The secretion of HCO_3^- was also stimulated by exposing the mucosa to 50~200 mM HCl (rat) or 50 mM HCl (mouse) for 10 min. The effects of indomethacin, N^G-nitro L-arginine methyl ester (L-NAME), ONO-8711 (an EP1 antagonist) (Aoi et al., 2004), FR172357 (a bradykinin B2 antagonist) [19], capsazepine (a TRPV1 antagonist), or the chemical ablation of capsaicin-sensitive afferent neurons were examined on the secretion of HCO_3^- induced by the above agents or mucosal acidification. Indomethacin (5 mg/kg), ONO-8711 (10 mg/kg) or FR172357 (1 mg/kg) was given s.c. 30 min or i.v. 15 min before each treatment, while L-NAME (20 mg/kg) was given s.c. 3 hr before because this agent was previously shown to acutely increase HCO_3^- secretion through a neural reflex due to an increase in blood pressure [20-22]. Capsazepine (2.5 mg/ml) was applied to the chamber for 20 min, starting from 10 min before the capsaicin or acid treatment [13], or applied for 20 min followed by an i.v. injection of bradykinin 10 min later. The chemical ablation of capsaicin-sensitive afferent neurons was achieved with repeated s.c. injections of capsaicin (total dose; 100 mg/kg) once daily for 3 days, 2 weeks before the experiment [3, 5].

MEASUREMENT OF MUCOSAL PGE_2 AND PGI_2 LEVELS: Mucosal PGE_2 and PGI_2 (6-keto PGF_{1a}) levels in the stomach were measured after the application of capsaicin (0.3 mg/ml) for 10 min. The stomach was removed 30 later, weighed, and put in a tube containing 100% methanol plus 0.1 M indomethacin [23]. The samples were then minced with scissors, homogenized, and centrifuged at 12000 g for 10 min at 4°C. The supernatant of each sample was used to measure PGE_2 and 6-keto PGF_1 α levels by EIA with PGE_2^- and 6-keto PGF_1 α-kits (Cayman Chemical Co., Ann Arbor, MI).

PREPARATION OF DRUGS: The drugs used in the present study were urethane (Tokyo kasei, Tokyo, Japan), capsaicin and bradykinin (Nacalai Tesque, Kyoto, Japan), prostaglandin E_2 (PGE_2: Funakoshi, Tokyo, Japan), capsazepine, N^G-nitro L-arginine methyl ester (L-NAME), and indomethacin (Sigma Chemicals, St. Louis, Mo, USA), ONO-8711 (Ono Pharmaceutical Co., Osaka, Japan), NOR-3 [(±)- (E)-ethyl-2- [(E)-hydroxyimino]-5-nitro-3-hexeneamine] (Dojindo, Kumamoto, Japan), omeprazole (Astra Zeneca, Möndal, Sweden), FR172357, and terbutaline (Buricanyl^R, Fujisawa, Osaka, Japan), and aminophylline (Neophylline^R, Eizai, Tokyo, Japan). Capsaicin was dissolved in a Tween 80-ethanol solution (10% ethanol, 10% Tween, and 80% saline, w/w: Wako, Osaka, Japan) for the s.c. injection, while it was suspended in a 0.5% carboxymethylcellulose solution (CMC: Nacalai Tesque) for the topical application. PGE_2 or NOR-3 was first dissolved in absolute ethanol or dimethyl sulfoxide (DMSO), respectively, and diluted with saline to the desired concentrations. Omeprazole was suspended in a 0.5% CMC solution. Other agents were dissolved in saline. Each agent was prepared immediately before use and given in a volume of 0.5 ml per 100 g body weight in the case of the i.p. or s.c. administration, in a volume of 0.1 ml per 100 g body weight in the case of the i.v. administration, or applied topically to the chamber in a volume of 2 ml per rat or 0.7ml per mice. Control animals received saline or CMC instead of active agents.

STATISTICS: Data are presented as the mean±SE from 4~8 rats or mice per group. Statistical analyses were performed using a two-tailed Dunnett's multiple comparison test, and values of $p<0.05$ were regarded as significant.

3. Results

3.1. Stimulation by capsaicin and mucosal acidification of HCO_3^- secretion in the rat stomach

Capsaicin (0.03~0.3 mg/ml) applied to the chamber for 10 min increased the secretion of HCO_3^- in a dose-dependent manner, and this effect was significant at a dose of 0.1 mg/ml or greater (Figure 1). The stimulatory effect of capsaicin (0.3 mg/ml) on HCO_3^- was significantly attenuated by the chemical ablation of capsaicin-sensitive afferent neurons as well as the prior administration of indomethacin (5 mg/kg, s.c.) or L-NAME (20 mg/kg, s.c.) (Figure 2). The action of capsaicin was also potently inhibited by the co-application of capsazepine, the TRPV1 antagonist. However, neither the EP1 antagonist, ONO-8711 (10 m/kg, s.c.) nor the bradykinin B2 antagonist, FR172357 (1 mg/kg, i.v.) had any effect on HCO_3^- secretion in response to capsaicin.

The secretion of HCO_3^- was also increased in a concentration-dependent manner when the mucosa was acidified following its exposure to 50~200 mM HCl for 10 min (Figure 3). The response to 200 mM HCl was significantly prevented by indomethacin, L-NAME, ONO-8711, and capsaicin pretreatments (Figure 4). However, acid-induced HCO_3^- secretion in the stomach was not affected by either capsazepine or FR172357.

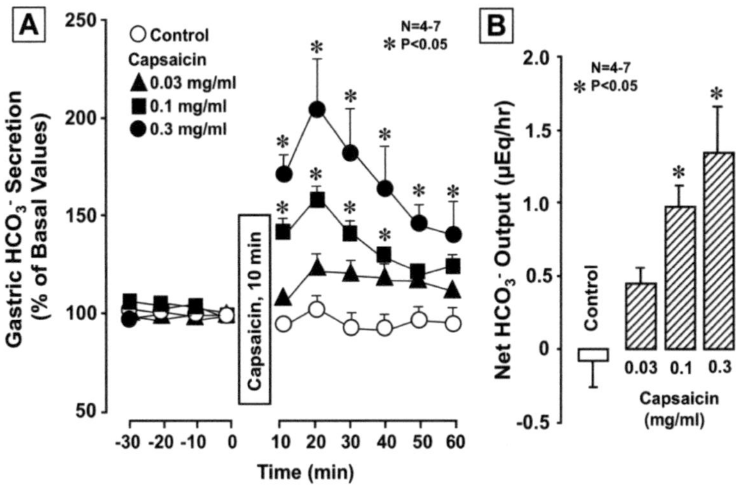

Figure 1. Effects of capsaicin on gastric HCO_3^- secretion in anesthetized rats. Capsaicin (0.03~0.3 mg/ml) was applied to the chamber for 10 min. In Figure A, data are presented as a % of basal values and represent the mean±SE of values determined every 10 minutes from 4~7 rats. Figure B shows the total net HCO_3^- output for 1 hr after the capsaicin treatment, and data are presented as the mean±SE for 4~7 rats. *Significantly different from the control, at P<0.05.

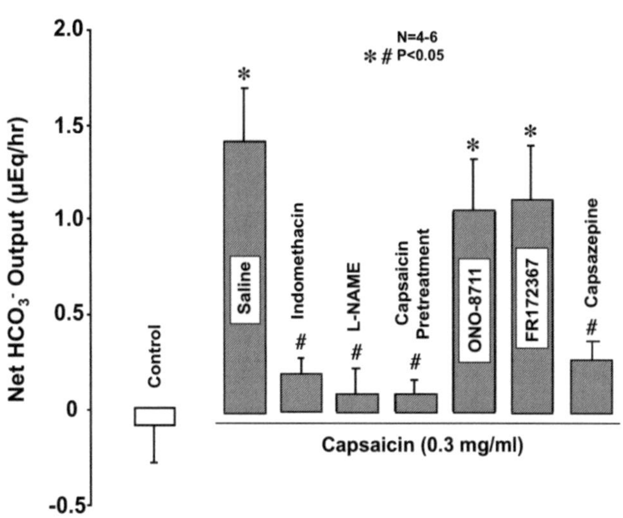

Figure 2. Effects of the pretreatment with various agents and capsaicin on gastric HCO_3^- secretion induced by capsaicin in anesthetized rats. Capsaicin (0.3 mg/ml) was applied to the chamber for 10 min. Indomethacin (5 mg/kg), ONO-8711 (10 mg/kg), or L-NAME (10 mg/kg) was administered s.c. 1 or 3 hr before capsaicin, respectively. FR172357 (1 mg/kg) was administered i.v. 15 min before the mucosal application of capsaicin. Capsazepine (2.5 mg/ml) was applied to the chamber for 20 min, starting 10 min before the capsaicin treatment. The chemical ablation of sensory neurons (capsaicin pretreatment) was achieved with 3 consecutive s.c. injections of capsaicin (total dose: 100 mg/kg) 2 weeks before the experiment. The figure shows the total net HCO_3^- output for 1 hr after the capsaicin treatment, and data are presented as the mean±SE from 4~6 rats. Significantly different at P<0.05; *from the control; # from saline.

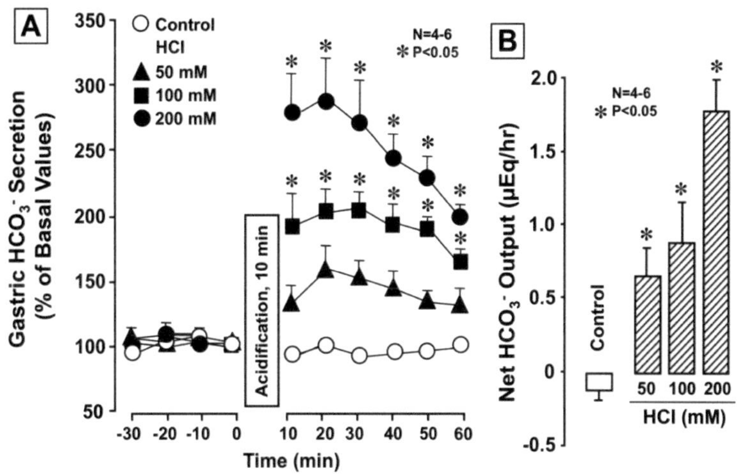

Figure 3. Effects of mucosal acidification on gastric HCO_3^- secretion in anesthetized rats. Acidification was achieved by exposing the mucosa to 50~200 mM HCl for 10 min. In Figure A, data are presented as a % of basal values and represent the mean±SE of values determined every 10 minutes from 4~6 rats. Figure B shows the total net HCO_3^- output for 1 hr after acidification, and data are presented as the mean±SE for 4~6 rats. *Significantly different from the control, at P<0.05.

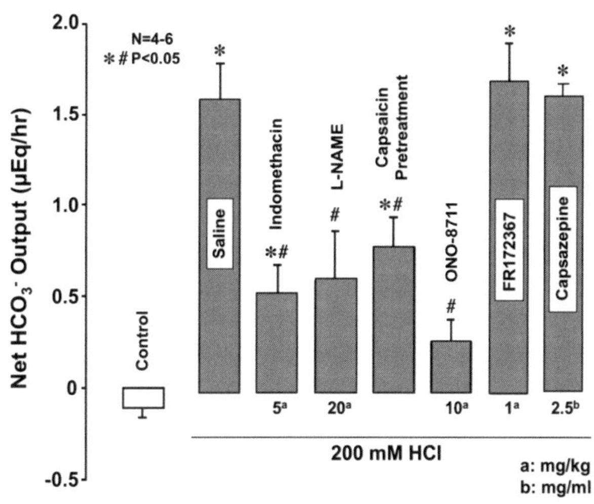

Figure 4. Effects of the pretreatment with various agents and capsaicin on gastric HCO_3^- secretion induced by mucosal acidification in anesthetized rats. Acidification was achieved by exposing the mucosa to 200 mM HCl for 10 min. Indomethacin (5 mg/kg), ONO-8711 (10 mg/kg), or L-NAME (10 mg/kg) was administered s.c. 1 or 3 hr before acidification, respectively. FR172357 (1 mg/kg) was administered i.v. 15 min before mucosal acidification. Capsazepine (2.5 mg/ml) was applied to the chamber for 20 min, starting 10 min before the capsaicin treatment. The chemical ablation of afferent neurons (capsaicin pretreatment) was achieved with 3 consecutive s.c. injections of capsaicin (total dose: 100 mg/kg) 2 weeks before the experiment. The figure shows the total net HCO_3^- output for 1 hr after the capsaicin treatment, and data are presented as the mean±SE for 4~6 rats. Significantly different at P<0.05; *from the control; # from saline.

3.2. Effect of capsaicin and mucosal acidification on PGE_2 and 6-keto PGF_1 α levels in the rat stomach

The intragastric application of capsaicin (0.3 mg/ml) for 10 min did not affect the amount of PGE_2, but significantly increased that of 6-keto PGF_1 α to approximately 2.8-fold that of the control level (data not shown). In contrast, the acidification of the gastric mucosa significantly stimulated the production of PGs and increased PGE_2 or 6-keto PGF_1 α levels to approximately 2 or 3-fold that of basal levels, respectively.

3.3. Stimulation by PGE_2, NOR-3, and bradykinin of HCO_3^-secretion in the rat stomach

The intravenous administration of PGE_2 (1 mg/kg) increased the secretion of HCO_3^- in the stomach, and this response was equivalent to that induced by capsaicin at 0.3 mg/ml (Figure 5). The NO donor, NOR-3 (3 mg/ml), which was applied topically to the mucosa for 10 min, also increased HCO_3^- secretion. Neither indomethacin, L-NAME, nor FR172357 significantly affected the increase in HCO_3^- secretion in response to PGE_2 (data not shown). Gastric HCO_3^- secretion was also stimulated by the i.v. administration of bradykinin (30 μg/kg), reached a maximal value of 160% that of the basal level; however, this effect was less potent than that of capsaicin or acidification and completely disappeared after 1 hr (Figure 6). The stimulatory effect of bradykinin on HCO_3^- was significantly antagonized by FR172357 and attenuated by the prior administration of indomethacin or L-NAME. In addition, the stimulatory effect of bradykinin was almost completely blocked by the chemical ablation of capsaicin-sensitive afferent neurons, but was not significantly affected by pretreatment with capsazepine.

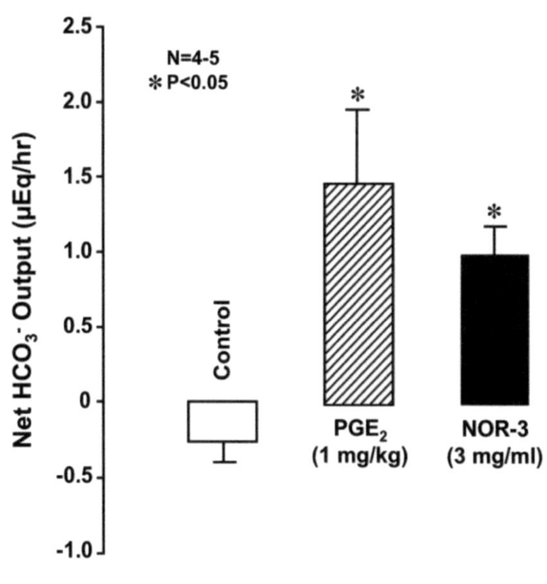

Figure 5. Effects of PGE_2 and NOR-3 on gastric HCO_3^- secretion in anesthetized rats. PGE_2 (1 mg/kg) was administered i.v., while NOR-3 (3 mg/ml) was applied to the chamber for 10 min. Data represent the total net HCO_3^- output for 1 hr after the administration of PGE_2 or NOR-3 and are presented as the mean±SE for 4-5 rats. *Significantly different from the control, at $P<0.05$.

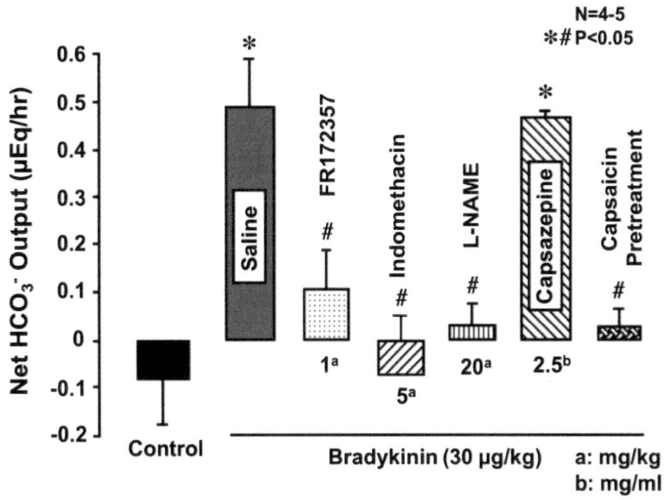

Figure 6. Effects of bradykinin on gastric HCO_3^- secretion in anesthetized rats. Bradykinin (30 μg/kg) was administered i.v. after basal HCO_3^- secretion had been stabilized. Indomethacin (5 mg/kg) was administered s.c. 1 hr before bradykinin, while FR172357 (1 mg/kg) was given i.v. 15 min before. L-NAME (20 mg/kg) was administered s.c. 3 hr before bradykinin. Capsazepine (2.5 mg/ml) was applied for 20 min to the chamber 10 min before the administration of bradykinin. The chemical ablation of sensory neurons (capsaicin pretreatment) was achieved with 3 consecutive s.c. injections of capsaicin (total dose: 100 mg/kg) 2 weeks before the experiment. Data show the total net HCO_3^- output for 1 hr after the capsaicin treatment and are presented as the mean±SE for 4~5 rats. Significantly different at $P<0.05$; *from the control; # from bradykinin+saline.

3.4. Effect of capsaicin on HCO_3^- secretion in wild-type and IP-receptor knockout mice

We previously demonstrated the importance of PGI_2/IP receptors in the HCO_3^- stimulatory action of capsaicin in the duodenum [16]. Since capsaicin also stimulated HCO_3^- secretion in the stomach, in an indomethacin-inhibitable manner, we attempted to identify the type of prostanoid receptor involved in capsaicin-induced responses in the stomach using EP1-, EP3-, and IP-receptor knockout mice, in comparison with those induced by mucosal acidification.

The mouse stomach spontaneously secreted HCO_3^- at a rate of 0.1-0.3 μEq/10 min. Capsaicin (0.3 mg/ml), which was applied to the chamber for 10 min, increased the gastric secretion of HCO_3^- in wild-type mice, and the same effect was also observed in EP1-or EP3-receptor knockout mice, but was absent in mice lacking IP receptors (Figure 7). HCO_3^- secretion was also increased in wild-type mice following the exposure of the mucosa to 50 mM HCl for 10 min, and the same response was also observed in EP3 and IP, but not EP1 receptor knockout animals (Figure 8). The response induced by either capsaicin or acidification in wild-type animals was significantly attenuated by the pretreatment with indomethacin.

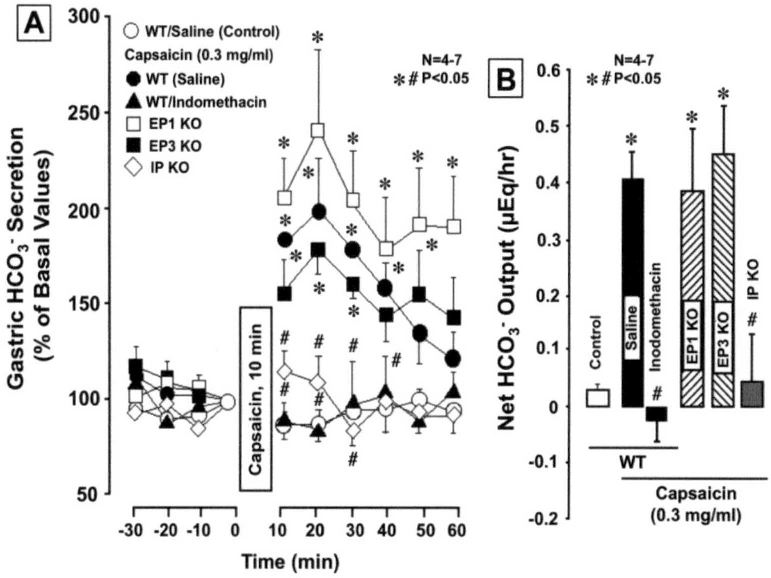

Figure 7. Effects of capsaicin on gastric HCO_3^- secretion in wild-type, and EP1-, EP3-, and IP-receptor knockout mice under urethane anesthesia. Capsaicin (0.3 mg/ml) was applied to the chamber for 10 min. In some wild-type mice, indomethacin (5 mg/kg) was given s.c. 1 hr before the capsaicin treatment. In Figure A, data are presented as a % of basal values and represent the mean±SE of values determined every 10 minutes from 4~7 rats. Figure B shows the total net HCO_3^- output for 1 hr after the capsaicin treatment, and data are presented as the mean±SE for 4~7 rats. Significantly different at $P<0.05$; *from control wild-type mice; # from wild-type mice treated with capsaicin+saline.

4. Commentary

The gastroduodenal mucosa responds to acidification by significantly increasing the secretion of HCO_3^-, which, in collaboration with mucus, contributes to the mucosal tolerance of luminal acid [1]. We previously reported that the intraluminal application of capsaicin stimulated the secretion of HCO_3^- in these tissues by activating capsaicin-sensitive afferent neurons [4, 5, 15, 16]. The present study confirmed that both acid and capsaicin increased HCO_3^- secretion in the stomach, which was mediated by these afferent neurons, and clearly showed the difference in their modes of action in terms of sensitivity to TRPV1 and prostanoid receptors. Furthermore, we observed the involvement of endogenous PGs and NO in the stimulatory action of capsaicin in the stomach, which was consistent with previous findings in the duodenum [21].

TRPV1 is a nonselective cation channel that responds to protons as well as capsaicin [6]. The binding sites of capsaicin are located on the intracellular site of the receptor protein [24], whereas the target of protons is thought to be located on the extracellular surface of the receptor protein [25]. When the TRPV1 antagonist, capsazepine was applied to the mucosa together with capsaicin or acid in the present study, it completely blocked the increase in gastric HCO_3^- secretion induced by capsaicin, but not acid, in spite of both responses being mediated

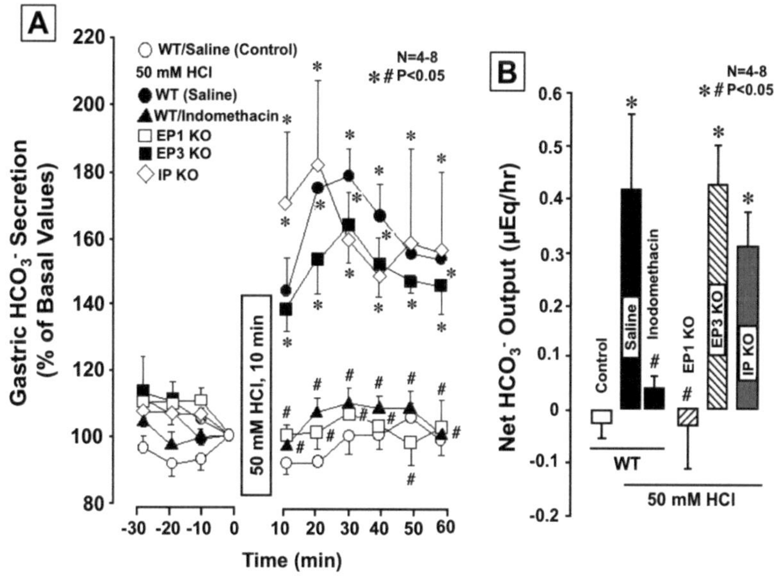

Figure 8. Effects of mucosal acidification on gastric HCO_3^- secretion in wild-type, and EP1-, EP3-, and IP-receptor knockout mice under urethane anesthesia. Acidification was achieved by exposing the mucosa to 50 mM HCl for 10 min. In some wild-type mice, indomethacin (5 mg/kg) was administered s.c. 1 hr before the capsaicin treatment. In Figure A, data are presented as a % of basal values and represent the mean±SE of values determined every 10 minutes from 4~8 rats. Figure B shows the total net HCO_3^- output for 1 hr after the capsaicin treatment, and data are presented as the mean±SE for 4~8 rats. Significantly different at P<0.05; * from control wild-type mice; # from wild-type mice treated with 50 mM HCl+saline.

by capsaicin-sensitive afferent neurons. These results are consistent with our previous findings in the duodenum, in which capsazepine significantly mitigated the response induced by capsaicin, but not mucosal acidification [13]. Akiba et al [26] reported that acid in the lumen induced a mucosal hyperemic response in the rat duodenum in a capsazepine-sensitive manner, and suggested that luminal acid may be an endogenous ligand for duodenal TRPV1. McIntyre et al [27] described pharmacological differences between the human and rat TRPV1 and demonstrated that capsazepine blocked the response of human, but not rat TRPV1 to low pH. The reason for these different results between studies currently remains unclear. The results of the present study do not exclude the involvement of TRPV1 in the acid-induced secretion of HCO_3^-; however, the target site of acid may differ from that of capsaicin, ie., the binding site inhibitable by capsazepine. Alternatively, acid may activate these afferent neurons through acid-sensing ionic channels (ASICs). This proposal has been supported by the recent findings in which the acid-induced duodenal HCO_3^- response was greater in female than male rats, with the different responses being parallel with the intensity of the expression of ASIC3, and ovariectomy suppressed the expression of ASIC3 in the duodenum and abolished such a gender difference in the HCO_3^- response [28].

Endogenous PGs are known to be particularly important in the local regulation of HCO_3^- secretion in the gastroduodenal mucosa. We previously demonstrated, using subtype-specific EP agonists and antagonists, that PGE_2 stimulated the secretion of HCO_3^- in the duodenum through EP3/EP4 receptors and in the stomach through EP1 receptors [15, 16, 29]. Many previous studies reported that mucosal acidification increased HCO_3^- secretion in these tissues, with a concomitant rise in mucosal PGE_2 levels [12, 13, 16]. Capsaicin also stimulated the secretion of HCO_3^- in the stomach in an indomethacin-inhibitable manner, which suggested the involvement of endogenous PGs. However, capsaicin was shown to increase PGE_2 production in the duodenum, but not in the stomach [13, 30]. Notwithstanding, this agent exhibited various effects in the stomach, such as mucosal protection and hyperemia, mediated by capsaicin-sensitive afferent neurons that also depended on endogenous PGs [4, 5, 31]. We confirmed that the intragastric application of capsaicin significantly enhanced the levels of 6-keto $PGF_1\alpha$, the PGI_2 metabolite, which was consistent with the findings reported in the mouse stomach [21, 31]. We previously demonstrated that the gastroprotective effects of capsaicin against HCl/ethanol were significantly attenuated by indomethacin in wild-type mice, but were completely absent in animals lacking IP receptors [30]. In the present study, capsaicin increased gastric HCO_3^- secretion in EP1-and EP3-receptor knockout mice, similar to wild-type mice, but did not in animals lacking IP receptors. These results strongly suggest that endogenous PGI_2 plays a supportive role in the action of capsaicin in the stomach, possibly by sensitizing sensory neurons through IP receptors.

However, HCO_3^- secretion induced by acidification remained unchanged in IP receptor knockout mice and was absent in animals lacking EP1 receptors. These results further support the response of HCO_3^- induced in the stomach by acidification and capsaicin, but depending on sensory neurons, being mediated by different mechanisms related to PG dependency; the former is mainly mediated by PGE_2 through EP1 receptors, while the latter depends on PGI_2/IP receptors. Similar results were obtained for the gastric hyperemic response induced by acid or capsaicin [31]. Although gastric hyperemic responses to these treatments were mitigated by the capsaicin pretreatment [2, 32], the response induced by acid required the presence of EP1 receptors [33], while that evoked by capsaicin required the presence of IP receptors [29]. Thus, it is not unreasonable to assume that the presence of different prostanoid receptors may be required for gastric HCO_3^- secretion in response to acid or capsaicin.

We found that capsaicin had no effect on the production of PGE_2, but significantly increased that of PGI_2 in the stomach. Capsaicin-sensitive afferent neurons are known to be abundantly at peri-vascular sites, and the stimulation by capsaicin releases CGRP/NO, resulting in an increase in mucosal blood flow [2]. Harada et al. [34] reported that the activation of these afferent neurons ameliorated ischemia/reperfusion-induced liver injury by limiting the inflammatory response through an enhancement in endothelial PGI_2 production, and suggested that the CGRP-induced activation of both endothelial NO synthase and cyclooxygenase-1 may be involved in this mechanism. Thus, it is possible that capsaicin increases endothelial PGI_2 production locally in the stomach when applied topically to the mucosa. The reason why capsaicin had different effects on the production of PGE_2 and PGI_2 in the stomach currently remains unknown.

The present study also showed that capsaicin-induced HCO_3^- secretion in the stomach was significantly attenuated by L-NAME, which suggesed the involvement of endogenous NO in this process, in addition to PGs. Several studies showed that CGRP, the dominant neurotransmitter of spinal afferents, had various pharmacological actions, such as vasodilation, that were mediated by endogenous NO [2, 3, 35]. We demonstrated that the NO donor, NOR-3 stimulated gastric HCO_3^- secretion in the present study, and this was consistent with our previous findings in the duodenum [12]. Nishihara et al [36] reported that capsaicin increased the release of CGRP and NO in the rat stomach. Although we did not measure NO release in the stomach following the capsaicin treatment, it is assumed that capsaicin activated primary afferent neurons, with the assistance of PGI_2, to liberate CGRP, which in turn stimulated NO release, resulting in an increase in gastric HCO_3^- secretion.

Bradykinin is also known to activate nociceptive-like afferent neurons through metabotropic G protein-coupled bradykinin B2 receptors [37, 38]. A previous study showed that binding to B2 receptors activated an intracellular signaling cascade, which led to the opening of TRPV1 channels [39]. We found that bradykinin itself stimulated the secretion of HCO_3^- in the stomach in the present study. Furthermore, this response was attenuated not only by FR172357, the B2 antagonist, but also by indomethacin and L-NAME, which suggested the involvement of both PGs and NO in the response of HCO_3^- to bradykinin. The stimulatory effect of bradykinin was also significantly mitigated by the chemical ablation of capsaicin-sensitive afferent neurons, but was not affected by capsazepine, a TRPV1 antagonist. The stimulatory effect of bradykinin on HCO_3^- secretion is assumed to be partly mediated by sensory neurons via B2 receptors, but not through the interaction with TRPV1, in addition to endogenous PGs. Since bradykinin also potentiates the activation of TRPV1 by capsaicin through the hydrolysis of endogenous posphatidylinositol-4, 5-bisphosphate in a phospholipase C-dependent manner [39, 40], it is possible that capsaicin-induced gastric HCO_3^- secretion may be affected by the B2 receptor antagonist. However, the present study showed that the responses induced by capsaicin and acidification were not significantly affected by FR172357, which suggests that endogenous bradykinin has no role in these responses. The reason for these results has yet to be elucidated and is currently under investigation in our laboratory.

5. Summary

Capsaicin is assumed to stimulate the secretion of HCO_3^- in the stomach mediated by endogenous PGs and NO, as well as capsaicin-sensitive afferent neurons, but not bradykinin B2 receptors. Mucosal acidification also increased gastric HCO_3^- secretion through sensory neurons mediated by both PGs and NO, similar to capsaicin; however, their modes of action differed in terms of capsazepine-sensitivity and prostanoid receptor-dependency (Figure 9). Although luminal H^+ played a modulator-type role in the physiological response mediated by capsaicin-sensitive afferent neurons in the stomach, it is likely that this action was not due to the interaction of H^+ with the capsazepine-sensitive site of TRPV1, but resulted from the activation of ASIC3.

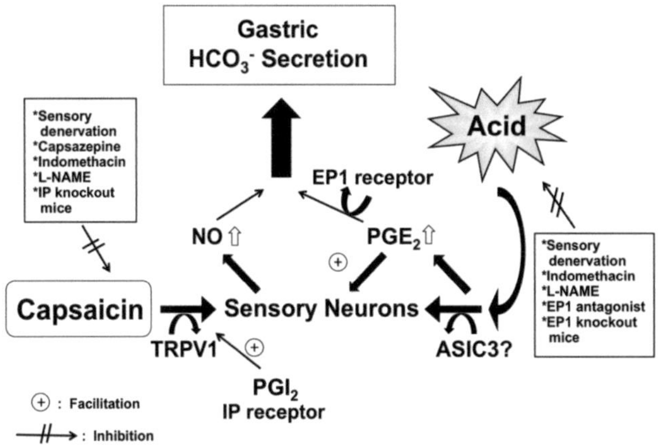

Figure 9. Mechanisms underlying stimulation of gastric HCO_3^- secretion induced by capsaicin and acid. Capsaicin stimulated HCO_3^- secretion in the stomach, essentially through capsaicin-sensitive afferent neurons via the activation of TRPV1, and this action was mediated with endogenous PGE_2/EP1 receptors and NO. Mucosal acidification also increased HCO_3^- secretion through the activation of sensory neurons as well as endogenous PGs and NO; however, this action did not result from an interaction between H^+ and the capsazepine-sensitive site of TRPV1, and depended on the PGI_2/IP receptor.

Acknowledgements

The authors are greatly indebted to Professor Shu Narumiya, Kyoto University Faculty of Medicine, for kindly supplying EP1, EP3, and IP receptor-knockout mice and Ono Pharmaceutical for supplying various EP agonists and antagonists. We also thank the undergraduate students at the Department of Pharmacology and Experimental Therapeutics, Kyoto Pharmaceutical University, Kyoto, Japan, for their technical collaboration.

Author details

Koji Takeuchi[1,2*] and Eitaro Aihara[1]

*Address all correspondence to: takeuchi@mb.kyoto-phu.ac.jp

1 Department of Pharmacology and Experimental Therapeutics, Kyoto Pharmaceutical University, Misasagi, Yamashina, Kyoto, , Japan

2 General Incorporated Association, Kyoto Research Center for Gastrointestinal Diseases, Karasuma-Oike, Kyoto, Japan

The authors declare no conflict of interest.

References

[1] Flemstrom G, Garner A. Gastroduodenal HCO_3^- transport: characteristics and proposed role in acidity regulation and mucosal protection. Am J Physiol 1982; 242: G183-93.

[2] Holzer P. Neural emergency system in the stomach. Gastroenterology 1998; 114: 823-39.

[3] Holzer P, Sametz W. Gastric mucosal protection against ulcerogenic factors in the rat mediated by capsaicin-sensitive afferent neurons. Gastroenterology 1986; 91: 975-87.

[4] Takeuchi K, Matsumoto J, Ueshima K, Okabe S. Role of capsaicin-sensitive afferent neurons in alkaline secretory response to luminal acid in the rat duodenum. Gastroenterology 1991; 101: 954-61.

[5] Takeuchi K, Ueshima K, Matsumoto J and Okabe S. Role of capsaicin-sensitive sensory nerves in acid-induced bicarbonate secretion in rat stomach. Dig Dig Sci 1992; 37: 737-43.

[6] Caterina MJ, Schumacher MA, Tominaga M, Rosen TA Levine JD, Julius D. The capsaicin receptor; a heat-activated ion channel in the pain pathway. Nature 1997; 389: 816-24.

[7] Clapham DE, Runnels LW, Strubing C. The TRP ion channel family. Nat Rev Neurosci 2001; 2: 387-96.

[8] Gunthorpe MJ, Benham CD, Randall A, Davis JB. The diversity in the vanilloid (TRPV) receptor family of ion channels. Trends Pharmacol Sci 2002; 23: 183-91.

[9] Merchant NB, Dempsey DT, Grabowski MW, Rizzo M, Ritchie WP Jr. Capsaicin-induced gastric mucosal hyperemia and protection: The role of calcitonin gene-related peptide. Surgery 1994; 116: 419-25.

[10] Ferreira J, Silva GL, Calixto JB. Contribution of vanilloid receptors to the overt nociception induced by B2 kinin receptor activation in mice. Br J Pharmacol 2004; 141: 787-94.

[11] Shin J, Cho H, Hwang SW, Jung J, Shin CY, Lee SY, Kim SH, Lee MG, Choi YH, Kim J, Haber NA, Reichling DB, Khasar S, Levine JD, Oh U. Bradykinin-12-lipoxygenase-VR1 signaling pathway for inflammatory hyperalgesia. PNAS 2002; 99: 10150-5.

[12] Sugamoto S, Kawauchi S, Furukawa O, Takeuchi K. Interactive roles of endogenous nitric oxide and prostaglandins in acid-induced bicarbonate response in rat duodenums. Dig Dis Sci 2001; 46: 1208-16.

[13] Kagawa S, Aoi M, Kubo Y, Kotani T, Takeuchi K. Stimulation by capsaicin of duodenal HCO_3^- secretion via afferent neurons and vanilloid receptors in rats. Comparison with acid-induced HCO_3^- response. Dig Dis Sci 2003; 48: 1850-6.

[14] Takeuchi K, Yagi K, Kato S, Ukawa H. Roles of prostaglandin E-receptor subtypes in gastric and duodenal bicarbonate secretion. Gastroenterology 1997; 113: 1553-9.

[15] Aoi M, Aihara E, Nakashima M, Takeuchi K. Participation of prostaglandin receptor EP4 subtype in duodenal bicarbonate secretion in rats. Am J Physiol 2004; 287: G96-103.

[16] Nakashima M, Aoi M, Aihara E, Takeuchi K. No role for prostacyclin IP receptors in duodenal HCO_3^- secretion induced by mucosal acidification in mice: Comparison with capsaicin-induced response. Digestion 2004; 70:16-25.

[17] Oida H, Namba T, Sugimoto Y, Ushikubi F, Ohishi H, Ichikawa A, Narumiya S. In situ hybridization studied of prostacyclin receptor mRNA expression in various mouse organs. Br J Pharmacol 1995; 116: 2828-37.

[18] Ushikubi F, Segi E, Sugimoto Y, Murata T, Matsuoka T, Kobayashi T, Hizaki H, Tuboi K, Katsuyama M, Ichikawa A, Tanaka T, Yoshida N, Narumiya S. Impaired febrile response in mice lacking the prostaglandin E receptor subtype 3. Nature 1998; 395: 281-4

[19] Asano M, Hatori C, Inamura N, Sawai H, Hirosumi J, Fujiwara T, Nakahara K. Effects of a nonpeptide bradykinin B2 receptor antagonist, FR167344, on different invivo animal models of inflammation. Br J Pharmacol 1997; 122: 1436-40.

[20] Takeuchi K, Ohuchi T, Miyake H, Okabe S. Stimulation by nitric oxide synthase inhibitors of gastric and duodenal HCO_3^- secretion in rats. J Pharmacol Exp Ther 1993; 266: 1512-9.

[21] Aihara E, Kagawa S, Hayashi M, Takeuchi K. ACE inhibitor and ATI antagonist stimulate duodenal HCO_3^- secretion mediated by a common pathway: Involvement of PG, NO and bradykinin. J Physiol Pharmacol 2005; 56: 391-406.

[22] Aihara E, Hayashi M, Yoshii K, Kobata A, Sasaki Y, Takeuchi K. Mechanisms involved in capsaicin-stimulated gastric HCO_3^- secretion: Comparison with mucosal acidification. J Pharmacol Exp Ther 315: 423-32, 2005

[23] Futaki N, Takahashi S, Yokoyama M, Arai I, Higuchi S, Otomo S. NS-938, a new antiinflammatory agent, selectively inhibits prostaglandin G/H synthase/cyclo-oxygenase (COX-2) activity in vitro. Prostaglandins 1994; 47: 55-9.

[24] Jordt SE, Tominaga M, Julius D. Acid potentiation of the capsaicin receptor determined by a key extracellular site. Proc Natl Acad Sci USA 2000; 97: 8134-9.

[25] Jung J, Hwang SW, Kwak J, Lee SY, Kang CJ, Kim WB, Kim D, Oh U. Capsaicin binds to the intracellular domain of the capsaicin-activated ion channel. J Neurosci 1999; 19: 529-38.

[26] Akiba Y, Guth PH, Engel E, Nastaskin I, Kaunitz JD. Acid-sensing pathways of rat duodenum. Am J Physiol 1999; 277: G268-74.

[27] McIntyre P, McLatchie LM, Chambers A, Phillips E, Clarke M, Savidge J, Toms C, Peacock M, Shah K, Winter J, Weerasakera N, Webb M, Rang HP, Bevan S, Fames IF. Pharmacological differences between the human and rat vanilloid receptor 1 (VR1). Br J Pharmacol 2001; 32: 1084-94.

[28] Takeuchi K, Ohashi Y, Kohmoto M, Oka H, Nomura Y, Aihara E. Gender difference in duodenal HCO_3^- response to mucosal acidification: Importance of up-regulation of ASIC3 by estradiol. Gastroenterology 2012; 142 (Supplement 1): S-202-S-203.

[29] Takeuchi K, Ukawa H, Araki H, Furukawa O, Kato S, Sugimoto Y, Ushikubi F, Ichikawa A, Narumiya S. Impaired duodenal bicarbonate secretion integrity in mice lacking prostaglandin E receptor subtype EP3. Gastroenterology 1999; 117: 1128-35.

[30] Takeuchi K, Kato S, Takeeda M, Ogawa Y, Nakashima M, Matsumoto M. Facilitation by endogenous prostaglandins of capsaicin-induced gastric protection in rodents through EP2 and IP receptors. J Pharmacol Exp Ther 2003; 304: 1055-62.

[31] Boku K, Ohno T, Saeki T, Hayashi I, Katori M, Murata T, Narumiya S, Saigenji K, Majima M. Adaptive cytoprotection mediated by prostaglandin I_2 is attributable to sensitization of CGRP-containing sensory nerves. Gastroenterology 2001; 120: 134-43.

[32] Mimaki H, Kagawa S, Aoi M, Kato S, Tsutumi S, Kohama K, Takeuchi. Effect of lafutidine, a histamine H_2-receptor antagonist, on gastric mucosal blood 4flow and duodenal HCO_3^- secretion in rats: Relation to capsaicin-sensitive afferent neurons. Dig Dis Sci 2002; 47: 2696-703.

[33] Takeuchi K, Komoike Y, Takeeda M, Ukawa H. Gastric mucosal ulcerogenic responses following barrier disruption in knockout mice lacking prostaglandin EP1 receptors. Aliment Pharmacol Ther 2002; 16: 74-82.

[34] Harada N, Okajima K, Uchiba M, Katsuragi T. Ischemia/reperfusion-induced increase in the hepatic level of prostacyclin is mainly mediated by activation of capsaicin-sensitive sensory neurons in rats. J Lab Clin Med 2002; 139: 218-26.

[35] Lambrecht N, Burchert M, Respondek M, Muller KM, Peskar BM. Role of calcitonin gene-related peptide and nitric oxide in the gastroprotective effect of capsaicin in the rat. Gastroenterology 1993; 104: 1371-80.

[36] Nishihara K, Nozawa Y, Nakano M, Ajioka H, Matsuura N. Sensitizing effects of lafutidine on CGRP-containing afferent nerves in the rat stomach. Br J Pharmacol 2002; 135: 1487-94.

[37] McGuirk SM, Dolphin AC. G-protein mediation in nociceptive signal transduction: an investigation into the excitatory action of bradykinin in a subpopulation of cultured rat sensory neurons. Neuroscience 1992; 49: 117-28.

[38] Maubach KA, Grundy D. The role of prostaglandins in the bradykinin-induced activation of serosal afferents of the rat jejunum in vitro. J Physiol 1999; 515: 277-85.

[39] Chuang HH, Prescott ED, Kong H, Shields S, Jordt SE, Basbaum AI, Chao MV, Julius D. Bradykinin and nerve growth factor release the capsaicin receptor from PtdIns (4, 5) P2-mediated inhibition. Nature 2001; 411: 957-62.

[40] Premkumar LS, Ahern GP. Induction of vanilloid receptor channel activity by protein kinase C. Nature 2000; 408: 985-90.

Chapter 7

The Role of Capsaicin-Sensitive Afferent Nerves in Gastric Mucosal Protection Initiated Centrally or Peripherally under Experimental Conditions

K. Gyires

Additional information is available at the end of the chapter

http://dx.doi.org/10.5772/58573

1. Introduction

How can gastric mucosa resist to wide variety of endogenous (e.g. acid, pepsin, H. pylori) and exogenous (bacterial products, NSAIDs, alcohol, cytotoxic agents) mucosal challenges? Or how can it be explained that while the incidence of mucosal injury related to acid secretion is about 20% of the population, everybody secretes acid throughout the life [1]? And how can be answered the classic question of Davenport: why the stomach does not digest itself [2]?

Though accumulating data strongly suggest an apparent redundancy in the processes of gastric mucosal defense, several mediators, mechanisms, structural elements involved in mucosal protection have been identified, the precious mechanism has not been completely clarified yet and incompletely understood.

The aim of present work is to give a short overview on the protective mechanism of gastric mucosal protection, particularly on capsaicin sensitive afferent pathways and mediators released from sensory nerve endings and play a role in maintaining gastric mucosal integrity.

2. Gastric mucosal defense: mechanisms, mediators

Gastric mucosal defense to acid and other noxious stimulus involves both structural and functional components. Gastric mucosal barrier consists of the pre-epithelial mucus bicarbonate layer, an epithelial layer, and a post-epithelial layer. The pre-epithelial mucus bicarbonate layer consist of mucus gel, bicarbonat surfactant phospholipids, treofil peptides. Epithelial layer, and a post-epithelial layer involve blood vessels, non-epithelial cells and enteric nerves play a role in generation of different substances which are essential in maintaining mucosal integrity and gastric mucosal defense, e.g. bicarbonate, mucus, phospholipids, trefoil peptides, prostaglandins (PGs), heat shock proteins [reviews 3-5].

2.1. Mucosal barrier

The pre-epitehlieal layer protects the gastric mucosa from microscopic damage. This layer consists of mucus gel, bicarbonate and surfactant phospholipids, which cover the mucosal surface. It retains bicarbonate secreted by surface epithelial cells to maintain a neutral micro-environment [5-7].

Trefoil factor family (TFF) proteins are able to enhance mucosal barrier functions by stabilizing the mucus gel and promoting epithelial restitution [8, 9]. These small protease-resistant proteins have been demonstrated to be protective demonstrated in various ulcer models [10, 11], the exact molecular mechanism has not been clarified yet.

2.2. Prostaglandin

Though the term „cytoprotection" has been used first by Chaudhury and Jacobson [12] the classic definition of cytoprotection derives from Robert et al [13]; they suggested that cyto-protection refers to protection of gastric mucosa against chemically/ physically-induced acute gastric ulceration in doses much smaller than that reduce gastric acid secretion. According to their results prostaglandins fulfilled this criteria. Later Lacy and Ito [14] reported that the superficial layer, that is supposed to be highly involved in maintenance of mucosal barrier, is not preserved during prostaglandin-induced protective processes; this was the main argue against the term "cytoprotection".

Prostaglandins are synthesized from arachidonic acid by all nucleated cells, but the highest concentrations are found in gastrointestinal mucosa. Continuous synthesis of prostaglandins by gastrointestinal mucosa most likely represents a physiological process necessary to maintain cellular integrity and for this process prostaglandins serve as trophic factors [15, 16]. Subsequent studies proved that the maintenance of gastric mucosal blood flow and thus the prevention of ischemia are the key elements in the mucosal protective effect of prostaglandins [17]. Takeuchi et al. [18] suggested recently, that endogenous PGs also contribute to maintain-ing mucosal integrity after barrier disruption through an increase in mucosal blood flow, which occurs via sensory neurons by activation of the EP_1 receptor.

Inhibition of leukocyte adherence to the vascular endothelium and inhibition of apoptosis are additional actions that can result in prevention of gastric mucosal damage [19].

Different prostaglandin receptors are involved in different processes resulting in mucosal defense. The effects of PGE_2 on various gastric functions are mediated by different EP receptor subtypes; such as inhibition of acid secretion (EP_3) and motility (EP_1), stimulation of mucus secretion (EP_4) and $HCO3^-$secretion (EP_1), and an increase in mucosal blood flow (EP_2/EP_4). However, the presence of EP_1 receptors is essential to the protective action of PGE_2 [20].

http://dx.doi.org/10.5772/58573

2.3. Nitric oxide

Nitric oxide (NO) is a freely diffusible molecule, synthetized from L-arginine by the enzyme NO synthase, exerts its biological action on vascular smooth muscle by stimulating soluble guanylate-cyclase and the subsequent formation of cyclic guanosine-monophosphate, which results in vasodilation.

NO has been shown to participate in the regulation of gastric mucosal microcirculation both under resting and stimulated conditions, since inhibition of NO synthase significantly reduced both the resting and the gastric acid-induced increased gastric mucosal blood flow [21, 22]. In addition, inhibition of NO synthase increases gastric mucosal injury [23, 24], and the constitutive isoform of NO synthase is important in maintaining gastric mucosal integrity [25].

NO mediates the mucosal vasodilatation and gastroprotective effect of calcitonin gene-related peptide (CGRP), which is released from nerve terminals of primary sensory neurons and plays a crucial role in gastric emergency system [26-28].

2.4. Protein and non-protein sulfhydryls

Protein and non-protein sulfhydryls were suggested also as endogenous protective compounds [29, 30], and it was raised that the maintenance of a critical level of non-protein sulfhydryls in the gastric mucosa is important for the gastroprotective action - besides nitric oxide [31].

2.5. Hydrogen sulfid

H_2S like NO, is an important gaseous mediator of gastric mucosal protection [32], and inhibition of endogenous H_2S synthesis increases the susceptibility of the gastric mucosa to the damaging action of non-steroidal anti-inflammatory drugs (NSAIDs) [33]. On the other hand, exogenous H_2S donors can increase the resistance of the gastric mucosa to injury induced by NSAIDs [34].

The gastroprotective effect of H_2S involves several mechanisms, such as maintenance of gastric mucosal blood flow, stimulation of bicarbonate secretion, inhibition of pro-inflammatory cytokine expression/release stimulation of prostaglandin synthesis, reduced leukocyte-endothelial adherence, decreased reactive oxygen metabolite production and enhanced tissue repair [35].

2.6. Matrix metalloproteinases

Matrix metalloproteinases (MMPs) play a role both in the pathogenesis and in healing of peptic ulcers. These endopeptidases degrade extracellular matrix proteins and are essential for extracellular matrix remodeling and wound healing [36]. Experimentally their altered expression have been demonstrated in gastric ulcers induced by NSAIDs (indomethacin, naproxen) or ethanol [37, 38].

3. Activation of gastric mucosal protective processes by noxious stimulus

Noxious stimulus results in both generation of endogenous substance(s) that may counteract or attenuate the mucosal injury, and initiation of further protective mechanisms or formation of additional protective mediators that stimulate repair and restore mucosal integrity.

3.1. Hypoxia-inducible factor-1

Early phase of mucosal lesions is characterized by decrease of mucosal blood flow and the consequent hypoxia. However, activation of hypoxia-inducible factor-1, in response to hypoxia, induces trefoil factor family (TFF) gene expression in rat and human gastric epithelial cells. The consequent production of TFF peptides augment surface mucous barrier functions (see above) and stimulate epithelial restitution by increasing mucosal blood flow, migration of cells and restoration of barrier function [39, 40].

3.2. Antioxidant enzymes

Gastric mucosal injury is characterized by excessive production and/or decreased elimination of reactive oxygen species (ROS), that can induce tissue damage by promoting lipid peroxidation and increasing the production of inflammatory mediators and proinflammatory cytokines. Antioxidant enzymes, such as superoxide dismutase (SOD), catalase or glutathione are able to counteract the oxidative stress, for example, SOD converts superoxide radical anion ($O_2^{\cdot -}$) into less noxious hydrogen peroxide (H_2O_2) [39].

3.3. Heme oxygenase-1

Heme oxygenase-1 (HO-1), the inducible form of heme oxygenase, also exerts cytoprotective effect and its generation may be induced by oxidative stress, inflammatory cytokines or heavy metals [40]. HO-1 catalyzes the oxidative degradation of the pro-oxidant heme to antioxidant and cytoprotective carbon monoxide and biliverdin [41, 42]. The activity of HO-1 is also increased during the healing of gastric ulcers, which indicates its involvement in the mucosal repair processes [43].

3.4. Growth factors

In addition, several genes, encoding peptides, are also upregulated after mucosal damage in the gastrointestinal mucosa and stimulate the repair process. *Epidermal growth factor (EGF)* a potent stimulant of growth and repair when infused systemically. It inhibits gastric acid secretion, and has a cytoprotective effect on the gastrointestinal mucosa. On the other hand, EGF is one of the main peptides secreted by repair lineages of the gastrointestinal tract [44]. *Treofil factor family (TFF)* has both cytoprotective and stimulant effect on repair. Three members (TFF1/pS2, TFF2/SP, and TFF3/ITF) of the family are present in human gastrointestinal mucosa. They are produced rapidly at sites of injury and stimulate the repair process. Exogenous TFF2/SP exerts a cytoprotective action in indomethacin-induced ulcer model in rats [45]. *Transforming growth factor α (TGF-α)* is normally trophic both in vitro in different cell lines and in vivo

http://dx.doi.org/10.5772/58573

in the intestine of rats [46]. TGF-α decreased the gastric damage induced by ethanol or stress [47], and enhanced immunoreactive TGF-α was measured in gastric juice (within 30 minutes) following gastric instillation of hydrochloric acid. *Transforming growth factor β (TGF-ß)* is also involved in mucosal defense, but in contrast to other growth factors, it regulates the epithelial proliferation, it halts the proliferation of epithelial cells once they have left the crypts or glands. In addition, it is also a potent stimulant of cell migration [48-50]). *Hepatocyte growth factor (HGF)* is secreted as inactive precursor and than converted to an active form. HGF receptor was shown to be increased in the gastric mucosa after injury [51]. It was suggested that, the active HGF, produced in the stomach after injury, may stimulate the proliferation of gastric mucosal epithelial cells through increased number of HGF receptor. *Basic fibroblast growth factor (bFGF)* a potent stimulant of angiogenesis, and accelerates the healing of experimental gastric and duodenal ulcers in rats [52, 53]. In ulcerated human gastric mucosa, immunoreactive bFGF is upregulated [54], thought additional data suggest that bFGF mRNA expression is an early event after mucosal injury [55]. *Platelet derived growth factor (PDGF)* also stimulates angiogenesis. It was shown that PDGF (and bFGF) accelerated the healing of cysteamine induced duodenal ulcers in rats by stimulating angiogenesis and granulation tissue formation [56]. Furthermore, in experimental duodenal ulcer and colitis in rats (after a transitory reduction) of the concentrations of bFGF and PDGF increased in the healing phases both experimental lesions [57]. *Vascular endothelial growth factor (VEGF)* has dual role; in acute gastric ulcer it induced gastroprotective effect surprisingly by enhancing vascular permeability and the consequent perivascular dilution barrier towards gastric mucosal irritants [58]. On the other hand, in chronic duodenal ulcer VEGF stimulates granulation tissue formation and angiogenesis resulted in ulcer healing. In addition, upregulation of VEGF mRNA expression was observed after ethanol challenge [59].

3.5. Capsaicin-sensitive primary afferent neurons

When the gastric epithelium is exposed to acid back diffusion or any irritant, one of the most rapid and important responses is an increase in mucosal blood flow. The aim of this hyperemic response is to remove, dilute and buffer any back-diffusing injurious agent or acid. This response is mediated by primary sensory afferent neurons, namely if the mucosal barrier is disturbed or disrupted in the presence of luminal acid, the acid reaching the lamina propria stimulates spinal afferents. This stimulation will initiate the efferent-like function of primary afferents resulting in CGRP and NO formation and release that induces a prompt hyperaemia in the gastro-duodenal mucosa and bicarbonate (HCO_3^-) secretion [60-68].

3.5.1. Capsaicin-sensitive primary afferent neurons and transient receptor potential vanilloid-1 (TRVP1) receptors

Afferent neurons have a basic role in regulation of gastrointestinal functions, and also in gastric mucosal defense. Beside intrinsic sensory neurons which have their cell body within the gastrointestinal tract and originate in the myenteric or submucosal plexus, there are two groups of extrinsic sensory neurons: vagal and spinal afferents. 75-90% of the axons in vagus nerve are afferent fibers [69], and 9% of these afferent fibres are the capsaicin-sensitive afferent nerves [70], that originate in the jugular and nodose ganglia and project to medullary brain stem. The spinal afferents have their cell body in dorsal root ganglia and reach the stomach via spinal and splanchnic nerves.

The first evidence that suggested the prominent role of sensory nerves in gastric mucosal resistance was obtained by experiments when ablation of sensory nerve was shown to result in aggravation of mucosal lesions induced by hydrochloric acid, aspirin, indomethacin [review 71]. Moreover, Szolcsányi and Barthó described that stimulation of afferent nerves by capsaicin resulted in mucosal protection against acid induced mucosal injury [63, 71]. The role of sensory nerves in gastric mucosal defense was confirmed by the findings that capsaicin induces gastroprotective action following intragastric administration, both in experimental animals [71, 72] and in humans [73].

The protective action of capsaicin is due to its stimulatory effect on *capsaicin-sensitive* primary afferent neurons, since defunctionalisation of afferent neurons by high parenteral dose of capsaicin [74] abolished the gastroprotective effect of capsaicin [67, 71].

The action of capsaicin is mediated by capsaicin receptor which was cloned and named as transient receptor potential vanilloid-1 (TRVP1) [75], the specific sensor for capsaicin [76-79].

In the gastrointestinal tract, TRPV1 can be identified in intrinsic enteric neurons, extrinsic sensory neurons, epithelial and endocrine cells [80-84].

The acid-evoked hyperemia in the esophageal and duodenal mucosa is inhibited by the TRPV1 antagonist capsazepine or sensory denervation, suggesting that acid activates TRPV1 on sensory nerve fibers [85, 86]. As a result, activation of TRPV1-positive sensory nerve fibers are able to protect the esophageal, gastric and intestinal mucosa from a variety of injurious by stimulating mucosal microcirculation [61].

3.5.2. Peptide mediators of capsaicin sensitive primary afferent neurones

Apart from signaling to the CNS, TRPV1-expressing sensory nerve fibers when activated, peptide transmitters, such as CGRP, somatostatin and the tachykinins substance P (SP) and neurokinin, as well as well as nitrogen oxide (NO) and /or ATP can be released from the peripheral nerve endings of afferents nerves and can influence the gastrointestinal function [61, 87-89]. Peptide mediators of TRPV1-positive afferent neurons may induce wide variety of actions.

CGRP and substance P fibers innervate the mucosal and submucosal microvasculature [78, 90]. CGRP in rat stomach are located exclusively in extrinsic afferent fibers, most if not all, in spinal sensory afferent neurons [91-93]. Others also confirmed that CGRP, substance P, somatostatin were characteristic of *capsaicin-sensitive* DRG neurons [77, 78, 93-95], while CGRP was absent from vagal afferent neurons containing TRPV1 [91]. However, Suzuki et al. [96] demonstrated that the density of CGRP-immunreactive fibers in the mucosa was largely reduced also by vagotomy suggesting CGRP-immunreactive fibers to be of both vagal and spinal origin. The CGRP-and SP-immunreactive fibers were less influenced by vagotomy in the submucosal and muscular layers. Furthermore, major portion of SP-immunreactive fibers in the mucosa is of vagal origin, and in contrast to CGRP, SP-immunreactive fibers are not capsaicin sensitive. In contrast, others showed that capsaicin also induces the release of SP from guinea pig and rat stomach [97]. Sternini et al [93] suggested that while CGRP-containing nerve fibers arise exclusively from extrinsic neurons, SP-containing fibers are of both extrinsic and intrinsic originl.

The gastroprotective effect of both CGRP and capsaicin was blocked by $CGRP_1$ receptor antagonist, CGRP 8-37 [98]. However, not only $CGRP_1$ receptor may mediate gastroprotective effects, since $CGRP_1$ receptor antagonist failed to influence the effect of CGRP against aspirin-induced lesions [99]. CGRP/NO released from the nerve terminal of sensory afferents, induces gastroprotective effect not only by increasing mucosal microcirculation, but also by stimulation of mucin synthesis in the gastric corpus mucosa [100] and by reduction of myoelectrical activity in gastric smooth muscle [101].

On the other hand, TRPV1 activation has been found to exacerbate inflammation and tissue injury [76]. In addition, in the murine gastric mucosa, in ethanol-induced injury TRPV1-mediated release of neuronal substance P and subsequent formation of reactive oxygen species are involved in the development of mucosal damage
[102]. Moreover, colitis induced by dextran sulfate or trinitrobenzene sulfonic acid in rodents was attenuated by TRPV1 antagonist or TRPV1 knockout animals [103, 104]. TRPV1 receptors may also play a proinflammatory role in the ileitis elicited by *C. difficile* toxin A. Formation of endocannabinoids is supposed to be involved in this process, and endocannabinoids stimulate TRPV1, consequently, induce the release of substance P from sensory nerve fibers. Substance P activates enteric neurons and immune cells, which finally results in hypersecretion, inflammation, and mucosal damage [105].

How can CGRP mediate gastric mucosal protection? As mentioned above the gastric mucosa and submucosa are densely innervated by CGRP, which is localized in capsaicin-sensitive afferent fibers. The protective effect of CGRP was lost after blockade of the nitric oxide system, but not the prostaglandin system indicating that the vasodilator and the consequent gastroprotective effect of CGRP is due to NO, but not to PG release [106]. However, the role of prostaglandins in sensory nerve-mediated gastroprotection was suggested by the findings that indomethacin inhibited the mucosal protective effect of capsaicin [107]. Takeuchi et al [108] concluded that capsaicin exhibits gastric cytoprotection, essentially by stimulating sensory neurons, and this action is facilitated by endogenous prostaglandins through EP_2/IP receptors, probably sensitizing the sensory neurons to capsaicin.

Substance P, released also from afferent nerve fibers, do not mediate vasodilation in the rats stomach, neither the NK_1 or NK_2 antagonists influenced capsaicin-induced vasodilatation nor tachykinins dilated the submucosal arteries and increased gastric mucosal blood flow; on the contrary, substance P and neurokinin A induced constriction of submucosal veins [109, 110] and substance P was supposed to be involved in the pathomechanism of ethanol-induced gastric mucosal damage [111, 112]. However, others reported that substance P induce vasodilatation in vivo [113], and the effect could be attenuated by N^G-monomethyl-L-arginine – a

NO synthase inhibitor – suggesting the role of endogenous NO in the vasodilator response of substance P.

3.5.3. Role of capsaicin sensitive afferent nerves in action of peripherally acting gastroprotective agents

Capsaicin sensitive afferent fibers are also involved in the mucosal protective action of several gastroprotective agents. E.g. defunctionalisation of capsaicin-sensitive afferent nerves by pretreatment with a neurotoxic dose of capsaicin aggravates gastric ulcers in rats and antagonised the gastroprotective effect of capsaicin (10 mg/kg p. os) and lafutidine indicating that gastroprotective activity mediated by capsaicin-sensitive afferent nerves [114].

Similarly, the gastroprotective effect of different flavonoids against ethanol-lesions was reduced by a neurotoxic dose of capsaicin, or by pretreatment with NO synthase inhibitor N^{G}-nitro-L arginine, indicating that plant-originated flavonoids-induced gastroprotection probably due to enhancement of the expression of constitutive NO synthase and the release of CGRP from sensory afferent nerves [115].

EGF was shown to exert a protective role against ethanol-induced gastric mucosal injury (10-30 μg, intragastrically), possibly by dilating the gastric mucosal arterioles via capsaicin-sensitive afferent neurons involving CGRP and NO mechanisms. Namely, the protective effect of EGF was significantly inhibited by pretreatment with capsaicin desensitization, human $CGRP_1$ antagonist hCGRP 8-37, or the NO synthesis inhibitor, N^{ω}-nitro-L-arginine methyl ester [116].

Mozsik et al [117] suggested participation of vanilloid/capsaicin receptors, CGRP and substance P in gastric protection of omeprazole and omeprazole-like compounds.

Moreover, accumulating evidence indicates that capsaicin sensitive afferent fibers play a pivotal role not only acutely in gastroprotection, but also in ulcer healing. In chronic ulcer model, the acetic acid-induced model neurotoxic dose of capsaicin (100 mg/kg s.c.) significantly increased ulcer size, decreased gastric mucosal cell proliferation at the ulcer margin, angiogenesis in the granulation tissue and also gastric mucus content. In addition, the dramatic increase in elevation of EGF levels in salivary glands and serum was completely abolished by neurotoxic dose of capsaicin. The results suggest that capsaicin sensitive nerves contribute to gastroprotective and ulcer healing processes in the stomach probably by stimulation of EGF expression in salivary glands [118].

3.5.4. Role of capsaicin sensitive afferent fibers and in the action of centrally acting gastroprotective agents

Besides the periphery, gastric mucosal integrity can be regulated also by central mechanism. In the last decades increasing number of evidence suggested that central nervous system (CNS) has a pivotal role in regulation of gastric mucosal integrity. Different brain areas have been suggested to be involved in centrally induced gastroprotection. Among them, hypothalamus and dorsal vagal complex (DVC) seem to have a particularly important role and well defined interconnections between neuroendocrine hypothalamus and the central autonomic system have been described. Descending hypothalamic efferents carry feedback signals to viscerosensory and brainstem catecholaminergic neurons and regulatory inputs to parasympathetic (dorsal vagal nucleus) and sympathetic (thoracolumbar intermediolateral cell column) preganglionic neurons. These fibers arise mainly from neurons of the paraventricular, arcuate, perifornical, and dorsomedial nuclei and the lateral hypothalamus. Pathways between the hypothalamus and autonomic centers are bidirectional; the descending axons are mainly peptidergic (corticotropin-releasing hormone, vasopressin, oxytocin, somatostatin, enkephalin, pro-opiomelanocortin), while the ascending fibers are both peptidergic (enkephalin, neuropeptide Y, neurotensin, dynorphins) and catecholaminergic [119].

The first pharmacological evidence that neuropeptides by central mechanism are able to influence gastric mucosal lesions was provided by the experiments with bombesin. Bombesin, 14-amino acid peptide, inhibited the gastric lesions induced by cold-restraint stress, aspirin, indomethacin by intracisternal (i.c.) and/or intracerebroventricular (i.c.v.) injection [120, 121]. Several mechanism may be involved in the centrally induced mucosal protective effect of bombesin, such as the antisecretory effect [122], inhibition of gastric motor activity, and stimulation of protective processes (gastric mucus, bicarbonate secretion, gastric blood flow) [123].

In addition, neurotensin, β-endorphin, substance P, and somatostatin proved to be also protective given i.c. against cold restraint ulcer model. [124].

Cold restraint stress ulcer model is an acid dependent ulcer model [125]. As a next step, an acid independent model, the ethanol-induced ulcer model has been used to examine the gastroprotective effect of centally injected neuropeptides, where inhibiton of acid secretion is not likely to contribute to the gastric mucosal protective action. Several neuropeptides were injected either into dorsal motor nucleus of vagus (DMNV), i.c. or i.c.v. First, the effect of thyreotropin-releasing hormon (TRH) or its stable analogue RX-77368, injected in low (0-5-1.5 ng), non-secretory dose into the cisterna magna or DMNV was shown to protect the gastric mucosa against ethanol injury [126, 127].

Hereafter, additional neuropeptides proved to be gastroprotective given centrally, among others adrenomedullin [128] peptide YY [129] amylin [130], leptin, cholecystokinin [131], ghrelin [132], opioids, e.g. β-endorphin, deltorphin II, endomorphins [4, 133] nociceptin, nocistatin [134], TLQP-21, a VGF-derived peptide [135], substance P [136] and angiotensin II [137] (see reviews: [4, 127, 138]).

How can the centrally injected neuropeptide induce gastric mucosal protection in the periphery, in gastric mucosa? Convincing evidence suggest the role of vagal nerve in conveying the central stimulus to the periphery. TRH or its stable analogue RX-77368, injected in non-secretory dose into the cisterna magna or DMNV was the first peptide reported to protect the gastric mucosa against ethanol injury through stimulation of vagal cholinergic pathways, since both vagotomy and atropine reversed the gastroprotective effect. As a result of an intensive research additional neuropeptides e.g. amylin, adrenomedullin, neurotensin, opioid peptides, melatonin, ghrelin, leptin, as well as cannabinoids were shown to initiate gastroprotective effect given centrally (i.c.v., i.c. or DMNV), mostly by a vagal dependent mechanism [139-142] (see reviews: [4,127,138,143, 144]).

The mechanism of vagally mediated gastroprotective effect has been well documented by pharmacological studies, demonstrating that activation of vagal cholinergic pathways stimulates gastric prostaglandin and nitric oxide release and the effector function of capsaicin-sensitive afferent fibers containing CGRP [72, 126, 128,129, 145-147, reviews, 4, 127, 143, 144].

In addition, TRH injected intracisternally at low, gastroprotective dose, stimulates gastric splanchnic afferents as was shown by electrophysiological recording [148] and consequently the local effector function of capsaicin-sensitive splanchnic afferent nerves containing CGRP is activated [128, 149]. Pretreatment with high, neurotoxic dose of capsaicin (125 mg/kg sc.), which induces ablation of primary sensory neurons and the depletion of CGRP-containing fibers, pharmacological blockade of peripheral $CGRP_1$ receptors by hCGRP 8-37 and NO synthesis by NO-synthase inhibitor N^{ω}-nitro-L-arginine methyl ester blocked the increased gastric mucosal blood flow induced by i.c. injection of TRH [149-153]. The results indicate that the intact function of sensory fibers containing CGRP and NO is basically important for stimulation of gastric mucosal blood flow and the consequent gastroprotection [152], and the CGRP/NO-mediated gastric hyperemia plays a crucial role to withstand gastric mucosal damage [reviews 61, 154].

Moreover, additional action due to activation of vagal cholinergic pathway might contribute to the mucosal protective effect. Namely, acetylcholine released from efferent nerve terminal of vagal nerve in the periphery, activates $\alpha 7$ subunit-containing nicotinic receptors of macrophages and other immune cells which results in inhibition of the release of proinflammatory cytokines, consequently suppression of inflammation [155, 156].

As the above data suggest DVC has a basic role in the regulation of gastrointestinal functions. We wondered if activation of different receptor populations identified in DVC. e.g. *μ-opioid* receptors (in NTS and DMNV) [157], *cannabinoid receptors* (*CB_1*-receptors in NTS and DMNV and *CB_2*-receptors in NTS and brain stem neurons) [158, 159] *NK_1*-receptors in NTS and DMNV) [160, 161], angiotensin AT_1 receptors in in the NTS, area postrema and DMNV [162, 163] can influence gastric mucosal homeostasis. Our experimental results demonstrated that opioid peptides [4, 133], anandamide, 2-arachidonoyl glycerol (2-AG) endocannabinoids, ligands of cannabinoid CB_1 and CB_2 receptors [137, 142], as well as (SP) [136] given i.c.v. induced gastric mucosal protective effect against ethanol-induced lesions.

We wondered, if in the periphery, sensory neuropeptides, such as CGRP or somatostatin may be involved in the centrally-induced mucosal protective effect of endomorphin-2, endocannabinoids, such as anandamide, 2-AG and SP.

Conclusions on the involvement of CGRP in gastric mucosal protection have been established on pharmacological analysis by using a competitive peptide antagonist of $CGRP_1$ receptor, CGRP 8-37 or functional ablation of neuropeptides by neurotoxic dose of capsaicin [149, 152]. However, the gastric mucosal level of CGRP or somatostatin has not been determined following central administration of gastroprotective agents.

Therefore we aimed to determine how the gastric mucosal level of CGRP and somatostatin is influenced by the mucosal damaging agent ethanol, and by endomorphin-2, endocannabinoids and SP.

As Fig 1. shows that endomorphin-2 inhibited the ethanol-induced mucosal lesions in the rat, the maximal effect was induced by 0.1 pmol. The mucosal levels of CGRP and somatostatin were decreased in a significant manner following oral administration of ethanol (after 60 min), while i.c.v. injection of endomorphin-2 reversed the decreased levels of both CGRP and somatostatin.

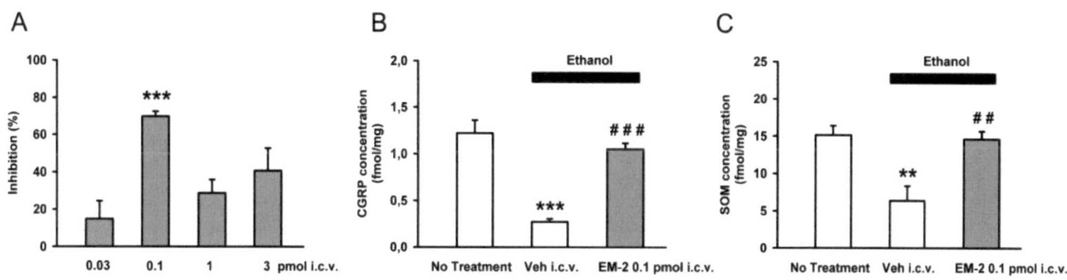

Adapted from Gyires et al. [4].

Figure 1. Panel A: The inhibitory effect of endomorphin-2 (EM-2) on the formation of ethanol-induced mucosal lesions in male Wistar rats. Acidified ethanol (2 ml concentrated HCl+98 ml absolute ethanol) was injected per os after 24 h food deprivation in a volume of 0.5 ml/rat. EM-2 was given intracerebroventricularly (i.c.v.) 10 minutes before the ethanol challenge in a volume of 10 µl in conscious rats. Mucosal lesions were evaluated macroscopically one hour after the administration of ethanol. Each column represents mean ± S.E.M., the number of rats was 5-10/group. ***p<0.001 compared to the respective control group (vehicle-treated rats) (One-way ANOVA, Newman-Keuls post hoc test). Panels B and C: The effect of EM-2 on the mucosal levels of calcitonin gene-related peptide (CGRP) and somatostatin. CGRP and somatostatin concentrations were determined from gastric mucosal tissue extract samples by means of radioimmunoassay (RIA). Peptide concentrations were calculated as the measured amount of peptide per wet tissue weight, expressed as fmol/mg. Detection limits of the assays were 2 fmol/ml (somatostatin) and 0.2 fmol/ml (CGRP). Each column represents mean ± S.E.M., the number of rats was 5/group. **p<0.01, ***p<0.001 compared to the absolute control group (no treatment), ##p<0.01, ###p<0.001 compared to vehicle (saline) i.c.v.+ethanol p.os-treated group (One-way ANOVA, Newman-Keuls post hoc test).

Similarly, anandamide and 2-AG inhibited the mucosal lesions in a dose dependent manner (though the protective effect of 2-AG was diminished in higher, 52.8 nmol dose), and both anandamide and 2-AG increased the ethanol-induced dramatic reduction of the mucosal CGRP and somatostatin levels in the gastroprotective doses (58, and 26 nmol, respectively) (Fig 2. 3.).

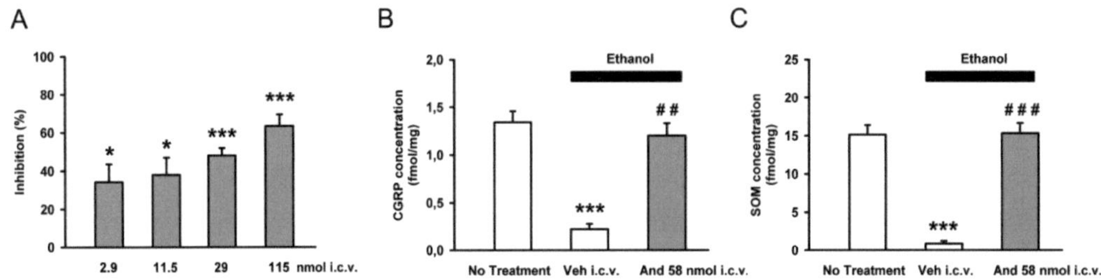

Adapted from Gyires et al. [137].

Figure 2. Panel A: The inhibitory effect of anandamide (And) on the formation of ethanol-induced mucosal lesions in male Wistar rats. Methods: see in the Legends of Fig. 1. Each column represents mean ± S.E.M., the number of rats was 5/group. *p<0.05, ***p<0.001 compared to the respective control group (vehicle-treated rats) (One-way ANOVA, Newman-Keuls post hoc test). Panels B and C: The effect of anandamide on the mucosal levels of calcitonin gene-related peptide (CGRP) and somatostatin. Methods: see in the Legends of Fig. 1. Each column represents mean ± S.E.M., the number of rats was 5/group. ***p<0.001 compared to the absolute control group (no treatment), ##p<0.01, ###p<0.001 compared to vehicle (ethanol diluted with saline) i.c.v.+ethanol p.os-treated group (One-way ANOVA, Newman-Keuls post hoc test).

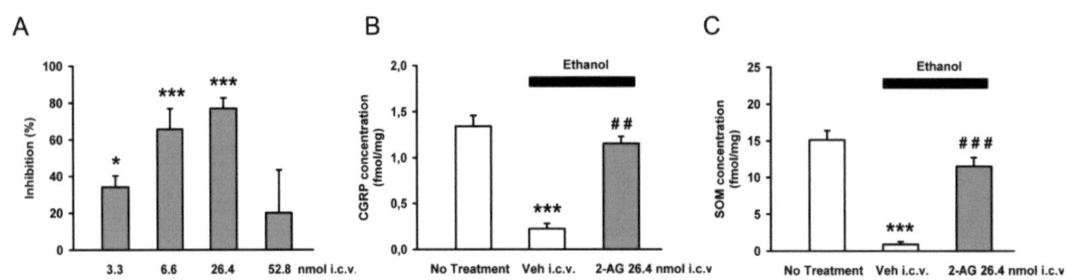

Adapted from Gyires et al. [137].

Figure 3. Panel A: The inhibitory effect of 2-arachidonoylglycerol (2-AG) on the formation of ethanol-induced mucosal lesions in male Wistar rats. Methods: see in the Legends of Fig. 1. Each column represents mean ± S.E.M., the number of rats was 5/group. *p<0.05, ***p<0.001 compared to the respective control group (vehicle-treated rats) (One-way ANOVA, Newman-Keuls post hoc test). Panels B and C: The effect of 2-AG on the mucosal levels of calcitonin gene-related peptide (CGRP) and somatostatin. Methods: see in the Legends of Fig. 1. Each column represents mean ± S.E.M., the number of rats was 5/group. ***p<0.001 compared to the absolute control group (no treatment), ##p<0.01, ###p<0.001 compared to vehicle (acetonitrile diluted with saline) i.c.v.+ethanol p.os-treated group (One-way ANOVA, Newman-Keuls post hoc test).

http://dx.doi.org/10.5772/58573

SP in pmolar dose range exerted mucosal protective action, the dose response curve proved to be bell shaped, similarly to 2-AG. However, though SP in gastroprotective doses also reversed the ethanol-induced reduction of CGRP mucosal level, it failed to counteract the reduced somatostatin level (Fig. 4.)

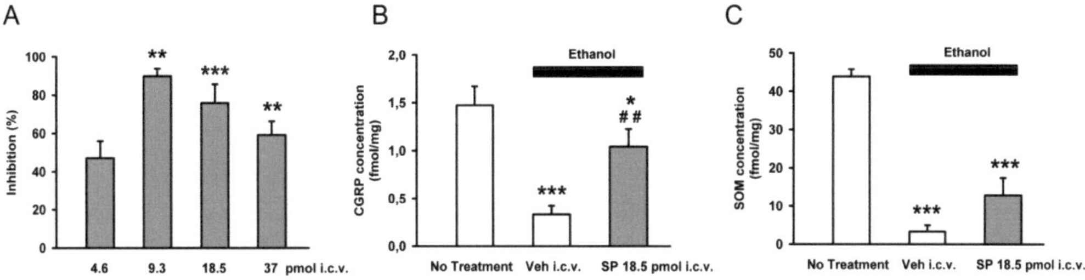

Adapted from Brancati et al. [136].

Figure 4. Panel A: The inhibitory effect of substance P (SP) on the formation of ethanol-induced mucosal lesions in male Wistar rats. Methods: see in the Legends of Fig. 1.. Each column represents mean ± S.E.M., the number of rats was 5/group. **p<0.01, ***p<0.001 compared to the respective control group (vehicle-treated rats) (One-way ANOVA, Newman-Keuls post hoc test). Panels B and C: The effect of SP on the mucosal levels of calcitonin gene-related peptide (CGRP) and somatostatin. Methods: see in the Legends of Fig. 1. Each column represents mean ± S.E.M., the number of rats was 5/group. *p<0.05, ***p<0.001 compared to the absolute control group (no treatment), ##p<0.01 compared to vehicle (saline) i.c.v.+ethanol p.os-treated group (One-way ANOVA, Newman-Keuls post hoc test).

Our experimental results provided direct evidence on the role of sensory neuropeptides in centrally initiated gastroprotective effect. It was shown that while ethanol decreased in a significant manner the mucosal CGRP and somatostatin concentration, the centrally injected endomorphin-2, endocannabinoids and SP were able to reverse the highly reduced mucosal levels of sensory neuropeptides supporting the concept on the role of sensory neuropeptides in centrally initiated gastroprotective effect.

4. Conclusion

The apparent redundancy in the mechanisms of gastric mucosal defense might be a potential answer to the question raised above: how can gastric mucosa resist to wide variety of endogenous and exogenous mucosal challenges. The redundancy can be observed in the wide scale of mediators involved in mucosal defense, in generation of endogenous substance(s) to noxious stimulus that may attenuate the mucosal injury and stimulate mucosal repair (for instance, peptide gene expression in gastrointestinal mucosal ulceration [164]), and can induce further protective mechanisms or formation of additional protective mediators.

In the early phase of mucosal injury when the gastric epithelium is exposed to acid or any irritant, one of the most rapid and important responses is the increase in mucosal blood flow to remove, dilute and buffer back-diffusing irritant or acid. In this process primary sensory afferent neurons activated by the back-diffusing acid play a crucial role, since sensory nerve endings can sense acid via acid sensing channel [60-68].

In addition, primary sensory afferent neurons are involved also in the actions of gastroprotective agents. Intensive studies revealed that gastric mucosal defense can be initiated also by central mechanism. Dorsal vagal complex is likely to have prominent role in centrally induced gastroprotective effect. Several neuropeptides, and their receptors e.g. *μ-opioid* receptors [157-159] NK_1-receptors [160, 161] angiotensin AT_1 receptors [162, 163] *TRH* receptors [126, 127, 165], neuropeptide Y receptors [166, 167] have been identified in this area, and activation of these receptors result in mucosal protection. Accumulating data suggest that in the periphery the final step in the chain of events of centrally initiated mucosal protective processes is the release of sensory neuropeptides, such as CGRP and partly somatostatin, from the capsaicin sensitive primary afferent neurons, as well as NO and prostaglandins. The process is likely to be vagal dependent, and biochemical and pharmacological studies have shown that vagal cholinergic pathway stimulates gastric prostaglandin and nitric oxide release. In addition, vagal muscarinic mediated release of prostaglandins, histamine and serotonin [147, 150] evoke sensory C-fiber excitation and a subsequent release of neuropeptides from sensory nerve endings.

However, sympathetic nervous system may also be involved in the centrally induced gastroprotective effect, since e.g. the gastroprotective effect of opioid peptides markedly decreased following i.c.v. administration of the catecholaminergic neurotoxin, 6-hydroxydopamine, that reduced the noradrenaline concentration in a significant manner in the NTS[138].

Tache [165] raised that that the redundancy of brain peptides may be linked with different pathophysiological conditions whereby they are recruited into the brain under stress, feeding or damage of the gastric mucosa. Further studies focusing to clarify the role of neuropeptide-interactions in gastroprotection, neuronal projections between brainstem autonomic centers and upper brain areas, additional pathway(s) that may convey central stimulus to the periphery, identification of additional peripheral mechanisms, signaling of peripheral insults of gastric mucosa to the CNS, are some of the opened questions that should be answered and consequently, the better understanding of the central regulation of gastric mucosal homeostatis may result in the development of new strategy and new concept in prevention/treatment of gastric mucosal injuries.

Acknowledgements

The author wish thank Dr. Viktória Tóth, Dr. Ágnes Fehér and Dr. Zoltán Zádori for their valuable help in preparation of the manuscript.

http://dx.doi.org/10.5772/58573

Author details

K. Gyires

Department of Pharmacology and Pharmacotherapy, Faculty of Medicine, Semmelweis University, Budapest, Hungary

References

[1] Sachs G, Chang HH, Rabon E, Schackman R, Lewin M, Saccomani G. A nonelectrogenic H+pump in plasma membranes of hog stomach. J Biol Chem 1976;(23) 7690-7698.

[2] Davenport HW. Why the stomach does not digest itself. Sci Am 1972;(1) 87-93.

[3] deFoneska A, Kaunitz JD. Gastroduodenal mucosal defense. Curr Opin Gastroenterol 2010;(6) 604-610.

[4] Gyires K, Nemeth J, Zadori ZS. Gastric mucosal protection and central nervous system. Curr Pharm Des 2013;19(1) 34-39.

[5] Laine L, Takeuchi K, Tarnawski A. Gastric mucosal defense and cytoprotection: bench to bedside. Gastroenterology 2008;(1) 41-60.

[6] Wallace JL. Prostaglandins, NSAIDs, and gastric mucosal protection: why doesn't the stomach digest itself? Physiol Rev 2008;(4) 1547-1565.

[7] Allen A, Flemstrom G. Gastroduodenal mucus bicarbonate barrier: protection against acid and pepsin. Am J Physiol Cell Physiol 2005;(1) 1-19.

[8] Hoffmann W. Trefoil factor family (TFF) peptides: regulators of mucosal regeneration and repair, and more. Peptides 2004;(5) 727-730.

[9] Hoffmann W. Trefoil factors TFF (trefoil factor family) peptide-triggered signals promoting mucosal restitution. Cell Mol Life Sci 2005;(24) 2932-2938.

[10] Farrell JJ, Taupin D, Koh TJ, Chen D, Zhao CM, Podolsky DK, et al. TFF2/SP-deficient mice show decreased gastric proliferation, increased acid secretion, and increased susceptibility to NSAID injury. J Clin Invest 2002;(2) 193-204.

[11] Konturek PC, Brzozowski T, Konturek SJ, Elia G, Wright N, Sliwowski Z, et al. Role of spasmolytic polypeptide in healing of stress-induced gastric lesions in rats. Regul Pept 1997;(1) 71-79.

[12] Chaudhury TK, Jacobson ED. Prostaglandin cytoprotection of gastric mucosa. Gastroenterology 1978;(1) 58-63.

[13] Robert A, Nezamis JE, Lancaster C, Hanchar AJ. Cytoprotection by prostaglandins in rats. Prevention of gastric necrosis produced by alcohol, HCl, NaOH, hypertonic NaCl, and thermal injury. Gastroenterology 1979;(3) 433-443.

[14] Lacy ER, Ito S. Microscopic analysis of ethanol damage to rat gastric mucosa after treatment with a prostaglandin. Gastroenterology 1982;(3) 619-625.

[15] Wallace JL, Granger DN. The cellular and molecular basis of gastric mucosal defense. FASEB J1996;(7) 731-740.

[16] Tarnawski A, et al. Cytoprotection of gastric and duodenal mucosa. Curr Med Lit Gastroenterol 1987;(6) 3.

[17] Guth PH, Paulsen G, Nagata H. Histologic and microcirculatory changes in alcohol-induced gastric lesions in the rat: effect of prostaglandin cytoprotection. Gastroenterology1984;(5) 1083-1090.

[18] Takeuchi K. Gastric cytoprotection by prostaglandin E2 and prostacyclin: relationship to EP1 and IP receptors. J Physiol Pharmacol 2014;(1) 3-14.

[19] Wallace JL, McKnight W, Reuter BK, Vergnolle N. NSAID-induced gastric damage in rats: requirement for inhibition of both cyclooxygenase 1 and 2. Gastroenterology 2000;(3) 706-714.

[20] Takeuchi K. Prostaglandin EP receptors and their roles in mucosal protection and ulcer healing in the gastrointestinal tract. Adv Clin Chem 2010;51 121-144.

[21] Moncada S, Palmer RM, Higgs EA. Nitric oxide: physiology, pathophysiology, and pharmacology. Pharmacol Rev 1991;(2) 109-142.

[22] Pique JM, Whittle BJ, Esplugues JV. The vasodilator role of endogenous nitric oxide in the rat gastric microcirculation. Eur J Pharmacol 1989;(2-3) 293-296.

[23] Guth PH. Current concepts in gastric microcirculatory pathophysiology. Yale J Biol Med 1992;(6) 677-688.

[24] Holzer P. Neural regulation of gastrointestinal blood flow. In: Johnson LR, ed. Physiology of the gastrointestinal tract. New York: Academic Press; 2006. p817-839.

[25] Tepperman BL, Whittle BJ. Endogenous nitric oxide and sensory neuropeptides interact in the modulation of the rat gastric microcirculation. Br J Pharmacol 1992;(1) 171-175.

[26] Kitagawa H, Takeda F, Kohei H. Effect of endothelium-derived relaxing factor on the gastric lesion induced by HCl in rats. J Pharmacol Exp Ther 1990;(3) 1133-1137.

[27] Pique JM, Esplugues JV, Whittle BJ. Endogenous nitric oxide as a mediator of gastric mucosal vasodilatation during acid secretion. Gastroenterology 1992;(1) 168-174.

[28] Holzer P, Livingston EH, Guth PH. Sensory neurons signal for an increase in rat gastric mucosal blood flow in the face of pending acid injury. Gastroenterology 1991;(2) 416-423.

[29] Nagy L, Nagata M, Szabo S. Protein and non-protein sulfhydryls and disulfides in gastric mucosa and liver after gastrotoxic chemicals and sucralfate: possible new targets of pharmacologic agents. World J Gastroenterol 2007;(14) 2053-2060.

[30] Szabo S, Nagy L, Plebani M. Glutathione, protein sulfhydryls and cysteine proteases in gastric mucosal injury and protection. Clin Chim Acta 1992;(1-2) 95-105.

[31] Ali AT. The role of nitric oxide and sulphydryls in gastric mucosal protection induced by sodium cromoglycate in rats. J Pharm Pharmacol 1995;(9) 739-743.

[32] Wallace JL. Physiological and pathophysiological roles of hydrogen sulfide in the gastrointestinal tract. Antioxid Redox Signal 2010;(9) 1125-1133.

[33] Fiorucci S, Antonelli E, Distrutti E, Rizzo G, Mencarelli A, Orlandi S, et al. Inhibition of hydrogen sulfide generation contributes to gastric injury caused by anti-inflammatory nonsteroidal drugs. Gastroenterology 2005;(4) 1210-1224.

[34] Wallace JL, Caliendo G, Santagada V, Cirino G. Markedly reduced toxicity of a hydrogen sulphide-releasing derivative of naproxen (ATB-346). Br J Pharmacol 2010;(6) 1236-1246.

[35] Wallace JL. Hydrogen sulfide: a rescue molecule for mucosal defence and repair. Dig Dis Sci 2012;(6) 1432-1434.

[36] Visse R, Nagase H. Matrix metalloproteinases and tissue inhibitors of metalloproteinases: structure, function, and biochemistry. Circ Res 2003;(8) 827-839.

[37] Kim SJ, Park YS, Paik HD, Chang HI. Effect of anthocyanins on expression of matrix metalloproteinase-2 in naproxen-induced gastric ulcers. Br J Nutr 2011;(12) 1792-1801.

[38] Swarnakar S, Ganguly K, Kundu P, Banerjee A, Maity P, Sharma AV. Curcumin regulates expression and activity of matrix metalloproteinases 9 and 2 during prevention and healing of indomethacin-induced gastric ulcer. J Biol Chem 2005;(10) 9409-9415.

[39] Davies GR, Simmonds NJ, Stevens TR, Grandison A, Blake DR, Rampton DS. Mucosal reactive oxygen metabolite production in duodenal ulcer disease. Gut 1992;(11) 1467-1472.

[40] Maines MD. The heme oxygenase system: a regulator of second messenger gases. Annu Rev Pharmacol Toxicol 1997;37 517-554.

[41] Bindu S, Mazumder S, Dey S, Pal C, Goyal M, Alam A, et al. Nonsteroidal anti-inflammatory drug induces proinflammatory damage in gastric mucosa through NF-kappaB activation and neutrophil infiltration: anti-inflammatory role of heme

oxygenase-1 against nonsteroidal anti-inflammatory drug. Free Radic Biol Med 2013; 456-467.

[42] Llesuy SF, Tomaro ML. Heme oxygenase and oxidative stress. Evidence of involvement of bilirubin as physiological protector against oxidative damage. Biochim Biophys Acta 1994;(1) 9-14.

[43] Guo JS, Cho CH, Wang WP, Shen XZ, Cheng CL, Koo MW. Expression and activities of three inducible enzymes in the healing of gastric ulcers in rats. World J Gastroenterol 2003;(8) 1767-1771.

[44] Wright NA, Pike C, Elia G. Induction of a novel epidermal growth factor-secreting cell lineage by mucosal ulceration in human gastrointestinal stem cells. Nature 1990; (6253) 82-85.

[45] Playford RJ. Peptides and gastrointestinal mucosal integrity. Gut 1995;(5) 595-597.

[46] Goodlad RA, Lee CY, Ghatei MA, et al. Differential effects of EGF and TGF-alpha on gastrointestinal epithelial cell proliferation [abstract]. Proc Nutr Soc 1993;(32)185.

[47] Romano M, Polk WH, Awad JA, Arteaga CL, Nanney LB, Wargovich MJ, et al. Transforming growth factor alpha protection against drug-induced injury to the rat gastric mucosa in vivo. J Clin Invest 1992;(6) 2409-2421.

[48] Playford RJ, Marchbank T, Chinery R, Evison R, Pignatelli M, Boulton RA, et al. Human spasmolytic polypeptide is a cytoprotective agent that stimulates cell migration. Gastroenterology 1995;(1) 108-116.

[49] Dignass A, Lynch-Devaney K, Kindon H, Thim L, Podolsky DK. Trefoil peptides promote epithelial migration through a transforming growth factor beta-independent pathway. J Clin Invest 1994;(1) 376-383.

[50] Dignass AU, Podolsky DK. Cytokine modulation of intestinal epithelial cell restitution: central role of transforming growth factor beta. Gastroenterology 1993;(5) 1323-1332.

[51] Tsujii M, Kawano S, Tsuji S, Ito T, Hayashi N, Horimoto M, et al. Increased expression of c-met messenger RNA following acute gastric injury in rats. Biochem Biophys Res Commun 1994;(1) 536-541.

[52] Satoh H, Shino A, Sato F, Asano S, Murakami I, Inatomi N, et al. Role of endogenous basic fibroblast growth factor in the healing of gastric ulcers in rats. Jpn J Pharmacol 1997;(1) 59-71.

[53] Szabo S, Folkman J, Vattay P, Morales RE, Pinkus GS, Kato K. Accelerated healing of duodenal ulcers by oral administration of a mutein of basic fibroblast growth factor in rats. Gastroenterology 1994;(4) 1106-1111.

[54] Hull MA, Brough JL, Powe DG, Carter GI, Jenkins D, Hawkey CJ. Expression of basic fibroblast growth factor in intact and ulcerated human gastric mucosa. Gut 1998;(4) 525-536.

[55] Florkiewicz RZ, Santos A,Tanoue K, et al. Gastric mucosal injury stimulates bFGF and its receptor gene expression and triggers CUG-initiated translation of 20.7 and 21.7 kDa bFGF isoforms [abstract]. Gastroenterology 1995;(108) 725.

[56] Vattey P, Gambier E, Morales RE, et al. Effect of orally-administered platelet-derived growth factor (PDGF) on healing of chronic duodenal ulcers and gastric secretion in rats [abstract]. Gastroenterology 1991;(100) 180.

[57] Szabo S, Sandor ZS, Al-Bassam J, et al. Despite different etiologies, virtually identical changes in local bFGF, PDGF and VEGF levels in duodenal ulceration and ulcerative colitis indicate similarities in healing [abstract]. Gastroenterology 1998;(114) 300.

[58] Szabo S, Vincze A, Sandor Z, Jadus M, Gombos Z, Pedram A, et al. Vascular approach to gastroduodenal ulceration: new studies with endothelins and VEGF. Dig Dis Sci 1998;(9) 40-45.

[59] Jones MK, Itani RM, Wang H, Tomikawa M, Sarfeh IJ, Szabo S, et al. Activation of VEGF and Ras genes in gastric mucosa during angiogenic response to ethanol injury. Am J Physiol 1999;(6-1) 1345-1355.

[60] Holzer P. Efferent-like roles of afferent neurons in the gut: Blood flow regulation and tissue protection. Auton Neurosci 2006;(1-2) 70-75.

[61] Holzer P. Neural emergency system in the stomach. Gastroenterology 1998;(4) 823-839.

[62] Akiba Y, Nakamura M, Nagata H, Kaunitz JD, Ishii H. Acid-sensing pathways in rat gastrointestinal mucosa. J Gastroenterol 2002;133-138.

[63] Szolcsanyi J, Bartho L. Capsaicin-sensitive afferents and their role in gastroprotection: an update. J Physiol Paris 2001;(1-6) 181-188.

[64] Aihara E, Sasaki Y, Ise F, Kita K, Nomura Y, Takeuchi K. Distinct mechanisms of acid-induced HCO3-secretion in normal and slightly permeable stomachs. Am J Physiol Gastrointest Liver Physiol 2006;(3) 464-471.

[65] Holzer P. Local microcirculatory reflexes and afferent signalling in response to gastric acid challenge. Gut 2000; 46-48.

[66] Li DS, Raybould HE, Quintero E, Guth PH. Calcitonin gene-related peptide mediates the gastric hyperemic response to acid back-diffusion. Gastroenterology 1992;(4-1) 1124-1128.

[67] Holzer P, Livingston EH, Saria A, Guth PH. Sensory neurons mediate protective vasodilatation in rat gastric mucosa. Am J Physiol 1991;(3-1) 363-370.

[68] Tashima K, Nakashima M, Kagawa S, Kato S, Takeuchi K. Gastric hyperemic response induced by acid back-diffusion in rat stomachs following barrier disruption--relation to vanilloid type-1 receptors. Med Sci Monit 2002;(5) 157-163.

[69] Berthoud HR, Neuhuber WL. Functional and chemical anatomy of the afferent vagal system. Auton Neurosci 2000;(1-3) 1-17.

[70] Gabella G, Pease HL. Number of axons in the abdominal vagus of the rat. Brain Res 1973;(2) 465-469.

[71] Holzer P. Sensory neurons in the stomach. In: Pierangelo G., Holzer P. (eds.) Neurogenic inflammation. Boca Raton, Florida: CRC Press LLC; 1996. p141-149.

[72] Holzer P, Lippe IT. Stimulation of afferent nerve endings by intragastric capsaicin protects against ethanol-induced damage of gastric mucosa. Neuroscience 1988;(3) 981-987.

[73] Mozsik G, Szolcsanyi J, Domotor A. Capsaicin research as a new tool to approach of the human gastrointestinal physiology, pathology and pharmacology. Inflammopharmacology 2007;(6) 232-245.

[74] Jancso G, Kiraly E, Jancso-Gabor A. Pharmacologically induced selective degeneration of chemosensitive primary sensory neurones. Nature 1977;(5639) 741-743.

[75] Caterina MJ, Schumacher MA, Tominaga M, Rosen TA, Levine JD, Julius D. The capsaicin receptor: a heat-activated ion channel in the pain pathway. Nature 1997;(6653) 816-824.

[76] Holzer P. Transient receptor potential (TRP) channels as drug targets for diseases of the digestive system. Pharmacol Ther 2011;(1) 142-170.

[77] Holzer P. Capsaicin: cellular targets, mechanisms of action, and selectivity for thin sensory neurons. Pharmacol Rev 1991;(2) 143-201.

[78] Szallasi A, Blumberg PM. Vanilloid (Capsaicin) receptors and mechanisms. Pharmacol Rev 1999;(2) 159-212.

[79] Szolcsanyi J. Forty years in capsaicin research for sensory pharmacology and physiology. Neuropeptides 2004;(6) 377-384.

[80] Paterson WG, Miller DV, Dilworth N, Assini JB, Lourenssen S, Blennerhassett MG. Intraluminal acid induces oesophageal shortening via capsaicin-sensitive neurokinin neurons. Gut2007(10):1347-52.

[81] Ward SM, Bayguinov J, Won KJ, Grundy D, Berthoud HR. Distribution of the vanilloid receptor (VR1) in the gastrointestinal tract. J Comp Neurol 2003;(1) 121-135.

[82] Holzer P. TRPV1 and the gut: from a tasty receptor for a painful vanilloid to a key player in hyperalgesia. Eur J Pharmacol 2004;(1-3) 231-241.

[83] Ryu V, Gallaher Z, Czaja K. Plasticity of nodose ganglion neurons after capsaicin-and vagotomy-induced nerve damage in adult rats. Neuroscience 2010;(4) 1227-1238.

[84] Zhao H, Simasko SM. Role of transient receptor potential channels in cholecystokinin-induced activation of cultured vagal afferent neurons. Endocrinology 2010;(11) 5237-5246.

[85] Akiba Y, Ghayouri S, Takeuchi T, Mizumori M, Guth PH, Engel E, et al. Carbonic anhydrases and mucosal vanilloid receptors help mediate the hyperemic response to luminal CO2 in rat duodenum. Gastroenterology 2006;(1) 142-152.

[86] Akiba Y, Mizumori M, Kuo M, Ham M, Guth PH, Engel E, et al. CO2 chemosensing in rat oesophagus. Gut 2008;(12) 1654-1664.

[87] Maggi CA. Tachykinins and calcitonin gene-related peptide (CGRP) as co-transmitters released from peripheral endings of sensory nerves. Prog Neurobiol 1995;(1) 1-98.

[88] Mózsik Gy, Pár A, Pár G, Juricskay I, Figler M, Szolcsányi J. Insight into the molecular pharmacology to drugs acting on the afferent and efferent fibers of the vagal nerve in the gastric mucosal protection. In: Sikiric P., Seiwerth P., Mózsik Gy., Arakawa T., Takeuchi K. (eds.) Ulcer Research. Bologna: Monduzzi; 2004. p163-168.

[89] Pinter E, Helyes Z, Szolcsanyi J. Inhibitory effect of somatostatin on inflammation and nociception. Pharmacol Ther 2006;(2) 440-456.

[90] Sternini C, Reeve JR, Jr., Brecha N. Distribution and characterization of calcitonin gene-related peptide immunoreactivity in the digestive system of normal and capsaicin-treated rats. Gastroenterology 1987;(4) 852-862.

[91] Tan LL, Bornstein JC, Anderson CR. Neurochemical and morphological phenotypes of vagal afferent neurons innervating the adult mouse jejunum. Neurogastroenterol Motil 2009;(9) 994-1001.

[92] Green T, Dockray GJ. Characterization of the peptidergic afferent innervation of the stomach in the rat, mouse and guinea-pig. Neuroscience 1988;(1) 181-193.

[93] Sternini C. Enteric and visceral afferent CGRP neurons. Targets of innervation and differential expression patterns. Ann N Y Acad Sci 1992; 170-186.

[94] Hwang SJ, Oh JM, Valtschanoff JG. Expression of the vanilloid receptor TRPV1 in rat dorsal root ganglion neurons supports different roles of the receptor in visceral and cutaneous afferents. Brain Res 2005;(2) 261-266.

[95] Price TJ, Flores CM. Critical evaluation of the colocalization between calcitonin gene-related peptide, substance P, transient receptor potential vanilloid subfamily type 1 immunoreactivities, and isolectin B4 binding in primary afferent neurons of the rat and mouse. J Pain 2007;(3)263-272.

[96] Suzuki T, Kagoshima M, Shibata M, Inaba N, Onodera S, Yamaura T, et al. Effects of several denervation procedures on distribution of calcitonin gene-related peptide and substance P immunoreactive in rat stomach. Dig Dis Sci 1997;(6) 1242-1254.

[97] Kwok YN, McIntosh CH. Release of substance P-like immunoreactivity from the vascularly perfused rat stomach. Eur J Pharmacol 1990;(2-3) 201-207.

[98] Lambrecht N, Burchert M, Respondek M, Muller KM, Peskar BM. Role of calcitonin gene-related peptide and nitric oxide in the gastroprotective effect of capsaicin in the rat. Gastroenterology 1993;(5) 1371-1380.

[99] Evangelista S, Tramontana M, Maggi CA. Pharmacological evidence for the involvement of multiple calcitonin gene-related peptide (CGRP) receptors in the antisecretory and antiulcer effect of CGRP in rat stomach. Life Sci 1992;50(5) 13-18.

[100] Ichikawa T, Kusakabe T, Gono Y, Shikama N, Hiruma H, Kawakami T, et al. Nitric oxide synthase activity in rat gastric mucosa contributes to mucin synthesis elicited by calcitonin gene-related peptide. Biomed Res 2006;(3) 117-124.

[101] Mizuguchi S, Ohno T, Hattori Y, Kamata K, Arai K, Saeki T, et al. Calcitonin gene-related peptide released by capsaicin suppresses myoelectrical activity of gastric smooth muscle. J Gastroenterol Hepatol 2005;(4) 611-618.

[102] Gazzieri D, Trevisani M, Springer J, Harrison S, Cottrell GS, Andre E, et al. Substance P released by TRPV1-expressing neurons produces reactive oxygen species that mediate ethanol-induced gastric injury. Free Radic Biol Med 2007;(4) 581-589.

[103] Kihara N, de la Fuente SG, Fujino K, Takahashi T, Pappas TN, Mantyh CR. Vanilloid receptor-1 containing primary sensory neurones mediate dextran sulphate sodium induced colitis in rats. Gut 2003;(5) 713-719.

[104] Szitter I, Pozsgai G, Sandor K, Elekes K, Kemeny A, Perkecz A, et al. The role of transient receptor potential vanilloid 1 (TRPV1) receptors in dextran sulfate-induced colitis in mice. J Mol Neurosci 2010;(1) 80-88.

[105] McVey DC, Schmid PC, Schmid HH, Vigna SR. Endocannabinoids induce ileitis in rats via the capsaicin receptor (VR1). J Pharmacol Exp Ther 2003;(2) 713-722.

[106] Lambrecht N, Burchert M, Respondek M, Muller KM, Peskar BM. Role of calcitonin gene-related peptide and nitric oxide in the gastroprotective effect of capsaicin in the rat. Gastroenterology 1993;(5) 1371-1380.

[107] Brzozowski T, Drozdowicz D, Szlachcic A, Pytko-Polonczyk J, Majka J, Konturek SJ. Role of nitric oxide and prostaglandins in gastroprotection induced by capsaicin and papaverine. Digestion 1993;54(1) 24-31.

[108] Takeuchi K, Kato S, Takeeda M, Ogawa Y, Nakashima M, Matsumoto M. Facilitation by endogenous prostaglandins of capsaicin-induced gastric protection in rodents through EP2 and IP receptors. J Pharmacol Exp Ther 2003;(3) 1055-1062.

[109] Katori M, Ohno T, Nishiyama K. Interaction of substance P and leukotriene C4 in ethanol-induced mucosal injury of rat stomach. Regul Pept 1993;(1-2) 241-243.

[110] Matsumoto J, Takeuchi K, Okabe S. Characterization of gastric mucosal blood flow response induced by intragastric capsaicin in rats. Jpn J Pharmacol 1991;(2) 205-213.

[111] Karmeli F, Eliakim R, Okon E, Rachmilewitz D. Gastric mucosal damage by ethanol is mediated by substance P and prevented by ketotifen, a mast cell stabilizer. Gastroenterology 1991;(5-1) 1206-1216.

[112] Karmeli F, Eliakim R, Okon E, Rachmilewitz D. Somatostatin effectively prevents ethanol-and NSAID-induced gastric mucosal damage in rats. Dig Dis Sci 1994;(3) 617-625.

[113] Whittle BJ, Lopez-Belmonte J, Rees DD. Modulation of the vasodepressor actions of acetylcholine, bradykinin, substance P and endothelin in the rat by a specific inhibitor of nitric oxide formation. Br J Pharmacol 1989;(2) 646-652.

[114] Yamamoto H, Horie S, Uchida M, Tsuchiya S, Murayama T, Watanabe K. Effects of vanilloid receptor agonists and antagonists on gastric antral ulcers in rats. Eur J Pharmacol 2001;(2-3) 203-210.

[115] Zayachkivska OS, Konturek SJ, Drozdowicz D, Konturek PC, Brzozowski T, Ghegotsky MR. Gastroprotective effects of flavonoids in plant extracts. J Physiol Pharmacol 2005; 219-231.

[116] Matsumoto Y, Kanamoto K, Kawakubo K, Aomi H, Matsumoto T, Ibayashi S, et al. Gastroprotective and vasodilatory effects of epidermal growth factor: the role of sensory afferent neurons. Am J Physiol Gastrointest Liver Physiol 2001;(5) 897-903.

[117] Mozsik G, Peidl Z, Szolcsanyi J, Domotor A, Hideg K, Szekeres G, et al. Participation of vanilloid/capsaicin receptors, calcitonin-gene-related peptide and substance P in gastric protection of omeprazole and omeprazole-like compounds. Inflammopharmacology 2005;13(1-3) 139-159.

[118] Ma L, Chow JY, Wong BC, Cho CH. Role of capsaicin sensory nerves and EGF in the healing of gastric ulcer in rats. Life Sci 2000;(15) 213-220.

[119] Palkovits M. Interconnections between the neuroendocrine hypothalamus and the central autonomic system. Geoffrey Harris Memorial Lecture, Kitakyushu, Japan, October 1998. Front Neuroendocrinol 1999;(4) 270-295.

[120] Tache Y, Simard P, Collu R. Prevention by bombesin of cold-restraint stress induced hemorrhagic lesions in rats. Life Sci 1979;(18) 1719-1725.

[121] Hagiwara M, Watanabe H, Kanaoka R. Effects of intracerebroventricular bombesin on gastric ulcers and gastric glycoproteins in rats. J Pharmacobiodyn 1985;(10) 864-867.

[122] Tache Y, Vale W, Rivier J, Brown M. Brain regulation of gastric secretion: influence of neuropeptides. Proc Natl Acad Sci U S A 1980;(9) 5515-5519.

[123] Martinez V, Tache Y. Bombesin and the brain-gut axis. Peptides 2000;(11) 1617-1625.

[124] Hernandez DE, Nemeroff CB, Orlando RC, Prange AJ, Jr. The effect of centrally administered neuropeptides on the development of stress-induced gastric ulcers in rats. J Neurosci Res 1983;9(2) 145-157.

[125] Ephgrave KS, Cullen JJ, Broadhurst K, Kleiman-Wexler R, Shirazi SS, Schulze-Delrieu K. Gastric contractions, secretions and injury in cold restraint. Neurogastroenterol Motil 1997;(3) 187-192.

[126] Tache Y, Yoneda M. Central action of TRH to induce vagally mediated gastric cytoprotection and ulcer formation in rats. J Clin Gastroenterol 1993;(17) 58-63.

[127] Tache Y. Brainstem neuropeptides and vagal protection of the gastric mucosal against injury: role of prostaglandins, nitric oxide and calcitonin-gene related peptide in capsaicin afferents. Curr Med Chem 2012;19(1) 35-42.

[128] Kaneko H, Mitsuma T, Nagai H, Mori S, Iyo T, Kusugami K, et al. Central action of adrenomedullin to prevent ethanol-induced gastric injury through vagal pathways in rats. Am J Physiol 1998;(6-2) 1783-1788.

[129] Yang H, Kawakubo K, Tache Y. Intracisternal PYY increases gastric mucosal resistance: role of cholinergic, CGRP, and NO pathways. Am J Physiol 1999;(3-1) 555-562.

[130] Guidobono F, Pagani F, Sibilia V, Soglian A, Rapetti D, Netti C. The role of sensory neurons in the antiulcer effect of centrally injected amylin in rat. Peptides 2000;(10) 1537-1541.

[131] Brzozowski T, Konturek PC, Konturek SJ, Pierzchalski P, Bielanski W, Pajdo R, et al. Central leptin and cholecystokinin in gastroprotection against ethanol-induced damage. Digestion 2000;62(2-3) 126-142.

[132] Sibilia V, Pagani F, Rindi G, Lattuada N, Rapetti D, De L, V, et al. Central ghrelin gastroprotection involves nitric oxide/prostaglandin cross-talk. Br J Pharmacol 2008;(3) 688-697.

[133] Gyires K, Ronai AZ. Supraspinal delta-and mu-opioid receptors mediate gastric mucosal protection in the rat. J Pharmacol Exp Ther 2001;(3) 1010-1015.

[134] Zadori ZS, Shujaa N, Koles L, Kiraly KP, Tekes K, Gyires K. Nocistatin and nociceptin given centrally induce opioid-mediated gastric mucosal protection. Peptides 2008;(12) 2257-2265.

[135] Sibilia V, Pagani F, Bulgarelli I, Mrak E, Broccardo M, Improta G, et al. TLQP-21, a VGF-derived peptide, prevents ethanol-induced gastric lesions: insights into its mode of action. Neuroendocrinology 2010;92(3) 189-197.

[136] Brancati SB, Zadori ZS, Nemeth J, Gyires K. Substance P induces gastric mucosal protection at supraspinal level via increasing the level of endomorphin-2 in rats. Brain Res Bull 2013; 38-45.

[137] Gyires K, Ronai AZ, Zadori ZS, Toth VE, Nemeth J, Szekeres M, et al. Angiotensin II-induced activation of central AT1 receptors exerts endocannabinoid-mediated gastroprotective effect in rats. Mol Cell Endocrinol 2014;(2) 971-978.

[138] Gyires K. Analysis of the Effect of Different Neuropeptides in Gastric Mucosal Defense Initiated Centrally. In: Filaretova LP., Takeuchi K. (eds.) Cell/Tissue Injury and Cytoprotection/Organoprotection in the Gastrointestinal Tract: Mechanism, Prevention and Treatment. Basel: Karger; 2012. p161-169.

[139] Brzozowski T, Konturek PC, Pajdo R, Kwiecien S, Ptak A, Sliwowski Z, et al. Brain-gut axis in gastroprotection by leptin and cholecystokinin against ischemia-reperfusion induced gastric lesions. J Physiol Pharmacol 2001;(4-1) 583-602.

[140] Brzozowski T, Konturek PC, Sliwowski Z, Drozdowicz D, Kwiecien S, Pawlik M, et al. Neural aspects of ghrelin-induced gastroprotection against mucosal injury induced by noxious agents. J Physiol Pharmacol 2006; 63-76.

[141] Brzozowska I, Ptak-Belowska A, Pawlik M, Pajdo R, Drozdowicz D, Konturek SJ, et al. Mucosal strengthening activity of central and peripheral melatonin in the mechanism of gastric defense. J Physiol Pharmacol 2009; 47-56.

[142] Shujaa N, Zadori ZS, Ronai AZ, Barna I, Mergl Z, Mozes MM, et al. Analysis of the effect of neuropeptides and cannabinoids in gastric mucosal defense initiated centrally in the rat. J Physiol Pharmacol 2009; 93-100.

[143] Gyires K. Neuropeptides and gastric mucosal homeostasis. Curr Top Med Chem 2004;4(1) 63-73.

[144] Gyires K. Gastric mucosal protection: from prostaglandins to gene-therapy. Curr Med Chem 2005;12(2) 203-215.

[145] Holzer P, Pabst MA, Lippe IT, Peskar BM, Peskar BA, Livingston EH, et al. Afferent nerve-mediated protection against deep mucosal damage in the rat stomach. Gastroenterology 1990;(4) 838-848.

[146] Kato K, Matsuno Y, Matsuo Y, Shimamura M, Tanaka K, Murai I, et al. Role of mucosal prostaglandins in vagally-mediated adaptive cytoprotection in the rat. Gastroenterol Jpn 1992;(1) 1-8.

[147] Yoneda M, Tache Y. Central thyrotropin-releasing factor analog prevents ethanol-induced gastric damage through prostaglandins in rats. Gastroenterology 1992;(5) 1568-1574.

[148] Adelson DW, Wei JY, Yashar M, Lee TJ, Tache Y. Central autonomic activation by intracisternal TRH analogue excites gastric splanchnic afferent neurons. J Neurophysiol 1999;(2) 682-691.

[149] Kato K, Yang H, Tache Y. Role of peripheral capsaicin-sensitive neurons and CGRP in central vagally mediated gastroprotective effect of TRH. Am J Physiol 1994;(5-2) 1610-1614.

[150] Tanaka T, Guth P, Tache Y. Role of nitric oxide in gastric hyperemia induced by central vagal stimulation. Am J Physiol 1993;(2-1) 280-284.

[151] Saperas E, Mourelle M, Santos J, Moncada S, Malagelada JR. Central vagal activation by an analogue of TRH stimulates gastric nitric oxide release in rats. Am J Physiol 1995;(6-1) 895-899.

[152] Kiraly A, Suto G, Guth PH, Tache Y. Mechanisms mediating gastric hyperemic and acid responses to central TRH analog at a cytoprotective dose. Am J Physiol 1997;(1-1) 31-38.

[153] Tache Y, Yoneda M, Kato K, Kiraly A, Suto G, Kaneko H. Intracisternal thyrotropin-releasing hormone-induced vagally mediated gastric protection against ethanol lesions: central and peripheral mechanisms. J Gastroenterol Hepatol 1994;(9) 29-35.

[154] Kawano S, Tsuji S. Role of mucosal blood flow: a conceptional review in gastric mucosal injury and protection. J Gastroenterol Hepatol 2000; 1-6.

[155] Pavlov VA, Tracey KJ. The cholinergic anti-inflammatory pathway. Brain Behav Immun 2005;(6) 493-499.

[156] Wang H, Yu M, Ochani M, Amella CA, Tanovic M, Susarla S, et al. Nicotinic acetylcholine receptor alpha7 subunit is an essential regulator of inflammation. Nature 2003;(6921) 384-388.

[157] Mansour A, Fox CA, Burke S, Meng F, Thompson RC, Akil H, et al. Mu, delta, and kappa opioid receptor mRNA expression in the rat CNS: an in situ hybridization study. J Comp Neurol 1994;(3) 412-438.

[158] Partosoedarso ER, Abrahams TP, Scullion RT, Moerschbaecher JM, Hornby PJ. Cannabinoid1 receptor in the dorsal vagal complex modulates lower oesophageal sphincter relaxation in ferrets. J Physiol 2003;(1) 149-158.

[159] Van Sickle MD, Duncan M, Kingsley PJ, Mouihate A, Urbani P, Mackie K, et al. Identification and functional characterization of brainstem cannabinoid CB2 receptors. Science 2005;(5746) 329-332.

[160] Dixon MK, Nathan NA, Hornby PJ. Immunocytochemical distribution of neurokinin 1 receptor in rat dorsal vagal complex. Peptides 1998;19(5) 913-923.

[161] Lewis MW, Travagli RA. Effects of substance P on identified neurons of the rat dorsal motor nucleus of the vagus. Am J Physiol Gastrointest Liver Physiol 2001;(1) 164-172.

[162] Diz DI, Jessup JA, Westwood BM, Bosch SM, Vinsant S, Gallagher PE, et al. Angiotensin peptides as neurotransmitters/neuromodulators in the dorsomedial medulla. Clin Exp Pharmacol Physiol 2002;(5-6) 473-482.

[163] Lenkei Z, Palkovits M, Corvol P, Llorens-Cortes C. Distribution of angiotensin type-1 receptor messenger RNA expression in the adult rat brain. Neuroscience 1998;(3) 827-841.

[164] Wong WM. Peptide gene expression in gastrointestinal mucosal ulceration: ordered sequence or redundancy? Gut 2000;(46) 286-292.

[165] Tache Y, Yang H, Miampamba M, Martinez V, Yuan PQ. Role of brainstem TRH/TRH-R1 receptors in the vagal gastric cholinergic response to various stimuli including sham-feeding. Auton Neurosci 2006;(1-2) 42-52.

[166] Mahaut S, Dumont Y, Fournier A, Quirion R, Moyse E. Neuropeptide Y receptor subtypes in the dorsal vagal complex under acute feeding adaptation in the adult rat. Neuropeptides 2010;(2) 77-86.

[167] Wolak ML, DeJoseph MR, Cator AD, Mokashi AS, Brownfield MS, Urban JH. Comparative distribution of neuropeptide Y Y1 and Y5 receptors in the rat brain by using immunohistochemistry. J Comp Neurol 2003;(3) 285-311.

Chapter 8

Stable Gastric PentadecapeptideBPC 157, Somatosensory Neurons and Their Protection and Therapeutic Extensions — A Survey

Predrag Sikiric

Additional information is available at the end of the chapter

http://dx.doi.org/10.5772/58681

1. Introduction

Stable gastric pentadecapeptide BPC 157 (GEPPPGKPADDAGLV, M. W. 1419, a partial sequence of human gastric juice protein BPC, in all studies used peptide with 99% (HPLC) purity, freely soluble in water at pH 7. 0 and in saline), was always given alone, without any carrier, µg-ng dose ranges and ways of application, intraperitoneal, intragastrical, in drinking water or topically, at the site of injury. Besides, tested in therapy of inflammatory bowel disease (IBD) (PL 14736) in clinical phase II. (Ruenzi et al., 2005), and now in multiple sclerosis.

As prime importance, BPC 157 was found to be stable at least 24 hours in human gastric juice and consequently, because of its anti-ulcerogenic potential in different, but relevant ulcer models, suggested to be novel mediator of Robert's cytoprotection and adaptive cytoprotection (for review see, i. e., (Sikiric et al., 2010, 2011, 2012)), and thereby, exhibited a particular wound healing effect, and cell protecting ability. At the general level this may likely explain its strong effectiveness and LD1 not achieved.

Thereby, such kind of pathophysiologic importance along with unlimited applications of BPC 157 regimens contrasts with the evidence for standard peptides providing that regardless commonly acknowledged pathophysiologic importance at least in many occasions they need a carrier (one or more) to become effective and furthermore, that their application prefers to be local, at the site of injury, given into the injury defect (for review see, i. e., (Urist, 1996)). Therefore, pentadecapeptide BPC 157 certainly avoids a common scenario with standard peptides where their limited application in pharmacology could hardly acknowledge their suggested prime physiological importance (Sikiric et al., 2010, 2011, 2012, 2013, 2014; Seiwerth et al., 2014)

2. Methods

With BPC 157 given alone, without a carrier, BPC 157 application strategy (for review see, i. e., (Sikiric et al., 2010, 2011, 2012, 2013, 2014; Seiwerth et al., 2014)) considerably overrides the standard peptides and their use with different carriers (i. e., peptide+carrier(s) complex) to establish the therapeutic effect (thereby erroneously) ascribed to the given peptide. Therefore, the activity – methodology dilemma whereby it is difficult to identify the real active part in peptide+carrier complex (peptide, carrier, peptide+carrier complex or neither of them) or specify their particular contribution is not applicable to BPC 157 (for review see, i. e., Urist, 1996). Finally, in BPC 157 – standard peptides relation, apart from the evidence that this anti-ulcer peptide may be effective in both upper and lower GI tract injuries (for review see, i. e., (Sikiric et al., 2010, 2011, 2012)), and initial successful use in clinic (Ruenzi et al., 2005), involving also a particular sphincter function control (Sikiric et al., 2010, 2011, 2012), the key difference appears in the healing outside the GI tract. This may be also because since this evidence was based on clear demonstration that it also may interact with the general systems, i. e., the NO-system, providing endothelium protection and angiogenic effect (Seiwerth et al. 2014; Sikiric et al., 2014). And even more, important to counteract severe complications of advanced and poorly controlled IBD, this occurs even in severely impaired conditions. Notably, the final background was that it stimulated expression of early growth response 1 gene (egr-1) responsible for cytokine and growth factor generation and early extracellular matrix (collagen) formation (but also its repressor nerve growth factor 1-A binding protein-2 (naB2)) (Tkalcevic et al., 2007).

To this point, it should be noted that BPC 157 markedly improves the healing of both traumatic nerve (Gjurasin et al., 2010) and traumatic brain injury (Tudor et al., 2010), and therefore, exhibits particular neuroprotective ability. Likewise, it ameliorates encephalopathies that occur in severely intoxicated animals (Ilic et al., 2010, 2011, 2011).

In addition, BPC 157 has in general a very safe profile. As an illustration, single dose toxicity studies in mice treated by oral and i. v. routes revealed a LD_{50} of PL 14736 higher than 2000 mg/kg. No mice died during both studies and transient sedation was the only finding in the dose of 2000 mg/kg. In the 4-week repeated i. v. dosing toxicity studies in rats and dogs no morphological findings related to PL 14736 administration were found at any of doses studied. Macroscopical and histological examination of the organs and tissues sampled following 14-day intracolonic administration in rats and dogs did not reveal changes that could be attributed to treatment with PL 14736 (doses up to 25 mg/kg). The only finding, lesions at the area of colon application site in rats, also seen in the control animals, was primarily caused by mechanical trauma of the catheter used. No effect of PL 14736 on female fertility and early embryonal development was noted. No effect of PL 14736 in sensitization study and in acute eye irritation/corrosion study was noted. PL 14736 does not cause chromosomal aberrations in cultures of human lymphocytes, nor it is mutagenic in the AMES test (doses up to 5 mg/plate were tested). Repeated i. v. administration of 10-30 μg/kg/day to mice did not induce the induction of microsomal liver enzymes *in vitro*. Safety pharmacology of PL 14736 has been studied in anaesthetised dogs following intraduodenal administration of 10 and 100 μg/kg, with no significant effects on the cardiovascular and respiratory systems.

Based largely upon the use of neurotoxin capsaicin, peptidergic neurons have been postulated to be involved in a physiological protective system (Holzer, 1991,1991). Protection of the gastric mucosa from various forms of injury occurs with different peptides given centrally (Heiling et al., 1987; Hernandez, 1986; Hernandez et al., 1987) and/or peripherally (Evangelista et al., 1991; Takeuchi et al., 1979).

The integrity of capsaicin somatosensory neurons and their protection were suggested to be related to BPC 157 activity in nociception (Sikiric et al., 1993). Capsaicin-sensitive afferent neurons, regulators of vascular functions in many somatic and visceral tissues (Holzer, 1991, 1991), are involved in local blood flow regulation in gastrointestinal tract (Holzer, 1991, 1991; Szabo et al., 1985). The population of capsaicin-sensitive neurons is heterogenous and comprises most but not all primary afferent neurons with small cells body and unmyelinated (C fiber) axons and some afferent neurons with thinly myelinated (A-δ) axons (Holzer, 1991, 1991). Low doses of capsaicin (micrograms per kilogram range) appear to be protective to the mucosa (Holzer, 1991, 1991) since they induce a transient excitation. In contrast, systemic administration of high doses of capsaicin (miligrams per kilogram range) is deleterious, causing long-lasting damage to these neurons (Holzer, 1991). This effect is age-dependent, being even more pronounced in the adult rat when capsaicin is given to newborn animals (Jancsó et al., 1977).

Therefore, the possibility that BPC 157 causes mucosal protection trough capsaicin-sensitive nerves was challenged. The effect of BPC 157 on gastroprotection, in rats treated with capsaicin, was investigated. Because of the mentioned different susceptibility to capsaicin of the adult and newborn animals (Holzer, 1991; Jancsó et al., 1977), and to achieve better insight into a possible mechanism of BPC 157 activity against the background of near maximal neuronal damage, it was necessary to use two different methods to deactivate sensory neurons by capsaicin pretreatment (Holzer, 1991; Jancsó et al., 1977), one in adult rats, the other in newborn rats. Likewise, since the importance of prostaglandins in organoprotection is well known (Robert, 1979; Schmidt et al., 1991), these effects were investigated with and without prostaglandin synthesis inhibition by indomethacin (Sikiric et al., 1988).

Stable gastric pentadecapeptide BPC 157 is an originally anti-ulcer peptide implemented in inflammatory bowel disease trials, and now multiple sclerosis, LD1 could be not achieved recently largely reviewed (Sikiric et al., 2010, 2011, 2012, 2013, 2014; Seiwerth et al., 2014).

The integrity of capsaicin somatosensory neurons and their protection were suggested to be related to the activity of BPC 157 (Sikiric et al., 1996).

Therefore, from this viewpoint, the focus was on the gastroprotective effect of the pentadecapeptide BPC 157, on gastric lesions produced in rats by 96% ethanol, restraint stress, and indomethacin (Sikiric et al., 1996). The possible involvement of sensory neurons in the salutary actions of BPC 157 (10 micrograms/kg, 10 ng/kg intraperitoneally) was studied with capsaicin, which has differential effects on sensory neurons: a high dose in adult (125 mg/kg subcutaneously, 3 months old) or administration (50 mg/kg subcutaneously) to neonatal animals (age of the 7 days) destroys sensory fibers, whereas a low dose (500 micrograms/kg intraperitoneally) activates neurotransmitter release and protective effects on the mucosa (Table 1-4). In the absence of capsaicin, BPC 157 protected gastric mucosa against ethanol, restraint, and indomethacin application. In the presence of neurotoxic doses of capsaicin, the negative influence of capsaicin on restraint, ethanol, or indomethacin lesions consistently affected salutary activity of BPC 157. However, BPC 157 protection was still evident in the capsaicin-treated rats (either treated as adults or as newborns) in all of these assays. Interestingly, after neonatal capsaicin treatment, a complete abolition of BPC 157 gastroprotection was noted if BPC 157 was applied as a single nanogram-regimen, but the mucosal protection was fully reversed when the same dose was used daily. In line with the excitatory dose of capsaicin the beneficial effectiveness of BPC 157 appears to be increased as well (Table 4). Taken together, these data provide evidence for complex synergistic interaction between the beneficial effectiveness of BPC 157 and peptidergic sensory afferent neuron activity (Sikiric et al., 1996). In broader sense, this should be a basis for further suitable generalization that was evidenced with transected peripheral nerve, traumatic brain injury, and brain lesions and subsequent disturbances (somatosensory disorientation, seizures, catalepsy/stereotypies) induced by various agents applications (BobanBlagaic et al., 2005; Gjurasin et al., 2010;Ilic et al., 2010, 2011, 2011; Jelovac et al., 1998, 1999; Klicek et al., 2013; Sikiric et al., 1999;Tohyama et al., 2004; Tudor et al., 2010).

Particularly, the evidence that it both protected somatosensory neurons against capsaicin neurotoxicity and restored their function (Sikiric et al., 1996) suggests BPC 157 as an agent with neuroprotective properties (Sikiric et al., 1996). One extension could be the healing of rat transected sciatic nerve and improvement made by stable gastric pentadecapeptide BPC 157 (10 microg, 10ng/kg) applied shortly after injury intraperitoneally/ intragastrically /locally, at the site of anastomosis, or after non-anastomozed nerve tubing (7 mm nerve segment resected) (It is known that the spontaneous regenerative capabilities of the nerve stumps, as well as Schwann cells abilities to provide a permissive environment for axonal elongation, are insufficient when there is a 7 mm gap between nerve ends in rat, which also presents an obstacle for the standard therapy (Gold, 2000)) directly into the tube) (Gjurasin et al., 2010). Improvement was shown clinically (autotomy), microscopically/morphometrically and functionally (EMG, one or two months post-injury, walking recovery (sciatic functional index (SFI)) at weekly intervals). BPC 157-rats exhibited faster axonal regeneration: histomorphometrically (improved presentation of neural fascicles, homogeneous regeneration pattern, increased density and size of regenerative fibers, existence of epineural and perineural regeneration, uniform target orientation of regenerative fibers, and higher proportion of neural vs. connective tissue, all fascicles in each nerve showed increased diameter of myelinated fibers, thickness of myelin sheet, number of myelinated fibers per area and myelinated fibers as a percentage of the nerve transected area and the increased blood vessels presentation), electrophysiologically (increased motor action potentials), functionally (improved SFI), the autotomy absent. Thus, BPC 157 markedly improved rat sciatic nerve healing with particular point that severe autotomy – regularly present after transected sciatic nerve – was practically completely avoided in BPC 157-treated rats (Gjurasin et al., 2010).

The further extension could be the effect of BPC 157 after an induced traumatic brain injury (TBI) in mice by a falling weight. BPC 157 regimens (10 micrograms/kg, 10 ng/kg intraperitoneally) demonstrated a marked attenuation of damage with an improved early outcome and a minimal postponed mortality throughout a 24h post-injury period. Ultimately, the traumatic lesions (subarachnoidal and intraventricularhaemorrhage, brain laceration, haemorrhagic laceration) were less intense and consecutive brain edema had considerably improved. Given prophylactically (30 min before TBI) the improved conscious/unconscious/death ratio in TBI-mice was after force impulses of 0. 068 Ns, 0. 093 Ns, 0. 113 Ns, 0. 130 Ns, 0. 145 Ns, and 0. 159 Ns. Counteraction (with a reduction of unconsciousness, lower mortality) with both microg-and ng-regimens included the force impulses of 0. 068-0. 145 Ns. A higher regimen presented effectiveness also against the maximal force impulse (0. 159 Ns). Furthermore, BPC 157 application immediately prior to injury was beneficial in mice subjected to force impulses of 0. 093 Ns-TBI. For a more severe force impulse (0. 130 Ns, 0. 145 Ns, or 0159 Ns), the time-relation to improve the conscious/unconscious/death ratio was: 5 min (0. 130 Ns-TBI), 20 min (0. 145 Ns-TBI) or 30 min (0. 159 Ns-TBI) (Tudor et al., 2010)

3. Results

In conclusion, these results should be viewed with numerous compounds and neuroprotective strategies more extensively discussed, evaluated and reviewed elsewhere (Maas et al., 2005; Marklund et al., 2006). However, brain trauma results in brain damage and dysfunction from both primary injury (due to biomechanical effects) and subsequent secondary damage due to activation of pathophysiologic cascades (Muir, 2006), and this study with BPC 157 (Tudor et al., 2010) evidenced the preserved consciousness and reduced mortality immediately after trauma in pentadecapeptide BPC 157-mice and subsequently, markedly reduced mortality, lowered brain edema, lowered the number and size of haemorrhagic traumatic lacerations, and lowered the intensity of subarachnoidal bleeding with significantly less intraventricular-haemorrhage.

The additional extension could be the evidence that pentadecapeptide BPC 157 particularly attenuated neurotoxin 1-methyl-4-phenyl-1,2,3,6-tetrahydropyridine (MPTP) damage, including mortality (Sikiric et al., 1999)(of note, neuroprotection by immunophillin ligands lack the effect on MPTP-toxicity (Gold, 2000), significantly affected the dopamine system (Jelovac et al., 1998, 1999; Sikiric et al., 1999)(a system also implicated in the traumatic brain injury course) (Yan et al., 2001)and prevented/reversed catalepsy or stereotypy due to central dopamine system failure induced by various procedures (Jelovac et al., 1998, 1999; Sikiric et al., 1999). Accordingly, regional serotonin synthesis in the rat brain, assessed by α-methyl-L-tryptophan autoradiographic measurements showed that, BPC 157 given peripherally may readily cross the blood–brain barrier, affect region-specific brain 5-HT synthesis in rats leading to significantly increased synthesis in the substantianigra (compacta and reticulata) structure and counteract serotonin syndrome (BobanBlagaic et al., 2005; Tohyama et al., 2004). Very recently, BPC 157 counteracts cuprizone-brain damage and motoric disability (Klicek et al., 2013). An additional emphasize may be that BPC 157 largely interferes with different NSAIDs-toxicity, including their brain damages that appear subsequently their gastrointestinal and/or liver toxicity (Ilic et al., 2010, 2011, 2011).

Also, in addition to several other effects of BPC 157 (such as counteraction of acute and chronic gastric lesions, blood pressure modulation and prevention/reversal of chronic heart failure (Balenovic et al. 2009, 2012; Barisic et al., 2013)), BPC 157's antagonization of acute and chronic ethanol intoxication (Blagaic AB et al., 2004) was found to be an effect that is at least partly NO-dependent (Boban-Blagaic et al., 2006; Klicek et al., 2008; Lovric-Bencic et al., 2004; Sikiric et al., 1997).

One possible option of treatment (i. e., injury is often irreversible because inability of nerve tissue to regenerate and no therapeutic solution of this problem to date) is protection of secondary injury – zone of vascular and inflammatory reaction in nerve tissue to primary injury.

Taken together, the data providing the protection and rescue of the capsaicin neurotoxicity, and thereby, the evidence for complex synergistic interaction between the beneficial effectiveness of BPC 157 and peptidergic sensory afferent neuron activity (Sikiric et al., 1996) was useful,in a broader sense, for the further experiments. We argue that the significance of these beneficial effects (Sikiric et al., 1996) was confirmed by the healing effect of pentadecapeptide BPC 157 on transected and anastomosed as well as non-anastomosed rat sciatic nerve (Gjurasin et al., 2010). The final prove was provided from brain trauma studies resulting in brain damage and dysfunction from primary injury and subsequent secondary damage due to activation of pathophysiologic cascades, but the preserved consciousness and reduced mortality in pentadecapeptide BPC 157 treated along with lowered brain edema, lessened number and size of haemorrhagic traumatic lacerations, subarachnoidal bleeding and intraventricularhaemorrhage (Tudor et al., 2010).

Intesity of gastric lesions following 48h restraint stress		
	Adult	Newborn
Healthy	+++	
BPC 157 10ng	+/-	
BPC 157 10μg	+/-	
Capsaicin	+++	+++++
BPC 157 10ng + Capsaicin	++	+++
BPC 157 10μg + Capsaicin	+	+

Table 1. Long-term somatosensory neuron damage. Gastric lesions in 3-month-old adult rats following 48 hours restraint stress, treated with capsaicin two weeks (125 mg/kg subcutaneously) before or as neonates at 7 days old (50 mg/kg subcutaneously). BPC 157 (10 ng or 10 μg per kg intraperitoneally) treatment 1 hour before restraint; 16-20 rats per each experimental group.

Intesity of gastric lesions 24h after indomethacin application		
	Adult	Newborn
Healthy	+++	
BPC 157 10ng	+/-	
BPC 157 10µg	+/-	
Capsaicin 50mg		+++++
BPC 157 10ng + Capsaicin 50mg		++
BPC 157 10µg + Capsaicin 50mg		+

Table 2. Long-term somatosensory neuron damage. Gastric lesions in 3-month-old adult rats following subcutaneous application of 30 mg/kg of indomethacin, treated with capsaicin as neonates at 7 days old (50 mg/kg subcutaneously). BPC 157 (10 ng or 10 µg per kg intraperitoneally) treatment 1 hour before indomethacin application; 16-20 rats per each experimental group.

Intesity of gastric lesions following 96% ethanol application		
	Adult	Newborn
Healthy	+++	
BPC 157 10ng	+	
BPC 157 10µg	+	
Capsaicin	+++	+++
BPC 157 10ng + Capsaicin	+	+++
BPC 157 10µg + Capsaicin	+	++

Table 3. Long-term somatosensory neuron damage. Gastric lesions in 3-month-old adult rats 1 hour following intragastric application of 96% ethanol, treated with capsaicin two weeks (125 mg/kg subcutaneously) before or as neonates at 7 days old (50 mg/kg subcutaneously). BPC 157 (10 ng or 10 µg per kg intraperitoneally) treatment 1 hour before ethanol; 16-20 rats per each experimental group.

Excitation of somatosensory neurons in adult rats	
Healthy	+++++
BPC 157 10ng	++
BPC 157 10µg	++
Capsaicin 500µg	++++
BPC 157 10ng + Capsaicin 500µg	+
BPC 157 10µg + Capsaicin 500µg	+

Table 4. Excitation of somatosensory neurons. Gastric lesions in adult rats 1 hour following intragastric application of 96% ethanol, treated with capsaicin (low dose 500µg/kg, intraperitoneally) and/or BPC 157 (10 ng or 10 µg per kg intraperitoneally) 1 hour before ethanol; 16-20 rats per each experimental group.

Author details

Predrag Sikiric*

Address all correspondence to: Sikiric@mef. hr

Department of Pharmacology, Medical Faculty University of Zagreb, Zagreb, Croatia

References

[1] Balenovic D, Barisic I, Prkacin I, Horvat I, Udovicic M, Uzun S, Strinic D, Pevec D, Drmic D, Radic B, Bardak D, Zlatar M, Aralica G, LovricBencic M, SeparovicHanzevacki J, Romic Z, Sindic A, Seiwerth S, Sikiric P. Mortal Furosemide-Hypokalemia-Disturbances in Rats NO-System Related Shorten Survival by L-NAME. Therapy Benefit with BPC 157 Peptide More Than With L-Arginine. J Clin Exp Cardiolog. 2012; 3: 201doi:10. 4172/2155-9880. 1000201

[2] Balenovic D, Bencic ML, Udovicic M, Simonji K, Hanzevacki JS, Barisic I, Kranjcevic S, Prkacin I, Coric V, Brcic L, Coric M, Brcic I, Borovic S, Radic B, Drmic D, Vrcic H, Seiwerth S, Sikiric P. Inhibition of methyldigoxin-induced arrhythmias by pentadecapeptide BPC 157: a relation with NO-system. Regul Pept. 2009; 156(1-3): 83-89.

[3] Barisic I, Balenovic D, Klicek R, Radic B, Nikitovic B, Drmic D, Udovicic M, Strinic D, Bardak D, Berkopic L, Djuzel V, Sever M, Cvjetko I, Romic Z, Sindic A, Bencic ML, Seiwerth S, Sikiric P. Mortal hyperkalemia disturbances in rats are NO-system related. The life saving effect of pentadecapeptide BPC 157. Regul Pept. 2013; 181: 50-66.

[4] Blagaic AB, Blagaic V, Romic Z, SikiricP. The influence of gastric pentadecapeptide BPC 157 on acute and chronic ethanol administration in mice. Eur J Pharmacol. 2004; 499(3): 285-290.

[5] Boban Blagaic A, Blagaic V, Mirt M, Jelovac N, Dodig G, Rucman R, Petek M, Turkovic B, Anic T, Dubovecak M, Staresinic M, Seiwerth S, Sikiric P. Gastric pentadecapeptide BPC 157 effective against serotonin syndrome in rats.. Eur J Pharmacol. 2005; 512(2-3): 173-179.

[6] Boban-Blagaic A, Blagaic V, Romic Z, Jelovac N, Dodig G, Rucman R, Petek M, Turkovic B, Seiwerth S, Sikiric P. The influence of gastric pentadecapeptide BPC 157 on acute and chronic ethanol administration in mice. The effect of N(G)-nitro-L-arginine methyl ester and L-arginine. Med Sci Monit. 2006; 12(1): BR36-45.

[7] Evangelista S, Maggi CA. Protection induced cholecystokinin-8 (CKK-8) in ethanol-induced gastric lesions is mediated via vagal capsaicin-sensitive fibres and CCK-A receptors. Br J Pharmacol. 1991; 102: 119-122.

[8] Gjurasin M, Miklic P, Zupancic B, Perovic D, Zarkovic K, Brcic L, Kolenc D, Radic B, Seiwerth S, Sikiric P. Peptide therapy with pentadecapeptide BPC 157 in traumatic nerve injury.. Regul Pept. 2010; 160(1-3): 33-41.

[9] Gold BG. Neuroimmunophilin ligands: evaluation of their therapeutic potential for the treatment of neurological disorders. Expert Opin Investig Drugs. 2000; 9: 2331–2342.

[10] Heiling M, Murison R. Intracerebroventricular neuropeptide Y protects against stress-induced gastric lesions in rat. Eur J Pharmacol. 1987; 137:127-129.

[11] Hernandez DE. Neuroendocrine mechanisms of stress ulceration: Focus on thyrotropin releasing hormone (TRH). Life Sci. 1986;39:279-296.

[12] Hernandez DE, Nemeroff CB, Orlando RO, Prange AJ. Influence of brain peptides on the development of stress gastric ulcers. In: S Szabo, Gy Mózsik, editors. New Pharmacology of Ulcer Disease. Experimental and New Therapeutic Approaches. New York: Elsevier; 1987. pp. 375-386.

[13] Holzer P. Capsaicin: Cellular targets, mechanisms of action and selectivity for thin sensory neurons. Pharmacol Rev. 1991; 43:143-201.

[14] Holzer P. Peptidergic sensory neurons in the control of vascular functions: Mechanisms and significance in the cutaneous and splanchic vascular beds. Rev Physiol Biochem Pharmacol. 1991; 121: 49-146.

[15] Ilic S, Drmic D, Zarkovic K, Kolenc D, Coric M, Brcic L, Klicek R, Radic B, Sever M, Djuzel V, Ivica M, BobanBlagaic A, Zoricic Z, Anic T, Zoricic I, Djidic S, Romic Z, Seiwerth S, Sikiric P. High hepatotoxic dose of paracetamol produces generalized convulsions and brain damage in rats. A counteraction with the stable gastric pentadecapeptide BPC 157 (PL 14736). J Physiol Pharmacol. 2010; 61(2): 241-250.

[16] Ilic S, Drmic D, Zarkovic K, Kolenc D, Brcic L, Radic B, Djuzel V, Blagaic AB, Romic Z, Dzidic S, Kalogjera L, Seiwerth S, Sikiric P. Ibuprofen hepatic encephalopathy, hepatomegaly, gastric lesion and gastric pentadecapeptide BPC 157 in rats. Eur J Pharmacol. 2011; 667(1-3): 322-329.

[17] Ilic S, Drmic D, Franjic S, Kolenc D, Coric M, Brcic L, Klicek R, Radic B, Sever M, Djuzel V, Filipovic M, Djakovic Z, Stambolija V, Blagaic AB, Zoricic I, Gjurasin M, Stupnisek M, Romic Z, Zarkovic K, Dzidic S, Seiwerth S, Sikiric P. Pentadecapeptide BPC 157 and its effects on a NSAID toxicity model: diclofenac-induced gastrointestinal, liver, and encephalopathy lesions. Life Sci. 2011; 88(11-12): 535-542.

[18] Jancsó G, Király E, Jancsó-Gabor A. Pharmacologically induced selective degeneration of chemosensitive primary sensory neurones. Nature. 1977; 270: 741-743.

[19] Jelovac N, Sikiric P, Rucman R, Petek M, Marovic A, Perovic D, Seiwerth S, Mise S, Turkovic B, Dodig G, Miklic P, Buljat G, Prkacin I. Pentadecapeptide BPC 157 attenu-

ates disturbances induced by neuroleptics: the effect on catalepsy and gastric ulcers in mice and rats. Eur J Pharmacol. 1999; 379(1):19-31.

[20] Jelovac N, Sikirić P, Rucman R, Petek M, Perović D, Konjevoda P, Marović A, Seiwerth S, Grabarević Z, Sumajstorcić J, Dodig G, Perić J. A novel pentadecapeptide, BPC 157, blocks the stereotypy produced acutely by amphetamine and the development of haloperidol-induced supersensitivity to amphetamine. Biol Psychiatry. 1998; 43(7): 511-519.

[21] Klicek R, Sever M, Radic B, Drmic D, Kocman I, Zoricic I, Vuksic T, Ivica M, Barisic I, Ilic S, Berkopic L, Vrcic H, Brcic L, Blagaic AB, Coric M, Brcic I, Rokotov DS, Anic T, Seiwerth S, Sikiric P. Pentadecapeptide BPC 157, in clinical trials as a therapy for inflammatory bowel disease (PL14736), is effective in the healing of colocutaneous fistulas in rats: role of the nitric oxide-system. J Pharmacol Sci. 2008; 108(1): 7-17.

[22] Klicek R, Kolenc D, Suran J, Drmic D, Brcic L, Aralica G, Sever M, Holjevac J, Radic B, Turudic T, Kokot A, Patrlj L, Rucman R, Seiwerth S, Sikiric P. Stable gastric pentadecapeptide BPC 157 heals cysteamine-colitis and colon-colon-anastomosis and counteracts cuprizone brain injuries and motor disability. J Physiol Pharmacol. 2013; 64(5): 597-612.

[23] Lovric-Bencic M, Sikiric P, Hanzevacki JS, Seiwerth S, Rogic D, Kusec V, Aralica G, Konjevoda P, Batelja L, Blagaic AB. Doxorubicine-congestive heart failure-increased big endothelin-1 plasma concentration: reversal by amlodipine, losartan, and gastric pentadecapeptide BPC157 in rat and mouse. J Pharmacol Sci. 2004; 95(1): 19-26.

[24] Maas AI, Schouten JW, Teasdale GM. Neuroprotection. In: Reilly P, Bullock MR, editors. Head Injury. London: Hodder Arnold Publishers; 2005. pp. 406–440.

[25] Marklund N, Bakshi A, Castelbuono DJ, Conte V, McIntosh TK. Evaluation of pharmacological treatment strategies in traumatic brain injury. Curr Pharm Des. 2006; 12: 1645–1680.

[26] Muir KW. Glutamate-based therapeutic approaches: clinical trials with NMDA antagonists. Curr Opin Pharmacol. 2006; 6: 53–60.

[27] Robert A. Cytoprotection by prostaglandins. Gastroenterology. 1979; 77: 761-767.

[28] Ruenzi M, Stolte M, Veljaca M, Oreskovic K, Peterson J, Ulcerative Colitis Study Group. A multicenter, randomized, double blind, placebo-controlled phase II study of PL 14736 enema in the treatment of mild-to-moderate ulcerative colitis. Gastroenterology. 2005; 128: A584.

[29] Schmidt KL, Miller TA. Cytoprotection: Fact or fancy? The morphologic basis of gastric protection by prostaglandins. Exp Clin Gastroenterol. 1991; 1:119-132.

[30] Seiwerth S, Brcic L, Vuletic LB, Kolenc D, Aralica G, Misic M, Zenko A, Drmic D, Rucman R, Sikiric P. BPC 157 and blood vessels. Curr Pharm Des. 2014; 20(7): 1121-1125.

[31] Sikiric P, Gyires K, Seiwerth S, Grabarevic Z, Rucman R, Petek M, Rotkvic I, Turkovic B, Udovicic I, Jagic V, Mildner B, Duvnjak M, Danilovic Z. The effect of pentadecapeptide BPC 157 on inflammatory, non-inflammatory, direct and indirect pain and capsaicin neurotoxicity. Inflammopharmacology. 1993 ; 2:121-127.

[32] Sikiric P, Seiwerth S, Rucman R, Turkovic B, Rokotov DS, Brcic L, Sever M, Klicek R, Radic B, Drmic D, Ilic S, Kolenc D, Aralica G, Stupnisek M, Suran J, Barisic I, Dzidic S, Vrcic H, Sebecic B. Stable gastric pentadecapeptide BPC 157-NO-system relation. Curr Pharm Des. 2014; 20(7): 1126-1135.

[33] Sikiric P, Marovic A, Matoz W, Anic T, Buljat G, Mikus D, Stancic-Rokotov D, Separovic J, Seiwerth S, Grabarevic Z, Rucman R, Petek M, Ziger T, Sebecic B, Zoricic I, Turkovic B, Aralica G, Perovic D, Duplancic B, Lovric-Bencic M, Rotkvic I, Mise S, Jagic V, Hahn V. A behavioural study of the effect of pentadecapeptide BPC 157 in Parkinson's disease models in mice and gastric lesions induced by 1-methyl-4-phenyl-1,2,3,6-tetrahydrophyridine. J Physiol Paris. 1999; 93(6):505-512.

[34] Sikiric P, Rotkvic I, Mise S, Krizanac S, Gjuris V, Jukic J, Suchanek E, Petek M, Udovicic I, Kalogjera L, Geber J, Tucan-Foretic M, Duvnjak M, Philipp M, Balen I, Anic T. The influence of dopamine agonists and antagonists on indomethacin lesions in stomach and small intestine in rats. Eur J Pharmacol. 1988; 158: 61-67.

[35] Sikirić P, Seiwerth S, Grabarević Z, Rucman R, Petek M, Jagić V, Turković B, Rotkvić I, Mise S, Zoricić I, Gjurasin M, Konjevoda P, Separović J, Ljubanović D, Artuković B, Bratulić M, Tisljar M, Jurina L, Buljat G, Miklić P, Marović A. Beneficial effect of a novel pentadecapeptide BPC 157 on gastric lesions induced by restraint stress, ethanol, indomethacin, and capsaicin neurotoxicity. Dig Dis Sci. 1996; 41(8): 1604-1614.

[36] Sikirić P, Seiwerth S, Grabarević Z, Rucman R, Petek M, Jagić V, Turković B, Rotkvić I, Mise S, Zoricić I, Konjevoda P, Perović D, Jurina L, Separović J, Hanzevacki M, Artuković B, Bratulić M, Tisljar M, Gjurasin M, Miklić P, Stancić-Rokotov D, Slobodnjak Z, Jelovac N, Marović A. The influence of a novel pentadecapeptide, BPC 157, on N(G)-nitro-L-arginine methylester and L-arginine effects on stomach mucosa integrity and blood pressure. Eur J Pharmacol. 1997; 332(1): 23-33.

[37] Sikiric P, Seiwerth S, Brcic L, Sever M, Klicek R, Radic B, Drmic D, Ilic S, Kolenc D. Revised Robert's cytoprotection and adaptive cytoprotection and stable gastric pentadecapeptide BPC 157. Possible significance and implications for novel mediator. Curr Pharm Des. 2010; 16(10): 1224-1234.

[38] Sikiric P, Seiwerth S, Rucman R, Turkovic B, Rokotov DS, Brcic L, Sever M, Klicek R, Radic B, Drmic D, Ilic S, Kolenc D, Vrcic H, Sebecic B. Stable gastric pentadecapeptide BPC 157: novel therapy in gastrointestinal tract. Curr Pharm Des. 2011; 17(16): 1612-1632.

[39] Sikiric P, Seiwerth S, Rucman R, Turkovic B, Rokotov DS, Brcic L, Sever M, Klicek R, Radic B, Drmic D, Ilic S, Kolenc D, Stambolija V, Zoricic Z, Vrcic H, Sebecic B. Focus

on ulcerative colitis: stable gastric pentadecapeptide BPC 157. Curr Med Chem. 2012; 19(1):126-132.

[40] Sikiric P, Seiwerth S, Rucman R, Turkovic B, Rokotov DS, Brcic L, Sever M, Klicek R, Radic B, Drmic D, Ilic S, Kolenc D, Aralica G, Safic H, Suran J, Rak D, Dzidic S, Vrcic H, SebecicB. Toxicity by NSAIDs. Counteraction by stable gastric pentadecapeptide BPC 157. Curr Pharm Des. 2013; 19(1) : 76-83.

[41] Szabo S, Trier JS, Brown A, Schnoor J. Early vascular injury and increased vascular permeability in gastric mucosal injury caused by ethanol in the rat. Gastroenterology 1985; 88: 228-236.

[42] Takeuchi K, Johnson LR. Pentagastrin protects against stress ulcerations in rats. Gastroenterology. 1979; 76: 788-792.

[43] Tkalcević VI, Cuzić S, Brajsa K, Mildner B, Bokulić A, Situm K, Perović D, Glojnarić I, Parnham MJ. Enhancement by PL 14736 of granulation and collagen organization in healing wounds and the potential role of egr-1 expression. Eur J Pharmacol. 2007; 570(1-3): 212-221.

[44] Tohyama Y, Sikirić P, Diksic M. Effects of pentadecapeptide BPC157 on regional serotonin synthesis in the rat brain: alpha-methyl-L-tryptophan autoradiographic measurements. Life Sci. 2004 ;76(3): 345-357.

[45] Tudor M, Jandric I, Marovic A, Gjurasin M, Perovic D, Radic B, Blagaic AB, Kolenc D, Brcic L, Zarkovic K, Seiwerth S, Sikiric P. Traumatic brain injury in mice and pentadecapeptide BPC 157 effect. Regul Pept. 2010;160(1-3):26-32.

[46] Urist MR. The first three decades of bone morphogenetic protein. Osteologie. 1996; 4: 207-233.

[47] Yan HQ, Kline AE, Ma X, Hooghe-Peters EL, Marion DW, Dixon CE. Tyrosine hydroxylase, but not dopamine beta-hydroxylase, is increased in rat frontal cortex after traumatic brain injury. Neuroreport. 2001; 12(11): 2323-2327.

Chapter 9

Lafutidine Protects the NSAID-Induced Small Intestinal Lesions Mediated by Capsaicin-Sensitive Afferent Neurons

Kikuko Amagase and Koji Takeuchi

Additional information is available at the end of the chapter

http://dx.doi.org/10.5772/58604

1. Introduction

Nonsteroidal anti-inflammatory drugs (NSAIDs) such as indomethacin damage the small intestine as well as the stomach, although the ulcerogenic dose is much lower in the former [1-3]. Several factors such as intestinal hypermotility, enterobacteria, neutrophils, nitric oxide (NO), and inducible NO synthase (iNOS) are involved in the pathogenesis of these intestinal lesions [3-7], yet a deficiency of endogenous prostaglandins (PGs) due to cyclooxygenase (COX) inhibition is most important in the background for the intestinal ulcerogenic response to NSAIDs [8-10]. Recent clinical studies, using capsule endoscopes or double-balloon endoscopes, confirmed that NSAIDs damage the small intestine in patients at a higher incidence than previously thought. Unfortunately, antisecretory drugs such as proton pump inhibitors and histamine H_2 receptor antagonists are reported to be ineffective against NSAID-induced small intestinal damage [11,12] and even worsen the severity of these lesions [12], though these drugs prevent gastric ulcerogenic response to NSAIDs [13].

Capsaicin-sensitive sensory neurons are known to play an important role in modulating the gastric mucosal integrity [14]. It has previously been reported that stimulation of these sensory neurons by capsaicin prevented the occurrence of experimental colitis as well as indomethacin-induced intestinal ulceration in rats, while sensory deafferentation increased both the degree and incidence of the latter lesion model [11,15,16]. These findings suggest the role of capsaicin-sensitive sensory neurons in maintaining the integrity of the intestinal mucosa, similar to the gastric mucosa.

Lafutidine, a histamine H_2-receptor antagonist, has been shown to exhibit a potent gastroprotective activity in addition to gastric antisecretory action [17,18]. Onodera et al. [19] reported that the gastroprotective action of lafutidine was independent of its antisecretory effect and partially mediated by capsaicin-sensitive sensory neurons.

In the present report, we described the protective effect of lafutidine against NSAID-induced enteropathy and suggested the involvement of capsaicin-sensitive afferent neurons in this action.

2. Materials and methods

2.1. Animals

Male Sprague-Dawley rats (240~280 g; Nippon Charles River, Shizuoka, Japan) were used. Studies were carried out using four to eight animals without fasting in a conscious state, unless otherwise specified. All experimental procedures described here were approved by the Experimental Animal Research Committee of Kyoto Pharmaceutical University.

2.2. Induction of small intestinal lesions

Animals were given loxoprofen (60 mg/kg, p.o.) and killed 24 h later under deep ether anesthesia. The small intestine was excised, treated with 2% formalin for fixation of the tissue wall for 10 min and opened along the antimesenteric attachment. The area of macroscopically visible damage (mm^2) was measured under a dissecting microscope with square grids (x10), summed per tissue and used as a lesion score. Lafutidine (10 and 30 mg/kg), cimetidine (100 mg/kg) or famotidine (30 mg/kg) was given p.o. twice, 0.5 h before and 6 h after the administration of loxoprofen, while omeprazole (100 mg/kg) was given p.o. once, 0.5 h before loxoprofen. On the other hand, ablation of capsaicin-sensitive sensory neurons was performed by s.c. injection of capsaicin once daily for 3 consecutive days (total dose 100 mg/kg) 2 weeks before the experiment [20]. All capsaicin injections were done under ether anesthesia, and the rats were pretreated with terbutaline (0.1 mg/kg, i.m.) and aminophylline (10 mg/kg, i.m.) to prevent respiratory impairment. The effectiveness of the treatment was tested by examining the protective wiping movements of the eye.

2.3. Determination of enterobacterial counts

Enterobacteria were enumerated according to a method described by Deitch et al. [21]. Twenty-four hours after loxoprofen treatment (60 mg/kg, p.o.), the animals were killed under deep diethyl ether anesthesia, and the small intestines were excised. Aliquots of the homogenate of intestine were placed on blood agar and Gifu anaerobic medium agar (Nissui, Tokyo, Japan). Blood agar plates were incubated at 37°C for 24 h under aerobic conditions, whereas Gifu anaerobic medium agar plates were incubated for 24 h under standard anaerobic conditions (BBL Gas Pack Pouch Anaerobic System; BD Biosciences, San Jose, CA). Plates containing 10 to 300 colony-forming units (CFU) were examined for numbers of enterobacteria, and the data were expressed as log CFU per gram of tissue. Lafutidine (10 and 30 mg/kg) was given p.o. twice, 0.5 h before and 6 h after the administration of loxoprofen.

http://dx.doi.org/10.5772/58604

2.4. Determination of iNOS and Muc2 mRNA Expression by RT-PCR

Expression of iNOS and Muc2 mRNA in the small intestinal mucosa was measured by RT-PCR. The animals were killed under deep ether anesthesia 6 h after the administration of loxoprofen, and the small intestines were removed, frozen in acetone/dryice, and stored at-80°C prior to use. Tissue samples were pooled from 2 to 3 rats for extraction of total RNA, which was prepared by a single-step acid phenol-chloroform extraction procedure by use of Sepasol RNA-I (Nacalai Tesque, Kyoto, Japan). Total RNA primed by random hexadeoxy ribonucleotide was reverse-transcribed with the Rever Tra Ace-a (Toyobo, Osaka, Japan). An aliquot of the RT reaction product served as a template in 35 cycles of PCR with 0.5 min of denaturation at 95°C and 1 min of extension at 68°C by Advantage-2 (BD Biosciences, Palo Alto, CA, USA) on a thermal cycler (PC806; ASTEC, Fukuoka, Japan). A portion of the PCR mixture was electrophoresed in 1.8% agarose gel in TAE buffer, and the gel was stained with ethidium bromide and photographed (Bio Doc-It Imaging System; UVP, Upland, CA, USA). Lafutidine (30 mg/kg) was given p.o. twice, 0.5 h before and 6 h after the administration of loxoprofen.

2.5. Determination of mucus secretion in small intestine

The amount of mucus secreted in the small intestine was determined by periodic acid-Schiff (PAS) staining. Three hours after the administration of loxoprofen (60 mg/kg, p.o.), the animals were killed under deep diethyl ether anesthesia, and the small intestines were removed. The removed tissues were fixed in Carnoy's fluid (ethanol : acetic acid : chloroform=6 : 1 : 3) for 24 h, embedded in paraffin, and sectioned at a thickness of 6 μm. PAS staining was subsequently performed according to the conventional method. Lafutidine (30 mg/kg) was given p.o. with or without co-administration of loxoprofen. In the combined administration, this agent was given p.o. 30 min before the administration of loxoprofen.

2.6. Preparation of drugs

The drugs used were lafutidine, cimetidine, famotidine, loxoprofen, ampicillin (Shigma Chemicals, St. Louis, MO), and omeprazole. Lafutidine, cimetidine, famotidine, omeprazole or loxoprofen was suspended in a 0.5% hydroxy propyl cellulose solution (Wako). All drugs were prepared immediately before use and administered p.o. or s.c. in a volume of 0.5 ml/100 g body weight. Control animals received the vehicle alone.

2.7. Statistics

Data are presented as the mean±SE for four to eight rats per group. Statistical analyses were performed using the two-tailed Dunnett's multiple comparison test, and values of $P<0.05$ were considered significant.

3. Results

3.1. Effect of anti-secretory drugs on loxoprofen-induced small intestinal lesions

Orally administered loxoprofen (10-100 mg/kg) in normally fed rats dose-dependently produced multiple hemorrhagic lesions in the small intestine, mainly in the jejunum and ileum. The severity of these lesions induced by loxoprofen at 60 mg/kg was similar to that of the lesions produced by indomethacin at 10 mg/kg. When animals were pretreated with lafutidine (10 and 30 mg/kg) given p.o., this treatment dose-dependently prevented the development of intestinal lesions in response to loxoprofen (60 mg/kg), and the effect was significant at 30 mg/kg; the inhibition rate was around 50 % (Figure 1). By contrast, neither cimetidine (100 mg/kg) nor famotidine (30 mg/kg), given p.o., had significant effect on the intestinal ulcerogenic response to loxoprofen. Similarly, omeprazole (100 mg/kg, p.o.) did not affect the severity of loxoprofen-induced intestinal lesions.

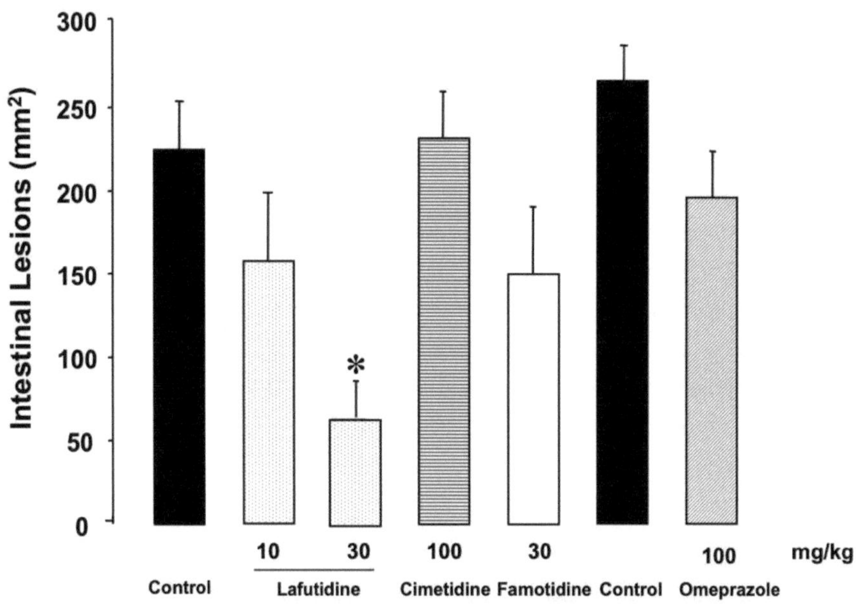

Figure 1. Effects of various agents on the intestinal lesions induced by loxoprofen in rats. Animals were given loxoprofen (60 mg/kg) p.o. and killed 24 h later. Lafutidine (10 and 30 mg/kg), cimetidine (100 mg/kg) or famotidine (30 mg/kg) was given p.o. twice, 30 min before and 6 h after administration of loxoprofen, while omeprazole (100 mg/kg) was given p.o. once, 30 min before. Data are presented as the mean±SE from 5~8 rats. *Significant difference from the corresponding control, at $P<0.05$. Data adapted after modification of ref. [26].

On the other hand, the severity of intestinal lesions induced by loxoprofen was significantly aggravated by chemical ablation of capsaicin-sensitive sensory neurons, about 1.4 times greater than the capsaicin nontreated animals (Figure 2). Lafutidine (30 mg/kg, p.o.) again significantly suppressed the intestinal ulcerogenic response to loxoprofen, but this effect was totally attenuated by sensory deafferentation, the lesion score was almost equivalent to the control value in the sensory deafferented animals.

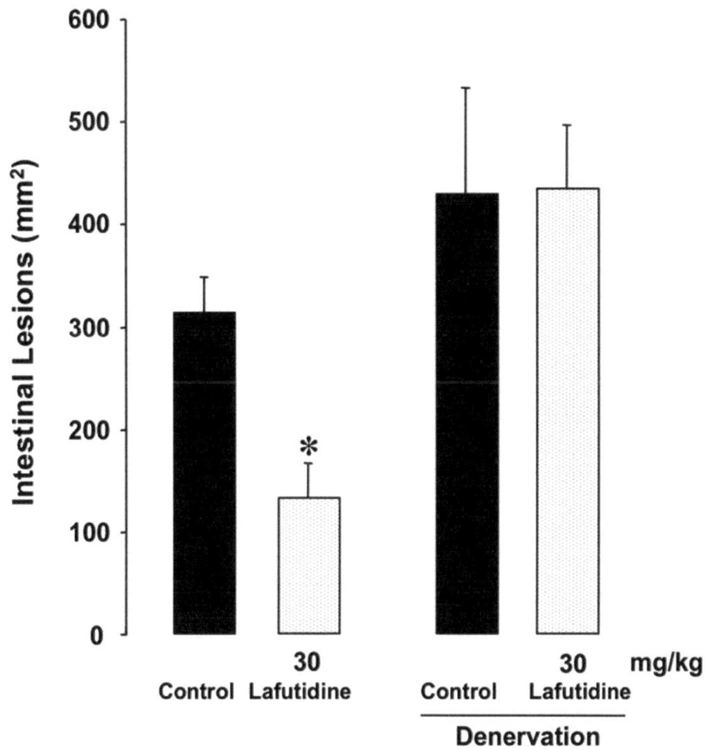

Figure 2. Effect of lafutidine on the intestinal lesions induced by loxoprofen in normal and sensory deafferented rats. Animals were given loxoprofen (60 mg/kg) p.o. and killed 24 h later. Sensory deafferentation was performed by 3 consecutive s.c. injections of capsaicin (total 100 mg/kg) 2 weeks before the experiment. Lafutidine (30 mg/kg) was given p.o. twice, 30 min before and 6 h after loxoprofen. Data are presented as the mean±SE from 6~7 rats. *Significant difference from control in normal rats, at $P<0.05$. Data adapted after modification of ref. [26].

3.2. Effect of lafutidine on mucosal invasion of enterobacteria caused by loxoprofen

Following oral administration of loxoprofen (60 mg/kg), the bacterial counts in both aerobic and anaerobic conditions were markedly increased compared to normal group, 24 h later (Table 1). Pretreatment of the animals with lafutidine (30 mg/kg) significantly prevented bacterial invasion in the mucosa following the administration of loxoprofen. The mucosal invasion of enterobacteria was also increased after loxoprofen treatment in sensory deafferented animals. The inhibitory effect of lafutidine on bacterial invasion was totally attenuated in the animals with sensory deafferentation.

	Numbers of Bacteria (Log CFU/g)	
	aerobic	anaerobic
Normal		
Control	6.79±0.99	7.62±0.56
Loxoprofen Na	9.51±0.42[a]	9.58±0.45[a]
+Lafutidine	7.88±0.34[b]	7.84±0.46[b]
Denervation		
Control	6.45±0.41	7.30±0.12
Loxoprofen Na	8.99±0.36[a]	9.30±0.19[a]
+Lafutidine	8.82±0.29	8.95±0.12

The animals were given loxoprofen (60 mg/kg, p.o.) and killed 24 h later. Lafutidine (30 mg/kg, p.o.) was given twice, 30 min before and 6 hr after the administration of sodium loxoprofen. Data are presented as the mean±SE from 4~5 rats. Significant difference at $P<0.05$; a) from the corresponding control, b) from loxoprofen in the normal group. Data adapted after modification of ref. [26].

Table 1. Effect of Lafutidine on Bacterial Counts in Rat Small Intestine

3.3. Changes in mucosal expression of iNOS and Muc2 mRNA

The iNOS mRNA expression was hardly detected in the normal intestinal mucosa, but markedly up-regulated after the administration of loxoprofen (60 mg/kg, p.o.) when examined 6 h later (Figure 3a). The up-regulation of iNOS expression following loxoprofen was markedly suppressed by pretreatment of the animals with lafutidine (30 mg/kg). Loxoprofen (60 mg/kg) similarly increased iNOS mRNA expression in sensory deafferented animals. In these animals, however, lafutidine did not affect the expression of iNOS mRNA in the small intestinal mucosa.

On the other hand, the expression of Muc2 mRNA was clearly detected in the normal intestinal mucosa, but apparently down-regulated after the administration of loxoprofen (60 mg/kg) when examined 6 h later (Figure 3b). The decrease in Muc2 expression caused by loxoprofen was almost totally reverted by pretreatment of lafutidine (30 mg/kg), but this effect was not observed in the animals with sensory deafferentation, similar to the inhibitory effect on the iNOS expression.

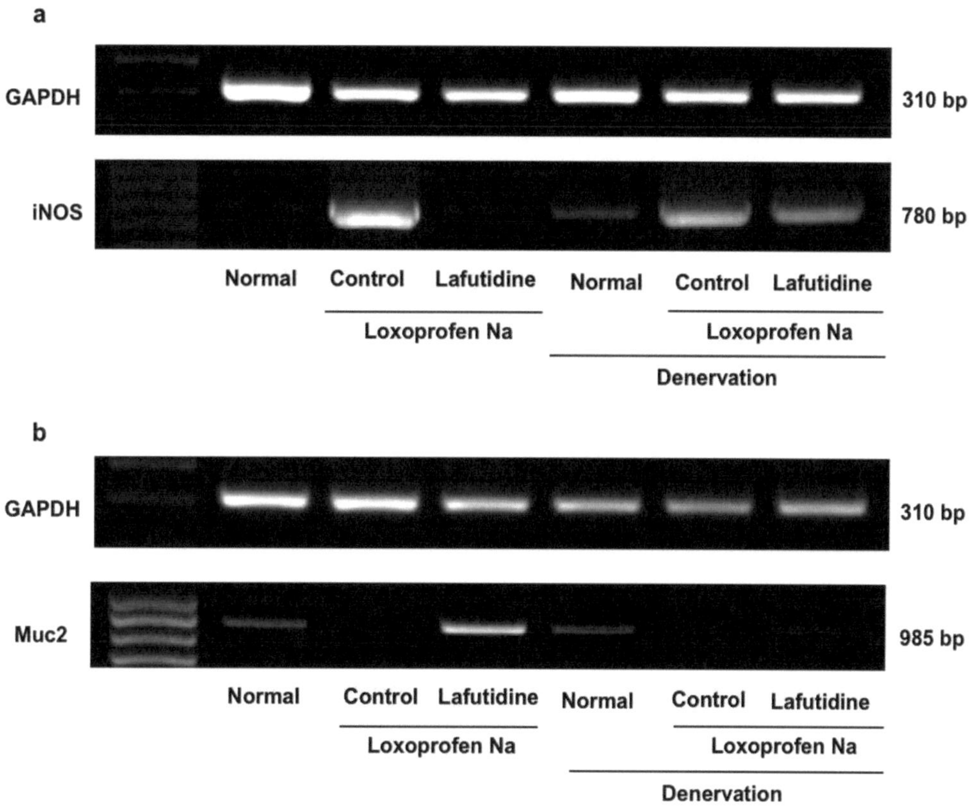

Figure 3. Effect of lafutidine on the expression of iNOS and Muc2 mRNAs in rat small intestine. Animals were given loxoprofen (60 mg/kg) p.o. and killed 6 h later. Sensory deafferentation was performed by 3 consecutive s.c. injections of capsaicin (total 100 mg/kg) 2 weeks before the experiment. Lafutidine (30 mg/kg) was given p.o. 30 min before the administration of loxoprofen. Data adapted after modification of ref. [26].

3.4. Effect of Lafutidine on PAS-Positive Substances in Small Intestine

In the normal intestinal mucosa, PAS-positive substances were observed over the surface epithelial cells and along the glands (Figure 4A). Loxoprofen (60 mg/kg, p.o.) apparently reduced the amount of PAS-positive substances in the epithelial cells as well as the glands (Figure 4B). However, the reduction in PAS staining was markedly restored when lafutidine (30 mg/kg) was administered prior to loxoprofen treatment (Figure 4C). In addition, lafutidine by itself increased the amount of PAS-positive substances in the mucosa compared to the control mucosa (Figure 4D).

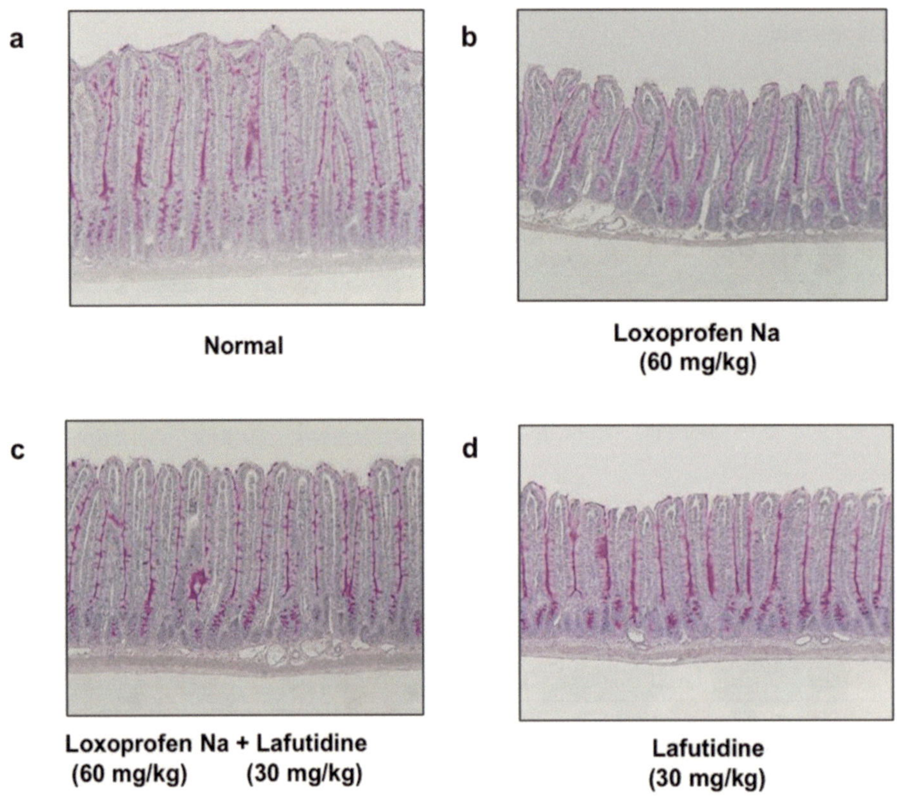

Figure 4. Microscopic observations of the rat small intestinal mucosa. The animals were given loxoprofen (60 mg/kg) p.o. and killed 3 h later. Lafutidine (30 mg/kg) was given p.o. 30 min before the administration of loxoprofen. Figures show; a: normal; b: loxoprofen alone; c: lafutidine plus loxoprofen; d: lafutidine alone. (PAS; x100). Data adapted after modification of ref. [26].

4. Commentary

The present study demonstrated that oral administration of loxoprofen induced multiple hemorrhagic lesions in the small intestine, similar to indomethacin [5], and that lafutidine protected these intestinal lesions, mediated by capsaicin-sensitive sensory neurons.

We confirmed that loxoprofen produced hemorrhagic lesions in the small intestine, and the severity of these lesions at 60 mg/kg was almost equivalent to that of the lesions generated by indomethacin. The onset of these lesions was accompanied by the mucosal invasion of enterobacteria and the up-regulation of iNOS expression, those events being similarly observed after indomethacin treatment. We also confirmed that the ulcerogenic response induced by loxoprofen in the small intestine was significantly prevented by pretreatment of the animals with dmPGE_2 as a supplement for PG deficiency or ampicillin as an antibiotic, the same was reported using the intestinal indomethacin-induced intestinal lesions [3-5].

Lafutidine is a histamine H_2-receptor antagonist with both antisecretory and gastroprotective action [17,18]. Onodera et al. [19] reported that the mucosal protective action of lafutidine was mediated by capsaicin-sensitive sensory neurons and independent of the antisecretory activity, because the action was not mimicked by cimetidine, another H_2-receptor antagonist, and was totally abolished by chemical deafferentation of sensory neurons. In the present study we observed that lafutidine protected the small intestine from loxoprofen-induced intestinal lesions. Certainly, this effect is not brought about by inhibition of gastric acid secretion, since omeprazole, an inhibitor of H^+/K^+ATPase, had no effect on this lesion model, similar to cimetidine. These drugs at the doses used (100 mg/kg) reportedly caused nearly a complete inhibition of acid secretion [22,23], supporting the idea that acid does not participate in the pathogenesis of loxoprofen-induced small intestinal lesions.

Lafutidine has been previously shown to prevent indomethacin-induced enteropathy and this effect was significantly attenuated by chemical ablation of capsaicin-sensitive sensory neurons [11]. Consistent with these findings, we found that lafutidine dose-dependently reduced the severity of intestinal lesions produced by loxoprofen and this action disappeared in the animals with sensory deafferentation. The peptidergic afferent innervation of the intestine has been demonstrated in various species of animals including the rat [14,24,25]. Several studies have demonstrated that stimulation of sensory neurons by capsaicin significantly prevented the occurrence of colitis as well as intestinal ulceration induced experimentally in rats [15,16]. We also noted that the ulcerogenic response to loxoprofen in the rat intestine was significantly aggravated by ablation of these sensory neurons. These results together with previous studies [11,15,16] strongly suggest that capsaicin-sensitive sensory neurons play a role in maintaining the mucosal integrity of the intestine against noxious stimuli, similarly in the stomach.

The intestinal ulcerogenic response to loxoprofen was also markedly suppressed by prior administration of ampicillin, an antibiotics, similar to that induced by indomethacin [26]. These findings were supported by the fact that NSAID-induced small intestinal lesions do not occur in germ-free animals or fasting animals [5,27], suggesting a major pathogenic role for entero-bacteria in these lesions. Because lafutidine significantly mitigated the bacterial invasion in the mucosa after loxoprofen treatment, this effect may account, at least partly, for the prophylactic effect of this agent against the intestinal lesions produced by loxoprofen. As mentioned earlier, the protective effect of lafutidine was almost totally attenuated by sensory deafferentation following capsaicin pretreatment. We also found in the present study that the suppression by lafutidine of the enterobacterial invasion following loxoprofen treatment was not observed in the sensory deafferented animals. Since mucus plays an important part in the innate host defense against intestinal pathogens and irritants, it is possible that a decreased mucus production/ secretion plays a role in the pathogenic mechanism of NSAID-induced intestinal damage by accelerating bacterial invasion in the mucosa. We have previously reported that indomethacin at an ulcerogenic dose reduced the amount of mucus secreted in the small intestine, in a PGE_2-sensitive manner, and this effect preceded bacterial invasion [10]. Lafutidine increased mucus secretion in the stomach, at least partly mediated by capsaicin-sensitive sensory neurons [28,29]. We observed in the present study that lafutidine by itself markedly increased levels of PAS-positive materials in the intestinal mucosa and reverted the reduced response to loxoprofen. Furthermore, it was found that lafutidine increased the expression of Muc2 mRNA in the small intestine and this response was totally mitigated by ablation of capsaicin-sensitive sensory neurons. Muc2, one of important mucin genes, plays an important role in the dimerization of secretory mucins, an essential step in the formation of the gastro-intestinal mucus-gels [30]. It is possible that lafutidine up-regulates Muc2 expression and mucus secretion through a sensory neuron-dependent mechanism and thereby increases the mucus gel thickness and hampers enterobacterial invasion in the mucosa.

Lafutidine prevented the up-regulation of iNOS expression in the small intestine, an important event in the occurrence of intestinal lesions caused by NSAIDs [2,31]. Boughton-Smith et al. [32] reported that bacterial endotoxin from E. coli enhanced the intestinal permeability though up-regulation of iNOS and overproduction of NO in the mucosa. Since lafutidine was found to prevent bacterial invasion, probably by up-regulating Muc2/mucus expression, it would be understandable that this agent suppressed the increase of iNOS expression in the small intestine following loxoprofen treatment. We previously reported that the mucosal protective drugs, such as irsogladine, rebamipide and teprenone, all significantly increased mucus secretion and suppressed bacterial invasion and iNOS expression, thereby reduced the severity of intestinal lesions produced by indomethacin [33]. These results together support a cause-effect relationship between changes in the above three events; ie., mucus secretion, bacterial invasion, and iNOS expression.

5. Summary

Lafutidine protects the small intestine against loxoprofen-induced lesions. This effect is not associated with inhibition of acid secretion due to the blockade of histamine H_2-receptors and appears to be mediated by capsaicin-sensitive sensory neurons. The exact mechanism underlying the intestinal protection by lafutidine remains unknown, yet it is assumed that lafutidine prevents the process of enterobacterial invasion in the mucosa by increasing the mucus gel layer through the up-regulation of Muc2 mRNA expression, and thereby suppresses iNOS induction, resulting in prevention of the occurrence of intestinal lesions following loxoprofen treatment.

Author details

Kikuko Amagase* and Koji Takeuchi

*Address all correspondence to: amagase@mb.kyoto-phu.ac.jp

Division of Pathological Sciences, Department of Pharmacology and Experimental Therapeutics, Kyoto Pharmaceutical University, Misasagi, Yamashina, Kyoto, Japan

The author declares no conflict of interest.

References

[1] Whittle BJR. Temporal relationship between cyclooxygenase inhibition, as measured by prostacyclin biosynthesis, and the gastrointestinal damage induced by indomethacin in the rat. Gastroenterology 80: 94-98, 1981

[2] Takeuchi K, Ueki S, Okabe S. Importance of gastric motility in the pathogenesis of indomethacin-induced gastric lesions in rats. Dig Dis Sci 31: 1114-1122, 1986

[3] Konaka A, Nishijima M, Tanaka A, Kato S, Takeuchi K. Nitric oxide, superoxide radicals and mast cells in pathogenesis of indomethacin-induced small intestinal lesions in rats. J Physiol Pharmacol 50: 25-38, 1999

[4] Takeuchi K, Miyazawa T, Tanaka A, Kato S, Kunikata T. Pathogenic importance of intestinal hypermotility in NSAID-induced small intestinal damage in rats. Digestion 66: 30-41, 2002

[5] Takeuchi K, Yokota A, Tanaka A, Takahira Y. Factors involved in upregulation of inducible nitric oxide synthase in rat small intestine following administration of nonsteroidal anti-inflammatory drugs. Dig Dis Sci 51: 1250-1259, 2006

[6] Yamada T, Deitch E, Specian RD, Perry MA, Sartor RB, Grisham MB. Mechanism of acute and chronic intestinal inflammation induced by indomethacin. Inflammation 17: 641-662, 1993

[7] Whittle BJR, Laszlo F, Evans SM, Moncada S. Induction of nitric oxide synthase and microvascular injury in the rat jejunum provoked by indomethacin. Br J Pharmacol 116: 2286-2290, 1995

[8] Wallace JL, McKnight W, Reuter BK, Vergnolle N. NSAID-induced gastric damage in rats: Requirement for inhibition of both cyclooxygenase 1 and 2. Gastroeneterology 119: 706-714, 2000

[9] Tanaka A, Araki H, Hase S, Takeuchi K. Inhibition of both COX-1 and COX-2 is required for development of gastric damage in response to nonsteroidal anti-inflammatory drugs. J Physiol Pari 95: 21-7, 2001

[10] Tanaka A, Hase S, Miyazawa T, Takeuchi K. Up-regulation of COX-2 by inhibition of COX-1: A key to NSAID-Induced intestinal damage. J Pharmacol Exp Ther 300: 754-761, 2002

[11] Kato S, Tanaka A, Kunikata T, Umeda M, Takeuchi K. Protective effect of lafutidine against indomethacin-induced intestinal ulceration in rats: Relation to capsaicin-sensitive sensory neurons. Digestion 61: 39-46, 2000

[12] Satoh H, Amagase K, Takeuchi K. Mucosal protective agents prevent exacerbation of NSAID-induced small intestinal lesions caused by antisecretory drugs in rats. J Pharmacol Exp Ther. 348: 227-35. 2014.

[13] Mashita Y, Taniguchi M, Yokota A, Tanaka A, Takeuchi K. Oral but not parenteral aspirin upregulates COX-2 expression in rat stomachs: A relationship between COX-2 expression and PG deficiency. Digestion 73: 124-132, 2006

[14] Holzer P: Neural emergency system in the stomach. Gastroenterology 114: 823-839, 1998

[15] Evangelista S, Meli A. Influence of capsaicin-sensitive fibers on experimentally induced colitis in rats. J Pharm Pharmacol 41: 574-575, 1989

[16] Goso C, Evangelista S, Tramontana M, Manzini S, Blumberg PM, Szallasi A. Topical capsaicin administration protects against trinitrobenzene sulfonic acid-induced colitis in the rat. Eur J Pharmacol 249: 185-190, 1993.

[17] Shibata M, Yamaura T, Inaba N, Onodera S, Chida Y, Ohnishi H. Gastric antisecretory effect of FRG-8813, a new histamine H_2 receptor antagonist, in rats and dogs. Eur J Pharmacol 235: 243-253, 1993

[18] Yamaura T, Shibata M, Inaba N, Onodera S, Chida Y, Ohnishi H. Effects of FRG-8813, a new type histamine H_2-receptor antagonist, on various experimental gastric and duodenal lesions in rats. Folia Pharmacol Japonica 99: 401-410, 1992

[19] Onodera S, Shibata M, Tanaka M. et al. Gastroprotective activity of FRG-8813, a novel histamine H_2-receptor antagonist, in rats. Jpn J Pharmacol 68: 161-173, 1995

[20] Tekeuchi K, Matsumoto J, Ueshima K, Okabe S. Role of capsaicin-sensitive afferent neurons in alkaline secretory response to luminal acid in the rat duodenum. Gastroenterlogy 101: 954-961, 1991

[21] Deitch EA, Ma L, Ma WJ, Grisham MB, Granger DN, Specian RD, Berg RD. Inhibition of endotoxin-induced bacterial translocation in mice. J Clin Invest 84: 36-42, 1989

[22] Yamazaki S, Kawamura M, Kitsukawa M, Ando K, Nitta I, Tobe A, Okabe S. Effects of MCI-727, a new antiulcer agent, on various gastric and duodenal lesions in experimental animals. Jpn J Pharmacol. 55: 415-424, 1991

[23] Yamamoto O, Okada Y, Okabe S. Effects of a proton pump inhibitor, omeprazole, on gastric secretion and gastric and duodenal ulcers or erosions in rats. Dig Dis Sci 29: 394-401, 1984

[24] Koch TR, Carney JA, Go VLW. Distribution and quantitation of gut neuropeptides in normal intestine and inflammatory bowel diseases. Dig Dis Sci 32: 369-376, 1987

[25] Sternini C, Reeve JR, Brecha N. Distribution and characterization of calcitonin gene-related peptide immunoreactive activity in the digestive system of normal and capsaicin-treated rats. Gastroenterology 93: 852-862, 1987

[26] Amagase K, Ochi A, Sugihara T, Kato S, Takeuchi K. Protective effect of lafutidine, a histamine H2 receptor antagonist, against loxoprofen-induced small intestinal lesions in rats. J. Gastroenterol. Hepatol., 25: S111-S118, 2010

[27] Yamada T, Deitch E, Specian RD, Perry MA, Sartor RB, Grisham MB. Mechanism of acute and chronic intestinal inflammation induced by indomethacin. Inflammation 17: 641-662, 1993

[28] Ichikawa T, Ishihara K, Saigennji K, Hotta K. Effect of acid inhibitory antiulcer drugs on mucin biosynthesis in the rat stomach. Eur J Pharmacol 251: 107-111, 1994

[29] Kagoshima M, Kodaira H, Tanaka M, Shimada H. Effect of FRG-8813, a new histamine H_2-receptor antagonist, on gastric mucus production in rats (in Japanese). Folia Pharmacol Japonica 106: 385-392, 1995

[30] van Klinken BJ, Einerhand AW, Büller HA, Dekker J. The oligomerization of a family of four genetically clustered human gastrointestinal mucins. Glycobiology 8: 67-75, 1998

[31] Whittle BJ, László F, Evans SM, Moncada S. Induction of nitric oxide synthase and microvascular injury in the rat jejunum provoked by indomethacin. Br. J. Pharmacol. 116: 2286-2290, 1995

[32] Boughton-Smith N, Evans SM, Laszlo F, Whittle BJR, Moncada S: The induction of nitric oxide synthase and intestinal vascular permeability by endotoxin in the rat. Br J Pharmacol 110: 1189-1195, 1993

[33] Kamei K, Kubo Y, Kato N, Hatazawa R, Amagase K, Takeuchi K. Prophylactic effect of irsogladine maleate against indomethacin-induced small intestinal lesions in rats. Dig Dis Sci 53: 2657-2666, 2008

Section 5

Observations with Capsaicin in the Human Gastrointestinal Tract

Chapter 10

Capsaicin-Sensitive Afferent Nerves and the Human Gastrointestinal Tract

Gyula Mózsik, András Dömötör, József Czimmer,
Imre L. Szabó and János Szolcsányi

Additional information is available at the end of the chapter

http://dx.doi.org/10.5772/58360

1. Introduction

Capsaicin is an active ingredient of red pepper and paprika. These plants are well known and used in every day of the culinary practice for about 9000-9500 years.

It was an important discovery that the capsaicin (capsaicin, dihydrocapsaicin, nordihydrocapsaicin and other capsaicinoids) specifically modify the function of certain nerves, later named to capsaicin sensitive afferent nerves (Jancsó et al., 1967; 1968; 1970).

Capsaicin activates the capsaicin (vanilloid) receptor expressed a subgroup of primary afferent nociceptive neurons (Szolcsányi, 2004). The capsaicin receptor has been cloned (Caterina et al., 1997) and turned out to be a cation channel. It is gated besides capsaicin and other capsaicinoids (some vanilloids) by low pH, noxious heat and various pains – producing endogenous and exogenous chemicals. Thus, these sensory nerve endings equipped with these ion channels are prone to be stimulated in gastric mucosa.

The action of capsaicin on the capsaicin sensitive afferent nerves is dose dependent (Szolcsányi and Barthó, 1981; Szolcsányi, 1984; 1997; 2004; Abdel-Salam et al., 1999; 2001; Mózsik et al., 2001). Szolcsányi indicated four different stages of capsaicin action (depending on the dose and duration of the exposure of the compound): a. excitation (stage 1); b. sensory blocking effect (stage 2); c. long-term selective neurotoxin impairment (stage 3) and d. irreversible cell destruction (stage 4) (Szolcsányi, 1984). The stages 1 and 2 are reversible; meanwhile the stages 3 and 4 are irreversible compound-induced actions on the capsaicin sensitive afferent nerve. These stages of capsaicin actions can be detected in the gastrointestinal (GI) tract (Mózsik et al., 2001) in animal experiments.

The vagal nerve has a key-role in the development of GI mucosal damage and prevention (Mózsik et al., 1982). The potency of vagal nerve has been emphasized dominantly in the aggressive processes to GI mucosa (such as peptic ulcer disease, gastric mucosal damage, etc.) in both animal models and in human investigations. The „chemical" and „surgical" vagotomy widely used in the treatment of patients with peptic ulcer disease in the years up to middle of 1970 (Karádi and Mózsik, 2000). By the other words, the primary aims of this therapy were to decrease the activity of vagal nerve at the level of efferent nerves in the target organs.

The application of capsaicin in the animal experiments was used as a specific tool to approach the group of primary afferent nociceptive neurons (Szolcsányi, 2004; Buck and Burks, 1986; Holzer, 1988; 1991; Szállasi and Blumberg, 1999, Holzer, 2013) involved in the different physiological, pathological processes and medical therapy in human healthy subjects and in patients with different GI disorders as well those treated with nonsteroidal anti-inflammatory drugs (NSAIDs).

Szolcsányi and Barthó (1981) were the firsts, who clearly indicated the beneficial and harmful effect of capsaicin in the peptic ulcer disease in rats on dependence of applied doses of capsaicin. Later, Holzer started with a very extensive research work with capsaicin in the field of gastroenterology (Holzer, 1998; 1999; Buck and Burks, 1986; Szállasi and Blumberg, 1999, Holzer, 2013). Our group also participated in the GI capsaicin research in animals experiments from 1980 (Mózsik et al., 1997) (the historical background see the chapter written by Szolcsányi, 2014).

Even new drug, Lafutidine, was developed in the medical treatment of GI mucosal damage (Ajioka et al., 2000; 2002; Onodera et al., 1995; 1999; Takeuchi, 2006). The Lafutidine is a histamin-2-receptor (H_2R) blocking compound showed typical capsaicin actions at the target organ.

The new and interesting results obtained with capsaicin application in animal experiments offered excellent tools to approach the different events of human GI physiology, pathology and pharmacology and to produce new drug or new drug combinations in human healthy subjects and patients with different GI and other diseases (myocardial infarction, thrombophylia, rheumatoid arthritis, chronic pain killer use).

We started clinical studies with capsaicin from 1997 (Mózsik et al., 1999; Debreceni et al., 1999; Mózsik et al., 2004a; 2004b; 2005) and these studies incorporated the different regulatory mechanisms of capsaicin in the human stomach, gastric mucosal preventive effects of capsaicin(noids) on the NSAID-induced gastric mucosal damage, chronic gastritis with Helicobacter pylori (H. pylori) positive and negative gastritis (with and without eradication treatment). We performed immuno-histochemical examinations of capsaicin receptor (TRPV1), calcitonin-gene-related peptide (CGRP), substance P (SP) in the human GI mucosa of patients with various GI disorders, took significant steps in the development of capsaicin containing drug and drug combinations (with aspirin, diclofenac, Naproxen), including the preparation of protocols for human phase I. examinations [and to carried out these examinations after the receiving permission from the National Institute of Pharmacy (Budapest, Hungary) and National Clinical Pharmacological and Ethical Committee of Hungary].

http://dx.doi.org/10.5772/58360

These studies were carried out as propective, randomized and multiclinical studies of human healthy subjects and in patients with various gastrointestinal disorders including gastric mucosal damage produced by application of NSAIDs or H. pylori infection.

The aims of this review are: (1) to give a short summary on the actions of capsaicin on the human gastrointestinal tract (dominantly on the stomach), (2) to indicate some details of gastroprotective actions of capsaicin in human healthy subjects; (3) to demonstrate the capsaicin-induced gastric protective effects against the NSAID-(selective and non-selective COX inhibitor) induced gastric microbleedings in human healthy subjects; (4) to prove the independency of TRPV1 and CGRP expression from the presence of the H. pylori positive or negative chronic gastritis, the efficacy of successfully carried out eradication treatment in patients with H. pylori positive gastritis in patients; 5. to indicate the clinical pharmacological problems of plant origin capsaicin in humans (in term of drug processing); (6). to point out that the gastroprotective effects of capsaicin (given orally in stimulatory doses of capsaicin on the capsaicin-sensitive afferent nerves) to human healthy subjects, and as treatment to patients who are under chronic NSAID use (like patients with myocardial infarction, stroke, thrombophylia, rheumatic diseases, etc.).

In terms of classical pharmacology we would like to demonstrate clearly in the human observations that the applied doses of capsaicin stimulate the capsaicin-sensitive afferent nerve with a clear cut exclusion of the existence of capsaicin desensitation.

On the other hand, our research activity clearly demonstrates the different difficulties of capsaicin(oids) application as new gastroprotective drug for healthy subjects and for patients with different GI disorders and NSAIDs use in regards to toxicology plant cultivation, storage, chemical detection and standardization questions as well as permission requests from authorities needed prior the launch of industrial processing of plant-derived, orally applicable drug or drug combinations.

2. Materials and methods

The observations were carried out in 198 healthy human subjects aged 25-65 years (40± 10 years) and in 178 patients with various GI disorders (gastritis, erosion, ulcer, polyps, cancer and chronic inflammatory bowel diseases, polyps, precancerous states, colorectal cancer), aged ranged 25-75 years (45±10), 69 patients with chronic gastritis 39-68 years (mean: 56.4 years) (altogether 445 healthy persons and GI patients).

The observations were carried out at First Department of Medicine, Department of Pharmacology and Pharmacotherapy and Institute of Pharmaceutical Chemistry, University of Pécs, Hungary, in the Department of Gastroenterology of Petz Aladár Teaching Hospital, Győr, Hungary, in the Department of Gastroenterology of Markusovszky Hospital, Szombathely, Hungary (and their relevant Departments of Pathology), in Histopatology Ltd., Pécs, Hungary and at our industrial research partner (PannonPharma Ltd., Pécsvárad, Hungary).

The human healthy subjects and patients were included into the groups of different randomized, prospective studies (see later).

The classical human clinical pharmacological phase I examinations were carried out in 15 healthy males in each protocol (additionally up today, 30 human healthy subjects for human phase I examinations for aspirin plus capsaicin and diclofenac plus capsaicin) (some parts of these observations are presented by the book chapter written Mózsik et al., 2014).

The physical, laboratory, and iconographic examinations were normal in the healthy human subjects, in patients with various GI disorders.

The healthy persons were randomized into different groups of prospective, randomized and prospective studies for evaluation the effects of capsaicin on:

1. gastric basal acid secretion (BAO) (Mózsik et al., 1999, 2005);
2. changes in cations, anions, albumin concentration (and outputs) of gastric secretory responses (Mózsik et al., 2004a; 2005);
3. gastric emptying (Debreceni et al., 1999);
4. sugar (glucose) loading test (75 g given orally) (Dömötör et al., 2006b);
5. gastric transmucosal potential difference (GTPD) alone (Mózsik et al., 2005);
6. GTPD measurement after intragastric administration of ethanol and capsaicin application (Mózsik et al., 2005);
7. indomethacin-induced gastric microbleedings without and with capsaicin (Fisher and Hunt, 1976).

The different doses of capsaicin (1 – 8 μg/100 mL in saline solution) were intragastrically given to identify the ED_{50} values on the gastric basal acid secretion. These doses of capsaicin were used to determine direct action of capsaicin on the gastric transmucosal potential difference (GTPD) (without and with intragastric administration of ethanol) and indomethacin-induced gastric microbleedings.

The all of the healthy volunteers received capsaicin in doses with random allocation. In the observations to study the gastric emptying, sugar loading test, the effect of the ED_{50} value (400 μg intragastrically given) of capsaicin was tested.

The 178 patients with different GI disorders were studied by immunohistochemical examinations of biopsy samples. The histological diagnosis was established on the opinion of independent pathologist. The immunohistochemical examinations for capsaicin receptor, CGRP, SP were carried out on the same on paraffin-embedded tissues samples from which the classical histological diagnosis was established by the independent pathologist (Dömötör et al., 2005, 2006).

The patients with chronic gastritis (69 patients) were divided H. pylori positive and negative groups. Smaller group of patients with H. pylori infection were studied further after classical eradication treatment had been performed.

The observations were carried out according to the method of Good Clinical Practice (GCP). The studies were carried out from 1997 up to now, which were permitted by the Regional

http://dx.doi.org/10.5772/58360

Ethical Committee of University of Pécs, Hungary. Written informed consent was obtained from all participants.

The following main methods were used in the human observations:

2.1. Determination of gastric basal acid out (BAO)

Determination of gastric basal acid out (BAO) in human healthy subjects: After an overnight fasting, a nasogastric tube was introduced at 8.00 a.m., and the total gastric content was suctioned. Than the newly secreted gastric juice was suctioned every 15 min for 1 h (BAO). The healthy subjects received intragastrically capsaicin (100, 200, 400 and 800 μg ig.), atropine (0.1-1.0 mg sc.), Pirenzepine 25-50 mg, famotidine (20-40 mg orally), ranitidine (150-300 mg orally), cimetidine (100-1000 mg orally), Omeprazole (20 – 40 mg iv.) and Esomeprazole (20-40 mg orally) given for determinations their dose responses curves (Mózsik et al., 2005; 2007; Szabó et al., 2013).

Gastric acid secretion was measured by titration of gastric juice with 0.1 N NaOH to pH 7.0 (pH titrimeter, Radelkis, Budapest). The gastric acid outputs were expressed as mmol/h (means ± SEM).

2.2. Determination of affinity and intrinsic activity curves

Determination of affinity and intrinsic activity curves for drugs inhibiting BAO in healthy human subjects: The applied doses of drugs were expressed in molar values, which were used to determine the affinity and intrinsic activity curves of the different drugs by the method of Csáky (1969). For drawing the affinity and intrinsic activity curves the doses of various drugs were expressed in [-] molar values, which offered to analyze the drug actions on the BAO according to the classical molecular pharmacological methods. We identified the pD_2 values (necessary doses of drugs to produce 50 per cent inhibition on BAO values). The effect of atropine ($\alpha_{atropine}$=1.00) in case of identification of intrinsic activity curves for other drugs and capsaicin (Mózsik, 2006).

2.3. Chemical composition of gastric juice without and with capsaicin application

These observations were carried out in the same healthy human subjects. The concentrations of Na^+, $K^+$and calcium^{2+}in the gastric juice were measured flamephotometrically. The concentration of $Mg^{2+}$was measured by atomic absorption spectrophotometrically, the chloride concentration by colorimetric method, the protein content by the method of biuret reaction. The 400 μg of capsaicin (as ED_{50} value) was used in these studies.

2.4. Calculation of „parietal" and „ non-parietal" components of gastric secretory responses without and with capsaicin

The chloride linked to $H^+$and sodium was calculated for the determination of „parietal" (chloride linked to H^+) and „non-parietal" (linked to sodium) components of gastric BAO (Hollander, 1934).

2.5. Measurement of gastric transmucosal potential difference (GTPD)

GTPD was measured during endoscopy. The exploring mucosal electrode was passed through the biopsy channel of gastroscope and the reference electrode was placed on the volar surface of the left forearm. The electrodes were connected to a digital voltmeter (Radelkis, Budapest, Hungary, OP 211/1). GTPD measurements were done at the greater curvature of the gastric body and the results were expressed in –mV (without and with intragastrically administration of different doses of capsaicin) (Hossennbocus et al., 1975; Mózsik et al., 2005). Five mL capsaicin (300 mL/L, diluted in saline) was intragastrically applied and only saline solution was given to identify the baseline in GTPD. The ΔGTPD values were expressed in –mV, ΔGTPD max was calculated at five minutes after intragastric application of capsaicin.

2.6. Effect of capsaicin on ethanol-induced changes GTPD changes

The GTPD baseline was identified. Then ethanol (5 mL, 300 mL/L) was intragastrically given. The GTPD change was determined after the ethanol had been passed through the biopsy channel of gastroscope without and with capsaicin administration (given in different doses in the same pathway after 1 min of ethanol administration).

2.7. Measurements of gastric microbleeding produced by acute application of indomethacin (without and with capsaicin administration) in healthy human subjects

Non-selective COX inhibitor, indomethacin (IND) was used to induce gastric microbleeding. The extents of IND-induced gastric microbleeding were measured in healthy human subjects by the method of hemoglobin concentration in the gastric juice respecting the value of gastric emptying rate (Fisher and Hunt, 1976). The details of this method were described in one previous paper (Mózsik et al., 2005).

2.7.1. Baseline of gastric mucosal microbleedings in acute observations with human healthy subjects

The baseline of gastric microbleeding was measured in the gastric juice without application of any drug and/or capsaicin. The hemoglobin concentration was determined. The extent of gastric emptying was measured with application of phenol red into the stomach (by the method of Fisher and Hunt 1976; Nagy et al., 1984). The extent of gastric microbleeding was expressed in mL/day (means ±SEM), and this value was taken as baseline (used as control for other observations).

2.7.2. Capsaicin-induced acute mucosal protection on the IND-induced acute gastric microbleeding in healthy human subjects

The healthy human subjects received IND (3x25 mg given orally for a day), and the forthcoming day the gastric microbleeding was measured on forthcoming day, when these healthy human subjects also received 25 mg IND orally. The extent of gastric microbleeding was measured as mentioned above, and its value was expressed as mL/ day (means ± SEM).

2.8. Measurements of gastric emptying

The gastric emptying measurements were performed on two consecutive days by the same protocol, without capsaicin on first day and with capsaicin (400 μg orally given, ED_{50} value) on second day. The measurement procedure was the following. The healthy human subjects went on an overnight starvation and the observations were started at 8.00 a.m. In total, 100 mL of ^{13}C-octanoid acid (Izinta, Budapest, Hungary) was given for the gastric emptying measurements. This material was given in 200 mL physiological saline and 75 g glucose was added to the solution. The volunteers exhaled into a plastic bag with a volume of 0.5 L. The first air sample was considered as reference. Then, the volunteers swallowed the test solution and gave air samples in every 15 min. The IRIS performed the infrared spectroscopy (IRIS, Izinta, Budapest, Hungary) measurements and calculated the delta over base (DOB) values. This value was directly proportional to the ratio $^{13}CO_2$ and $^{12}CO_2$ (DOB is about $^{13}CO_2/^{12}CO_2$) in the air sample. When we respected the DOB values against to the time in the graph, we obtained a gastric emptying curve. On this curve, we could consider the following four parameters to characterize gastric emptying rate: 1. maximal value of DOB (DOB_{max} unit) (U); 2. the time at DOB_{max} (U/min); 3. the slope of the rising part of the curve (U/min) and 4. the time at 50% of area under curve ($AUC_{50\%}$, min). The DOB_{max} and slope are direct, meanwhile the time at DOB_{max} and the time at $AUC_{50\%}$ are inversely proportional to gastric emptying (Debreceni et al., 1999; Mózsik et al., 2004a).

2.9. Sugar loading test in healthy human subjects

The glucose (75 g) was orally given in 100 mL water. The plasma level of glucose was measured enzymatical (Boehringer, Germany). The plasma levels of insulin (μIU/mL) (Biochem Immunsystem), C peptide and glucagon (pg/mL) (Byk-Sangtect Diagnostic GmbH) were measured by RIA. The all measurements were carried out before and after administration repeatedly in every 15 mins for 4 h period (Dömötör et al., 2006b).

2.10. Immunohistochemical examinations in the gastric and large bowel mucosa in patients with various disorders

The classical pathological histological examinations were carried out by an independent pathologist for giving the histopathological diagnosis of patients (besides the classical laboratory, iconographic examinations).

The specific immunohistochemical examinations were used for the same biopsy specimens used for pathological examination. Specific antisera were used for detection of vanilloid (TRVP1) receptor (polyclonal anti-TRVP1, Abcam, Cambridge, UK), CGRP (polyclonal anti-CGRP, Abcam, Cambridge, UK) and SP (monoclonal anti SP, Abcam, Cambridge, UK).

The TRVP1 and CGRP positive and/or negativity was detected, meanwhile SP staining was evaluated by a semi-quantitave scale (Dömötör et. al., 2005).

2.11. Detection of Helicobacter pylori in patients with chronic gastritis

The presence of H. pylori was detected by ^{13}C-urea breath test (Izinta, Hungary) and with specific histological staining of biopsy specimens. The diagnosis of chronic gastritis was based on the classical pathological histology. The results of observations were expressed as means ± SEM. The unpaired and paired Student's *t* tests were used for the calculation of results between the identical observations. P value ≤ 0.05 was considered statistically significant.

2.12. Evaluation of capsaicin-stimulated gastric mucosal protection on IND-induced gastric microbleeding and capsaicin-produced gastric mucosal protection on the IND-induced gastric microbleeding before and after 2 weeks capsaicin treatment (based on randomized, prospective and multi-clinical study in healthy subjects) (Mózsik et al., 2004 a; 2005; 2007)

2.12.1. Measurement of gastric microbleeding before and after 2 weeks capsaicin treatment

The baseline in gastric microbleeding was measured and carried out as those under the point of 7.1. The gastric microbleeding was expressed in mL/ day (means ±SEM).

2.12.2. Measurement of IND-induced acute gastric microbleeding before and after 2-week capsaicin treatment

These measurements were carried out in healthy human subjects as those were written under 7.2. These healthy subjects received 3x25 mg IND for one day and 25 mg IND on the next day before the measurement of the extent of gastric microbleeding. The gastric microbleeding was expressed in mL/day (means ±SEM).

2.12.3. Measurement of capsaicin-induced acute gastric mucosal protection against the IND-induced acute gastric microbleeding before and after 2-week capsaicin treatment

The observations were carried out under the observational circumstances mentioned in 12.2, however, different doses of capsaicin (200 and 400 μg given orally) were used. Two hundred and 400 μg capsaicin were applied given orally before the measurement of IND-induced acute gastric microbleeding before and after 2-week capsaicin treatment.

2.12.4. Evaluation of capsaicin's effect by randomized, prospective, multi-clinical studies in patients with chronic Helicobacter pylori positive gastritis before and after eradication treatment to capsaicin-effect due to stimulation of capsaicin-sensitive neural afferentation (Lakner et al 2011)

These studies were carried out in 38 persons (including 20 healthy persons and 18 patients with H. pylori positive gastritis). The histologically normal controls were in ages: 41 to 67 years, mean: 52.1 years), meanwhile the ages of patients with chronic Helicobacter pylori infection were 39 to 68 years, mean: 56.4 years) (Lakner et al., 2011).

The presence of H. pylori was determined by the methods mentioned above.

The eradication therapy was involved a seven days treatment with double dose proton-pump inhibitor consisting of PPI (pantoprazole 2x40 mg/day), amoxicillin (1000 mg twice daily) and clarithromycin (500 mg twice daily), according to European guidelines (Malfertheiner et al., 2007). Following this one week of eradication period, the patients further treated with normal dose of PPI for other another week.

The gastroscopies, gastric biopsies, general and special immuno-histochemical examinations were carried out at the time of entry of patients into the eradication treatment, after the eradication treatment (Lakner et al., 2011).

2.13. Used drugs and compounds

Anticholinergic (atropine, Egis, Budapest, Hungary), antimuscarinic (Pirenzepine, Boehringer, Ingelheim, Germany) agents; [histamine H_2-receptor antagonists (Cimetidine, Pannon-Pharma, Hungary), ranitidine (Biogal-Teva, Hungary), famotidine (Richter Gedeon, Hungary)], proton pump inhibitors (PPI) [(Omeprazole, Astra-Zeneca, Sweden), Esomeprazole (Astra-Zeneca, Sweden)]; indomethacin (Chinoin, Budapest, Hungary) were used.

Capsaicin was applied in these studies obtained from Asian Herbex Ltd: Capsaicin USP as manufactured in Andhra Pradesh, India). The Drug Master File (DMF) is signed in the documentation of Drug and Food Administration (FDA) in the United States as only one capsaicin preparation for orally applicable preparate (" 17856 A II 26.10.2004 Asian Herbex Ltd. : Capsaicin USP as manufactured in Andhra Pradesh, India") (for further details, see Mózsik et al. 2009b).

2.14. Statistical evaluation of results

The results were expressed as means ± SEM. The paired and unpaired Student's t test and ANOVA test were used for the statistical analysis of the results. The results were taken to be significant when the P value was found ≤ 0.05. Special mathematical programs were applied for the evaluation of results of human phase I. examinations.

3. Results

3.1. Capsaicin-induced BAO in healthy human subjects

The capsaicin (given in doses of 100, 200,400 and 800 μg orally) dose-dependently inhibited the gastric acid output (Y=-0.13.X+1.164; r=0.97; n=16; $P < 0.001$) (Mózsik et al., 1999; Mózsik et al., 2005). The ED_{50} value of capsaicin was obtained as 400 μg/person on the gastric BAO (in case of administration of capsaicin in doses which stimulates the capsaicin-sensitive afferent nerves) (Figures 1 and 2) (Mózsik et al., 1999; 2005).

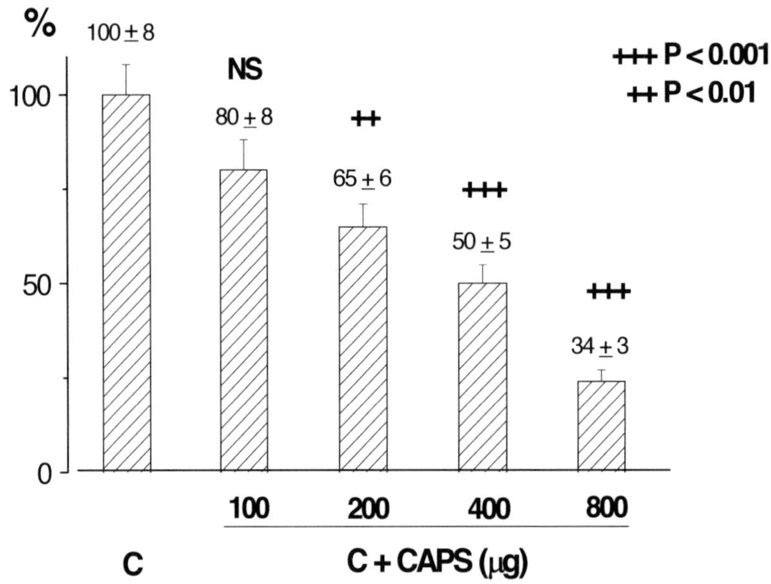

Figure 1. Capsaicin-induced inhibition on gastric basal acid output (BAO) in 16 human healthy subject. The results were expressed as per cent of untreated (control) group (means±SEM). The results of the mathematical analysis were expressed as control vs. capsaicin treated groups. Abbreviations: NS=not significant;++=P<0.01;+++=P<0.001 (Mózsik et al., J Physiol Paris 93:433-436, 1999).

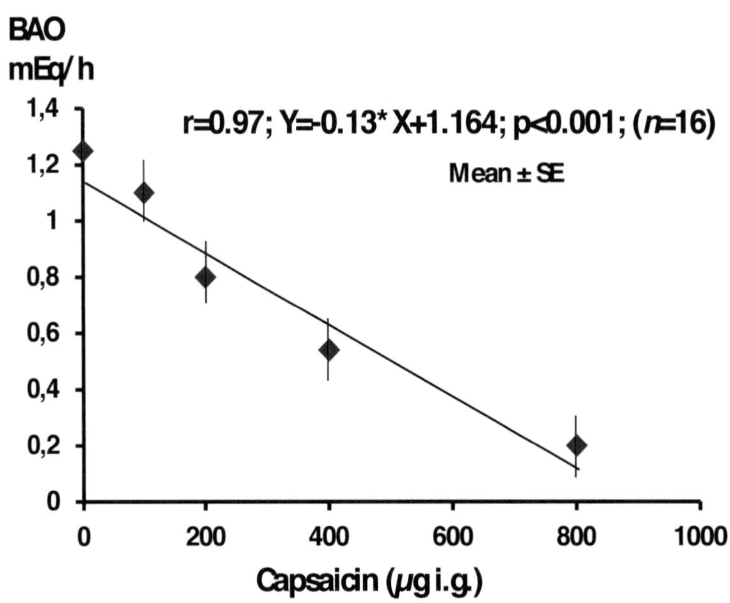

Figure 2. Inhibition of gastric acid basal output (BAO) by capsaicin in 16 healthy human subjects (after Mózsik et al.: World J Gastroenterol 11: 5180-83, 2005).

3.2. Affinity and intrinsic affinity curves for the capsaicin, muscarinic agents, H_2-receptor antagonists and proton pump inhibitors on BAO in healthy human subjects

The action of the compounds inhibiting the gastric basal acid secretion is presented by Figure 3. The curve indicates that no competitive actions of these drugs exist on the gastric basal acid output. The pD_2 values were calculated from the affinity curves obtained in the molecular pharmacological studies.

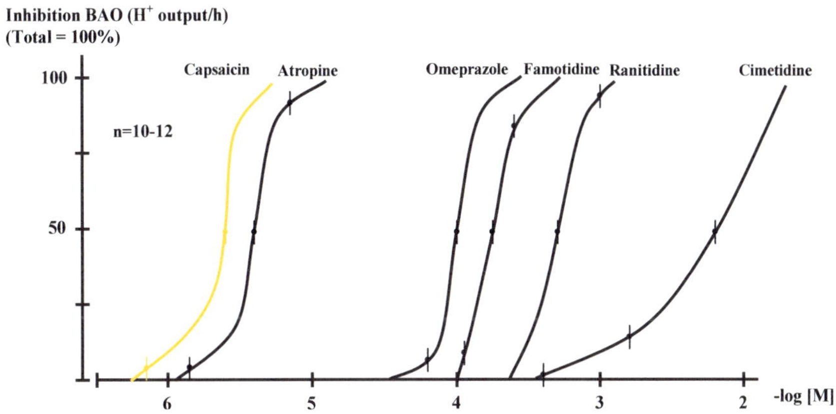

Figure 3. Affinity curves for drugs inhibitory actions of different antisecretory drugs on the gastric basal acid output (BAO) in human healthy subjects. The absolute values were calculated as H^+output/h, the presentations of curves expressed in per cent value (total=100%) (means ±SEM). (After Mózsik et al.: Inflammopharmacology 15: 232-45, 2007)

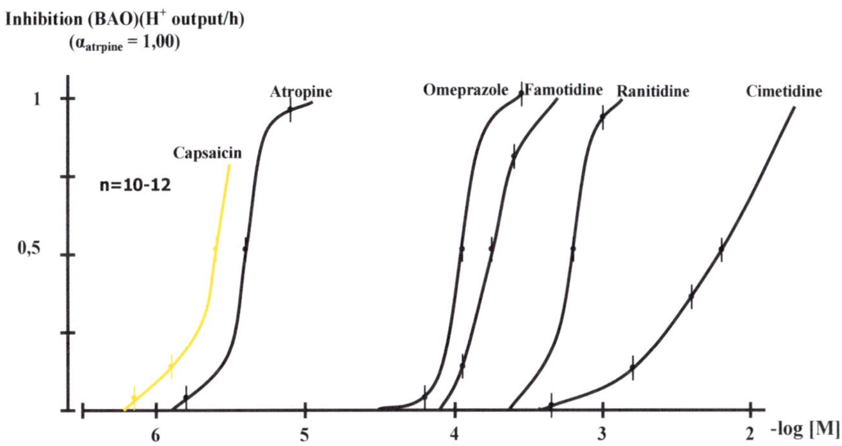

Figure 4. Intrinsic activity curves for the inhibitory drugs of different antisecretory drugs and capsaicin (given in stimulatory doses of capsaicin-sensitive afferent nerves) on the gastric acid basal output (BAO) in human healthy subjects, which were expressed to action of atropine (1.00) (α atropine) (means ±SEM). (After Mózsik et al.: Inflammopharmacology 15: 232-45, 2007).

The intrinsic activity curves for the drugs inhibiting the gastric basal acid outputs in healthy human subjects were calculated. The intrinsic activity ($\alpha_{atropine}$=1.00) was taken to be equal to 1.00, and the values for other drugs were expressed to action of atropine (Figure 4). The pA_2 values (50 % inhibition of intrinsic activity in [-] molar values) were calculated from the intrinsic activity curves.

For the molecular pharmacological understanding the background of the action of drugs, action the molecular weights, pD_2 values, of the intrinsic activity (in comparison to atropine action) and pA_2 values were calculated and presented in Table 1.

Compounds	M.W.	pD_2	Intrinsic activity	pA_2
Capsaicin	305,4	5,88	0,76	5,87
Atropine	289,38	5,40	1,00	5,40
Pirenzepine	424,34	3,93	0,89	3,93
Cimetidine	252,34	2,23	1,00	2,23
Ranitidine	314,41	3,33	1,00	3,33
Famotidine	337,43	3,77	1,00	3,77
Nizatidine	331,47	3,34	1,00	3,34
Omeprazole	345,42	3,97	1,00	3,97
Esomeprazole	345,42	3,97	1,00	3,97

Table 1. Summary of the affinity (pD_2) and intrinsic activity (expressed in value of $\alpha_{atropine}$=1,00)(pA_2) values of capsaicin, atropine, Pirenzepine, cimetidine, ranitidine, famotidine, Omeprazole and Esomeprazole on the gastric basal acid output (BAO) in healthy human subjects. (After Mózsik et al.: Inflammopharrmacology 15:232-45, 2007)

The Figures 3, 4 and Table 1 clearly indicate that the capsaicin acts in the smaller doses as those drugs acting on the muscarinic (atropine, Pirenzepine), H_2R receptor antagonists (cimetidine, ranitidine, fomatidine, nizatidine) and proton pump inhibitors (Omeprazole, Esomeprazole).

3.3. Changes in the „parietal" and „non-parietal" components of gastric secretory responses in healthy human subjects

The measurements of cations (H^+, sodium, potassium, calcium, magnesium) and of chloride offered the possibility to identify the „parietal" and „non-parietal" components of gastric secretion in humans without and with administration of different drugs (or compounds) (Hollander, 1934).

Using the Hollander's method for the calculation and evaluation of cations, chloride in the gastric juice indicated clearly the significant decrease of „parietal component" (Δ-18±2 mmol/L, P< 0.001) in association with significant increase of „ non-parietal component" (Δ+19±2 mmol/L, P < 0.001) of the gastric secretion after application of 400 μg (given orally) of capsaicin (n=10) (Mózsik et al., 2005).

http://dx.doi.org/10.5772/58360

H^+		Na^+		K^+		Ca^{2+}		Mg^{2+}	
A	B	A	B	A	B	A	B	A	B
43±3	25±1	73±4	89±2	13±1	8±0,6	0,98± 0,02	0,88± 0,01	0,49± 0,01	0,38± 0,01
P<0.001		P<0.001		P<0.001		P<0.001		P<0.001	
100±7	58±2	100±5	122±3	100±8	62±5	100±2	90±1	100±2	78±2

"parietal" component		"non-parietal" component		albumin (g/L)	
A	B	A	B	A	B
43±3	25±2	126±4	145±4	1,23±0,001	1,650 ±0.02
P<0.001		P<0.001		P<0.001	
100±7	58±5	100±3	115±3	100±1	131±2

Table 2. Chemical composition of gastric juice without (A) and with (B) application of capsaicin (ED_{50}=400 µg orally give) in healthy human subjects. The results are given as mmol/L or % (means ±SEM) (n=10). (After Mózsik et al.: World J Gastroenterol 11: 5080-84, 2005)

3.4. Changes of albumin level in the gastric juice after capsaicin administration in healthy human subjects

The albumin concentration increased from 1.24 ± 0.001 g/L vs. 1.63 ± 0.02 g/L (P < 0.001; n=10) after 400 µg capsaicin (i.g. given) application (Mózsik et al., 2005).

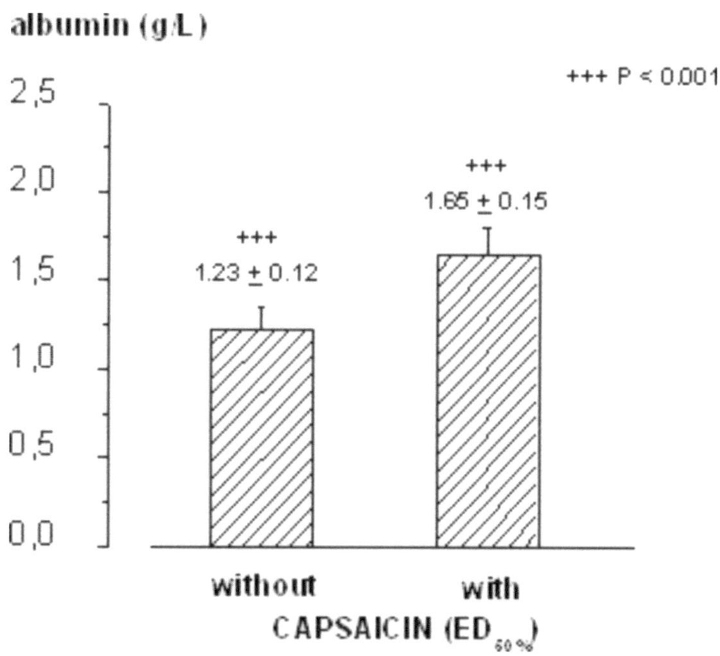

Figure 5. Changes in gastric mucosal proteins (albumin) in the gastric basal output (BAO), without and with capsaicin, in 10 healthy subjects (g/L) (means±SEM).

3.5. Action of capsaicin on the GTPD in the healthy human subjects

The capsaicin (given ig. in doses of 100, 200, 400 and 800 μg) dose-dependently increased the GTPD alone [Δ value from to baseline 10 (-mV)] (Mózsik et al., 2005).

When we applied capsaicin in double dose (800 μg intragastrically given) than we received the same increase in GTPD at the same time period (Hossenbocus et al., 1975; Mózsik et al., 2005) (Figure 6).

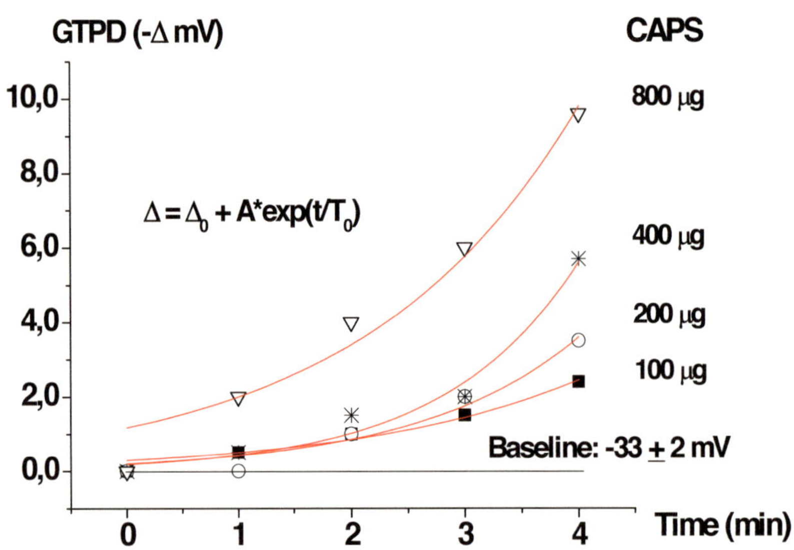

Figure 6. Capsaicin (CAPS) dose-dependent gastric mucosal protective effect of capsaicin on gastric transmucosal potential difference (GTPD) in 10 healthy subjects (after Mózsik et al., World J Gastroenterol 11:5180-5184, 2005).

3.6. Action of ethanol on GTPD in healthy human subjects

The intragastrically applied ethanol immediately and significantly decreased the GTPD [Δ 25 (-mV)] (Mózsik et al., 2005).

http://dx.doi.org/10.5772/58360

3.7. Preventive action of capsaicin on the ethanol-induced decrease of GTPD in healthy human subjects

The intragastrically applied capsaicin (given in doses of 100, 200, 400 and 800 μg) dose-dependently prevented the ethanol-induced decrease of GTPD in human healthy subjects (Mózsik et al., 2003; 2005).

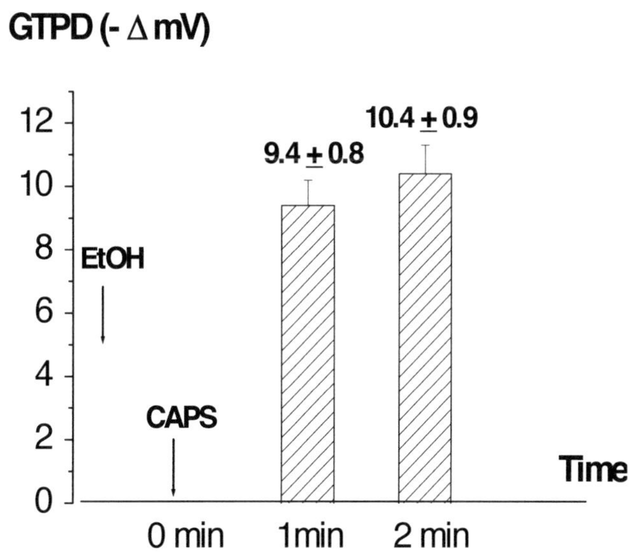

Figure 7. The ethanol (30 v/v in 5 ml intragastrically given) immediately the GTPD in the gastric mucosal surface (in comparison to baseline) (means±SEM) (n=14) (after Mózsik et al., World J Gastroenterol 11:5180-5184, 2005).

3.8. IND-induced acute gastric microbleeding and the acute gastric mucosal preventive effect of capsaicin on the IND-induced acute gastric mucosal damage in healthy human subjects (based on the results of prospective, randomized and multi-clinical study)

3.8.1. Extent of IND-induced acute gastric mucosal damage in healthy human subjects

The baseline of blood losing was 2.0 ± 0.2 mL/ day (n=14) without application of IND, which was increased to 8.1 ± 0.2 mL/day (n= 14; P< 0.001) after application of indomethacin.

3.8.2. Gastric mucosal preventive effect of capsaicin on the IND-induced acute gastric microbleeding in healthy human subjects

The capsaicin was given in doses of 200, 400 and 800 μg orally before the administration of indomethacin. The acutely applied capsaicin prevented by dose-dependent manner of IND-induced gastric microbleeding in healthy human subjects (Y=-0.0071*X+7.78; r=-0.98, n=14; *P*< 0.001) (Mózsik et al., 2005; Sarlós et al., 2003).

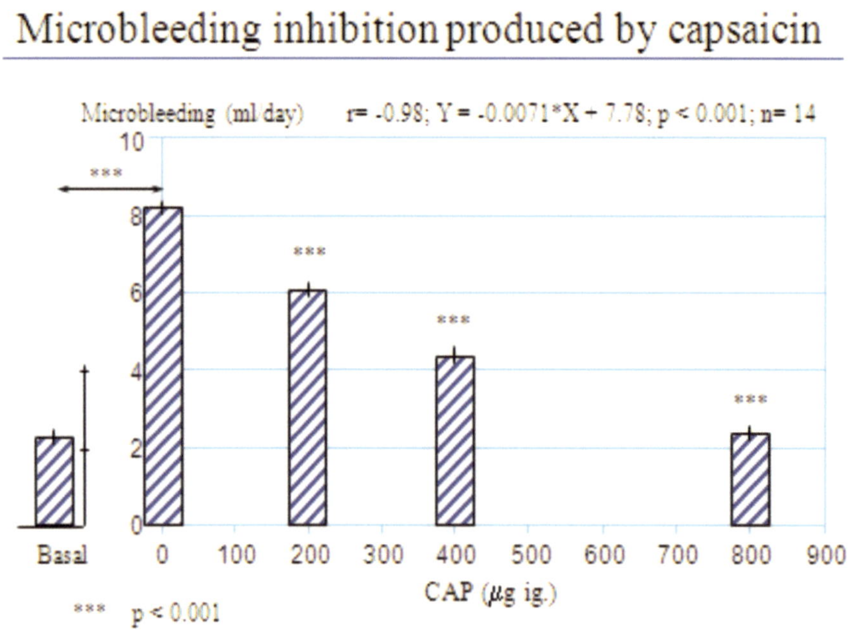

Figure 8. Gastric mucosal protection demonstrated by reduced microbleeding after capsaicin treatment of indomethacin (IND)-induced mucosal damage. (After Mózsik et al.: World J Gastroenterol 11.5180-83, 2005).

3.9. Effect of capsaicin on the gastric emptying in healthy human subjects

The capsaicin was intragastrically given in dose of ED_{50}, which increased significantly the gastric acid emptying: 1. Capsaicin (400 μg, ig=ED_{50})-induced changes in the maximal values of DOB_{max} decreased from 18±1 to 14±1 U (*P<0.01*); 2. the time to reach the DOB_{max} decreased from 148±13 to 70±12 min (*P<0.01*); 3. the slope (in U/min) increased from 0.11±0.01 to 14±0.001 (*P<0.001*); 4. the time to reach the AUC_{50} decreased from 115±10 to 80±8 (min) (n=10; P<0.01) (Debreceni et al., 1999).

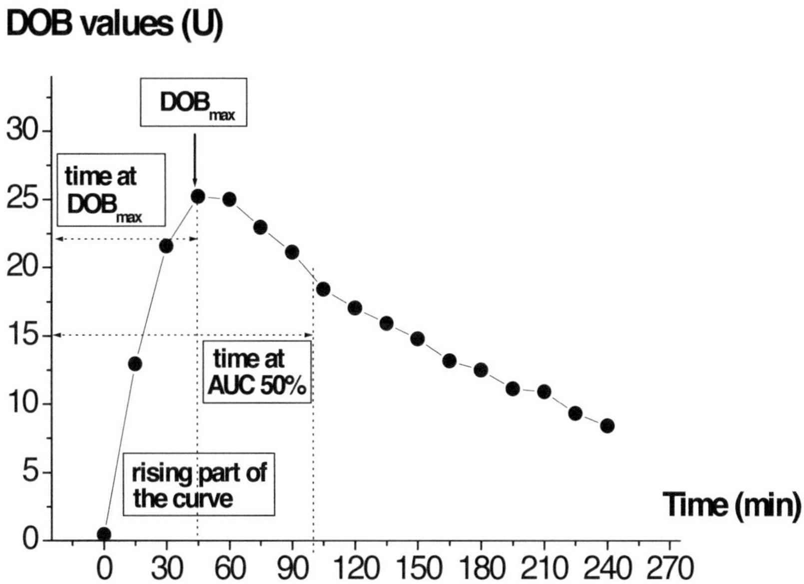

Figure 9. Typical curce obtained by the IRIS (infra-red-spectocsopy) measurement and calculated the delta over base (DOB) value. This value is directly proportional to ratio of $^{13}CO_2$ and $^{12}CO_2$ (DOB~$^{13}CO_2$/$^{12}CO_2$) in the air sample (Debreceni et al., J Physiol Paris 93: 455-460, 1999).

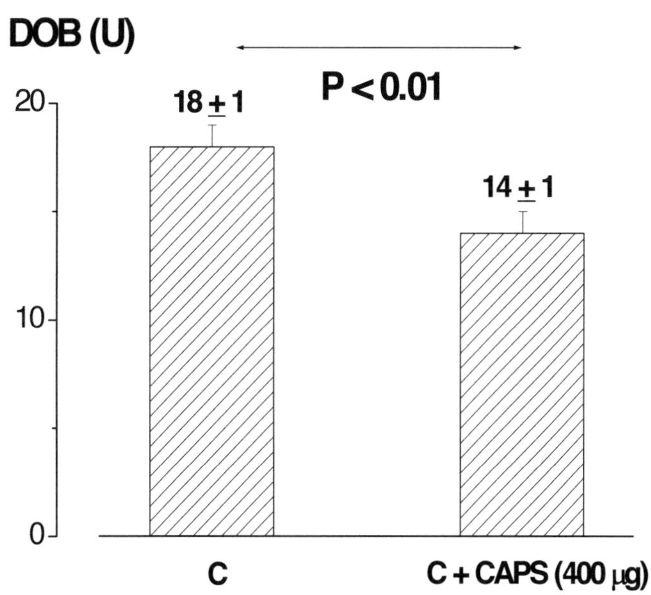

Figure 10. Capsaicin (400 µg ig.given)-induced changes in the maximal values of Delta Over Base (DOB max) (U) in 14 human healthy subjects (means±SEM) (Debreceni et al., J Physiol Paris 93:455-460, 1999).

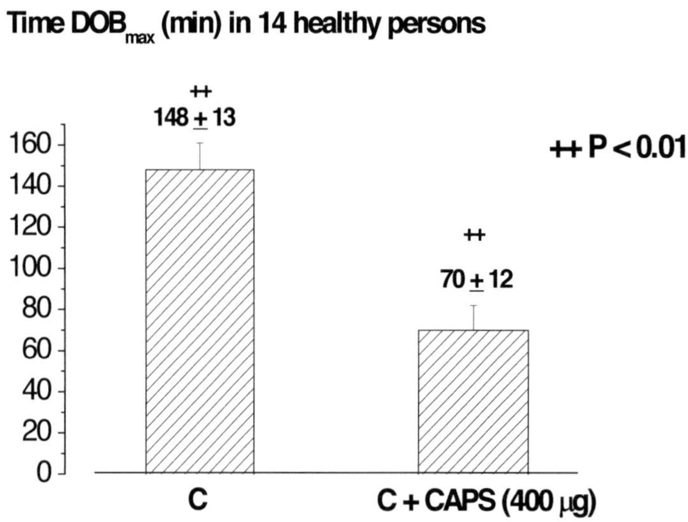

Figure 11. Capsaicin (400 μg ig. given)-induced changes in time to reach the value of DOB $_{max}$ (min) in 14 human healthy subjects (means±SEM) (Debreceni et al., J Physiol Paris 93:455-460, 1999).

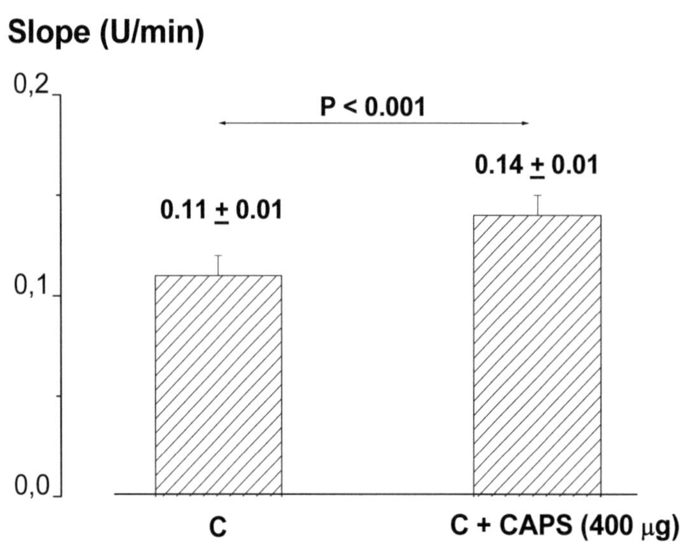

Figure 12. Capsaicin (400 μg ig. given)-induced changes in the slope in its rising part in 14 human healthy subjects (means±SEM) (Debreceni et al., J Physiol Paris 93:455-460, 1999).

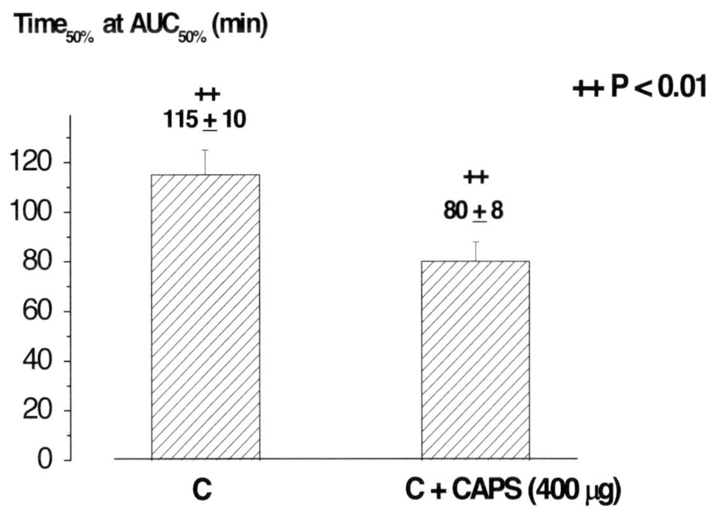

Figure 13. The time of 50% (in min) to rearch the **AUC** $_{50\%}$ in 14 healthy subjects (means±SEM) (U/min) in 14 human healthy subjects means±SEM) (Debreceni et al., J Physiol Paris 93:455-460, 1999).

3.10. Increased glucose absorption from small intestine and of glucagon release by capsaicin during the glucose loading test in healthy human subjects

During glucose loading test we measured the glucose absorption in the proximal part of the small intestine, insulin, C peptide, glucagon using the plasma level of glucose as markers substance (Dömötör et al., 2006).

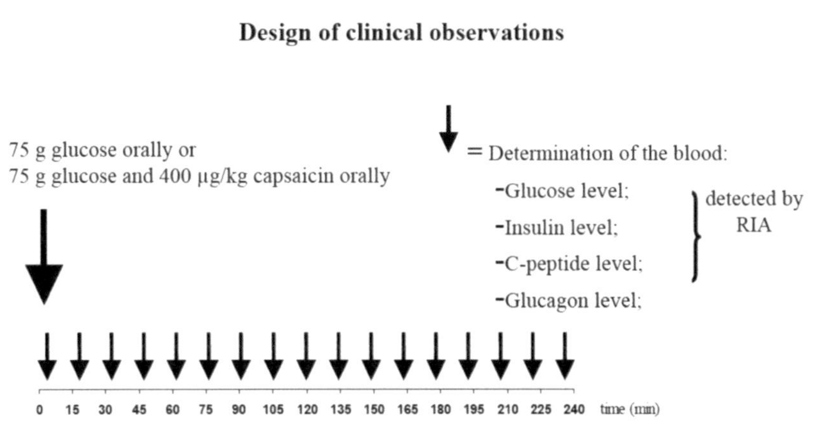

Figure 14. Design of clinical observations with glucose observation and utilization in 14 healthy human subjects without and with (400 µg, $ED_{50,}$ orally given) capsaicin application. The measurement of glucose, insulin, C-peptide, glucagon was carried out from the plasma level in every 15 min period from the glucose application to 4 h. (After Mózsik et al.: Inflammopharmacology 15:232-45, 2007).

The absorption of glucose from the small intestine and glucagon release increased by capsaicin administration; however no significant changes were obtained in neither insulin nor C peptide release under these observational circumstances (Figure 15).

The plasma levels of glucose increased significantly 30 to 150 min and the plasma level of glucagon increased from 90 to 180 min after capsaicin administration in human healthy subjects given 75 g glucose orally. The plasma levels of insulin and C peptide increased from 75 to 165 min after glucose administration; however, levels did not differ significantly.

3.11. Results of the immunohistochemical examinations in the human gastric and large bowel mucosa in healthy human subjects and in patients with different gastrointestinal disorders

3.11.1. Demonstration of capsaicin receptors, CGRP and SP in the human gastric and large bowel mucosa in healthy human subjects

The results of these observations were obtained in „ healthy human subjects", who had different functional complaints and the endoscopic examinations were carried out to exclude the presence of any histologically proven disease (the clinical histological examinations were carried out by the independent pathologist) and the opinion of pathologist gave normal histology.

The immunohistochemical examination demonstrated the presence of capsaicin (TRVP1) receptors in the gastric and large bowel mucosa obtained from biopsy samples. The location of capsaicin receptor could be demonstrated near the nerve endings, vascular vessel and in the epithelial layer (Figure 16) (Dömötör et al., 2005).The CGRP and SP could be observed in gastric mucosa and these parts of large bowel mucosa as well (Figure 17) (Dömötör et al., 2005).

3.11.2. Demonstration of capsaicin receptor, CGRP and SP in the gastric and large bowel mucosa in patients with different disorders

The preliminary results of these observations were published by Dömötör et al. (2005).

These patients went over the clinical endoscopic and pathological examinations. The original pathological diagnosis was given by an independent pathologist.

The capsaicin receptor, and released neuropeptides (CGRP and SP) could be detected in all types of patients with different disorders (Table 3). The results of these preliminary clearly indicated the following: 1. capsaicin could be demonstrated in patients with superficial gastritis, erosive gastritis, stomach polyps, stomach cancer, inflammation of large bowel disease, colon polyps with severe dysplasia and colorectal cancers.

The CGRP could be demonstrated in most of the all of the above mentioned diseases; meanwhile the SP could not be demonstrated in these diseases (Table 3).

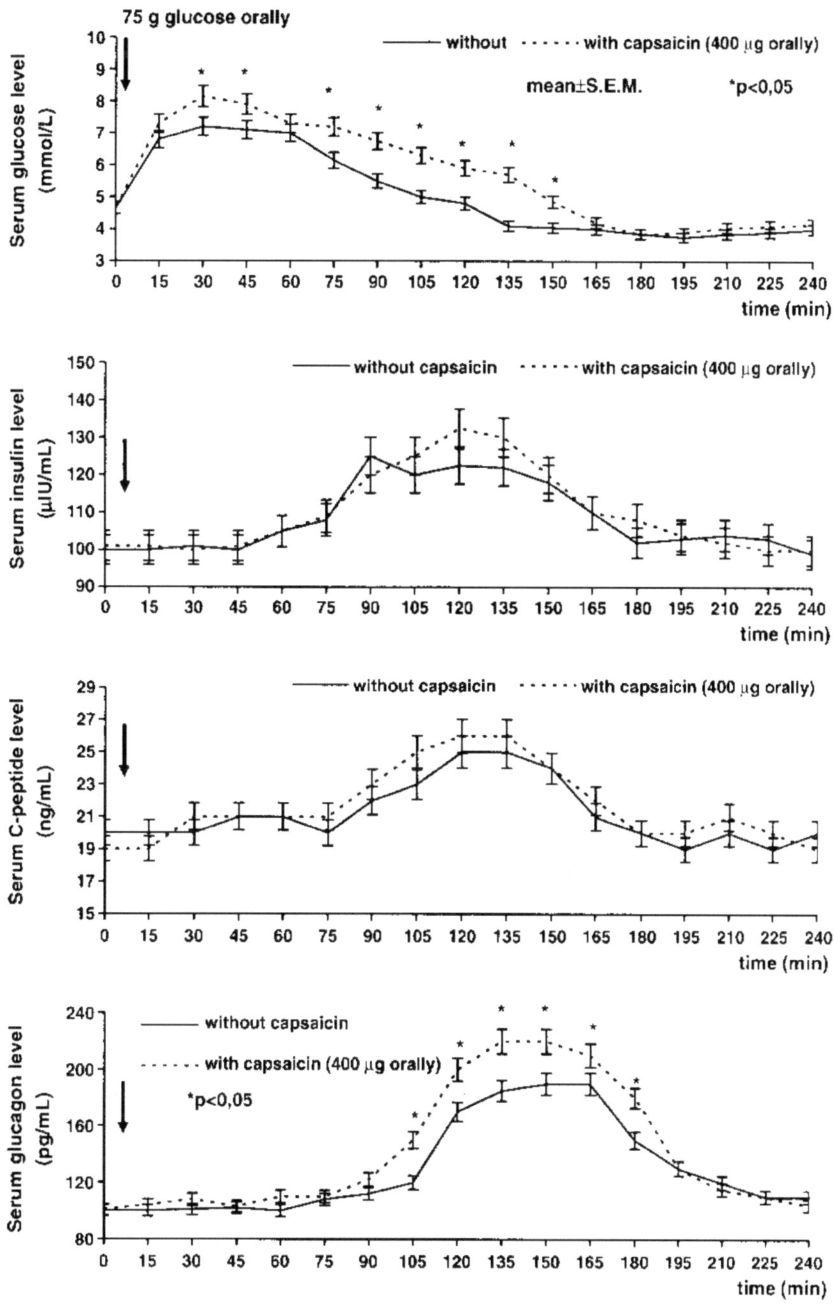

Figure 15. Changes in plasma level of glucose, insulin, C-peptide and glucagon after oral administration of glucose (75 g in 100 ml water) in 14 healthy human subjects. Capsaicin (400 μg) was orally given in gelatine capsule (Hungaropharma, Budapest, Hungary). The plasma levels of glucose, insulin, C-peptide and glucagon were measured every 15 min for 4 h. The results are expressed as means ±SEM. (After Dömötör et al.: Eur J Pharmacol 534: 280-83, 2006).

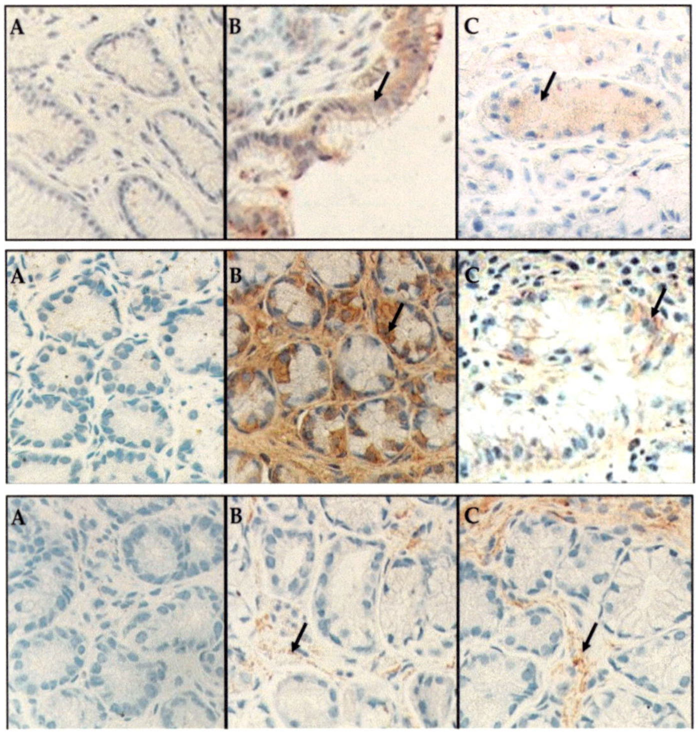

Figure 16. The immundistribution of TRPV1 (first row), CGRP (second row) and of SP (third row) in the gastric mucosa of a healthy subject (A) and of patient with H. pylori negative (B) and H. pylori positive (C) chronic gastritis. Arrows show the immunsigns in the mucosa. (After Mózsik et al.: Inflammopharmacology 15: 232-45, 2007).

STOMACH	TRPV1	CGRP	SP
Superficial gastritis	+	+	-
Erosive gastritis	+	+	-
Gastric ulcer	-/+	-/+	-/+
Polyp	+	+	-
Carcinoma	+	+	-
LARGE BOWEL	**TRPV1**	**CGRP**	**SP**
Inflammation	+	+	+
Polyp with moderate dysplasia	-	-	-
Poly with severe dysplasia	+ spot-like	-	-
Carcinoma	+ spot-like	+	-

*The signs of+or – indicate the trend of expression in the specific immunohistochemical examinations in the mucosa specimens (stomach and large bowel) in patient different disease.

Table 3. Immundistribution of capsaicin receptor (TRPV1), calcitonin-gene releted peptide (CGRP) and substance P (SP) in the gastric and large bowel mucosa of patients with different GI disorders. (After Mózsik et al.: Inflammopharmacology 15: 232-45, 2007)*

http://dx.doi.org/10.5772/58360

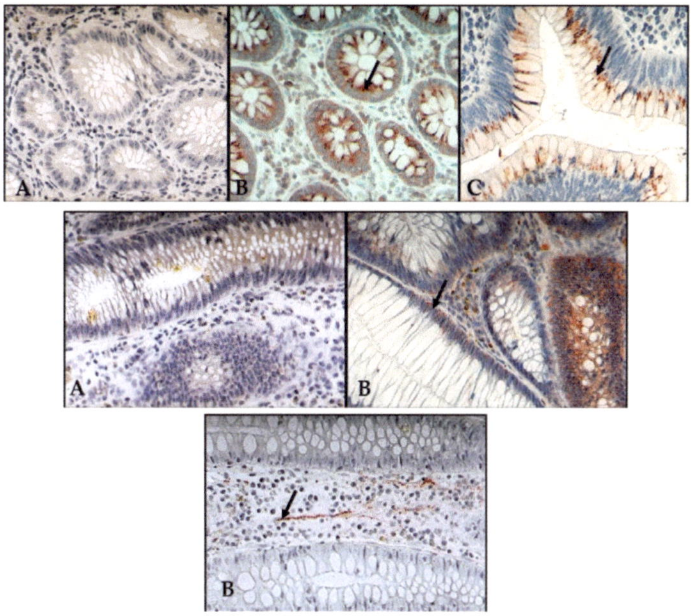

Figure 17. The immundistribution of TRPV1 (first line), CGRP (second line) and of SP (third line) in the colon mucosa of control person (A) and of patient with inflammatory bowel disease (B) and with severe dysplastic polyp (C). Arrows show the immunsigns in the mucosa. (After Mózsik et al.: Inflammopharmacology 15: 232-45, 2007)

3.12. Capsaicin receptor, CGRP and SP in the patients with Helicobacter positive and negative chronic gastritis

These observations were carried out in 57 patients with chronic gastritis (21 patients from them were H. pylori positive and 30 patients were H. pylori negative).

The expression of capsaicin receptors and CGRP increased in the gastric mucosa with both bacteria positive and negative chronic gastritis, meanwhile SP increased with a limited extent Determined by a semi quantitative scale (Dömötör et al., 2006a). The expression of TRVP1, CGRP, and SP increased significantly in the human gastric mucosa with chronic gastritis; however, no difference was obtained in their expression in patients with H. pylori positive and negative chronic gastritis (Dömötör et al., 2006a).

3.13. Measurements of the gastric microbleeding before and after 2-week capsaicin treatment: Testing of the changes in baseline, IND-induced acute gastric microbleeding and of capsaicin-stimulated gastric mucosal protective effect on the IND-induced acute gastric microbleeding in healthy human subjects (Figures 18 and 19)

3.13.1. Baseline before and after 2 weeks IND treatment without application of any drug and/or compound

The baseline of gastric microbleeding was detected 2.1 ± 0.1 vs. 2.0± 0.1 mL/day, before and after 2 weeks capsaicin treatment (without other drug /compound application).

3.13.2. Measurement of IND-induced acute gastric mucosal microbleeding – before and after 2 weeks capsaicin treatment – in healthy human subjects

The acute administration of IND significantly increased the extent of gastric microbleeding vs. baseline (without administration of IND) (*P<0.001*; n=14) in healthy human subjects before (baseline vs. IND., 2.1 ± 0.1 vs. 8.3 ± 0.2 mL/day) and after (baseline vs. IND., 2.0± 0.1 vs 7.8±0.3 mL/ day) 2 weeks capsaicin (3 x 400 μg orally given) treatment (Mózsik et al., 2005).

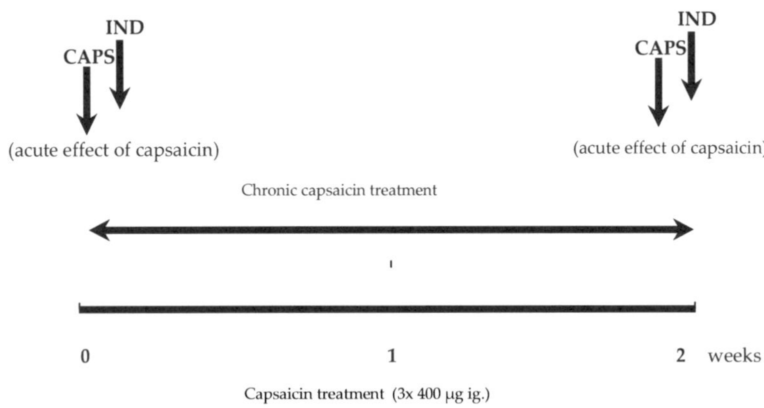

Figure 18. Clinical study design of a chronic capsaicin treatment in human healthy subjects. Abbreviations: CAPS: capsaicin, IND: indomethacin.

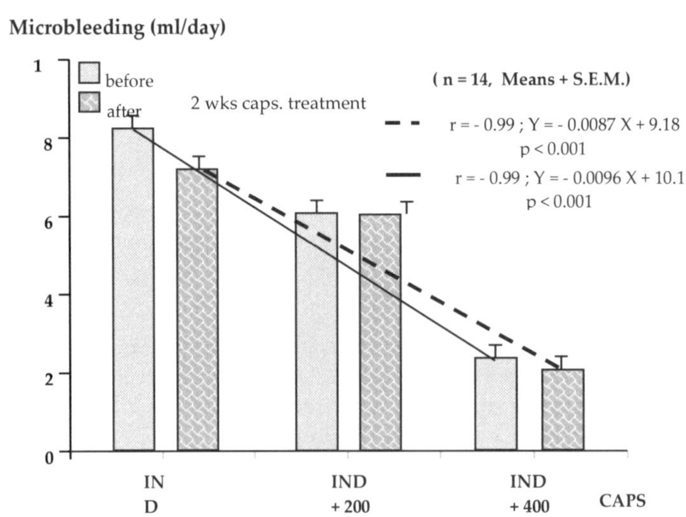

Figure 19. Capsaicin (given 200 and 400 μg ig.)-induced gastric mucosal preventive effects on indomethacin (3x25 mg ig.)-produced gastric mucosal microbleeding before and after a chronic capsaicin (3x400 μg i.g. for 2 weeks) in 14 human healthy subjects. The results were expressed as means ± SEM).

3.13.3. Measurement of acutely applied capsaicin-induced gastric mucosal protective effect on the IND-induced acute gastric microbleeding before and after 2 weeks capsaicin treatment in healthy human subjects

The intragastrically applied capsaicin dose–dependently prevented the IND-induced gastric mucosal damage (Mózsik et al., 2003; 2004a; 2005) – before (Y=-0.0087X+9.18, r=-0.99: *P<0.001*) and after (Y=-0.0096 X+10.1 ; r=-.0.99 ; *P<0.001*) 2 weeks capsaicin treatment – when the capsaicin was acutely and intragastrically given (in doses of 200 and 400 μg) before the one day IND treatment (see the description in the methods) (Mózsik et al., 2005).

3.14. Expression of capsaicin receptor, CGRP, and SP in patients with chronic gastritis

3.14.1. Capsaicin-sensitive afferentation in H. pylori positive and negative chronic gastritis

The symptoms of patient's suffering from chronic gastritis with or without H. pylori infection (20 H. pylori positive and 30 H. pylori negative) were nonspecific including epigastric discomfort, nausea, loss of appetite and vomiting. The patients underwent physical, laboratory, ultrasonographic, endoscopic and histological (including special immuno-histochemical) examinations. Twenty people with functional dyspepsia (all of them underwent the aforementioned medical, laboratory, iconographic and histological examinations and all of these examinations indicated negative results) were taken as healthy controls. The age of patients was 39 to 68 years; there were 22 males and 29 females with chronic gastritis, and ten males and ten females in the functional dyspepsia group.

The H. pylori infection was detected by ^{14}C urea breath test, rapid urease test, Warthinn-Starry silver staining and other specific histological examinations. The gastric tissue samples from the stomach and antrum were examined by an independent histologist and classified of chronic gastritis according to the Sydney System.

The immuno-histochemical studies were carried out on formalin fixed, paraffin embedded tissue samples of gastric mucosa using the peroxidase-labeled polymer method (Lab Vision Co., Fremont, USA). SP was detected by the NC1/34HL rat monoclonal antibody, the TRPV1 receptor and CGRP were labeled using polyclonal rabbit antisera (all from Alcam Ltd., UK, Cambridge).

3.14.2. Capsaicin-sensitive afferentation in H. pylori positive chronic gastritis before and after eradication treatment

These observations were carried out in 38 persons, including 20 healthy subjects and 18 patients with H. pylori positive gastritis. The age of persons with histologically intact gastric mucosa (controls) were 41 to 67 years (mean=52.2 years). The age of patients with chronic H. pylori positive gastritis (6 males, 12 females) was 39 to 68 years (mean=56.4 years).

The time period between the first and control gastroscopy was 6 weeks after the starting of the examinations. The biopsies were taken from the corpus and antrum of patients with chronic gastritis, before and after eradication treatment and from healthy subjects.

The H. pylori positive patients underwent 7-day eradication treatment with combination of double dose of PPI (pantoprazole 2x40 mg/ day), amoxicillin (1000 mg twice daily) and clarithromycin (500 mg twice daily) according to the European guidelines. After this one week combination treatment, the patients continued to take normal dose of PPI for another week.

The H. pylori infection was detected before and after treatment. The results of eradication treatment was successful in 89%, the gastric histology (by biopsy and by histology) indicated normal picture in 22% of cases, and 78 % of patients showed moderate gastritis.

The expression of TRPV1 and CGRP increased significantly in the gastric mucosa of patients with chronic gastritis – independently on the presence of H. pylori positive or negative status and of successful eradication treatment in patients with H. pylori positive gastritis), meanwhile no significant expression changes were obtained for SP in the gastric mucosa in these groups) (Dömötör et al., 2005; Lakner et al., 2012, Mózsik et al., 2011; 2013, Czimmer et al., 2013) (Figures 20, 21 and Table 4).

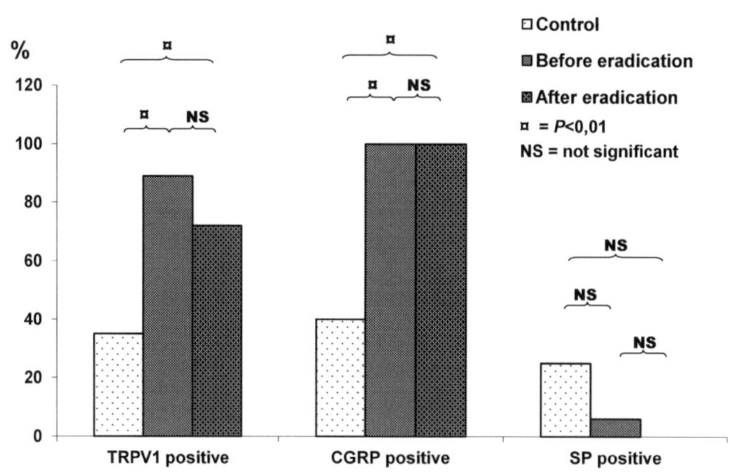

Figure 20. Changes in the immunhistochemical distribution of capsaicin receptor (TRPV1), CGRP and SP in patients with H. pylori positive chronic gastritis before and after eradication therapy. (After Lakner et al., World J Gastrointest Pharmacol Ther. 2: 36-41, 2011)

	TRPV1		CGRP		Substance P	
	Positive	Negative	Positive	Negative	Positive	Negative
Before eradication (n=18)	88,89 % (16)	11,11 % (2)	100 % (18)	0 % (0)	5,56 % (1)	94,44 % (17)
After eradication (n=18)	72,22% (13)	17,78% (5)	100 % (18)	0 % (0)	0 % (0)	100 % (18)
Control group (n=20)	35 % (7)	65 % (13)	40 % (8)	60 % (12)	75 % (15)	25 % (5)

Table 4. The summary of the changes in the immunhistochemical distribution of capsaicin receptor, calcitonin gene-related peptide and substance P in patient with chronic *H. pylori* positive gastritis before and after eradication therapy.

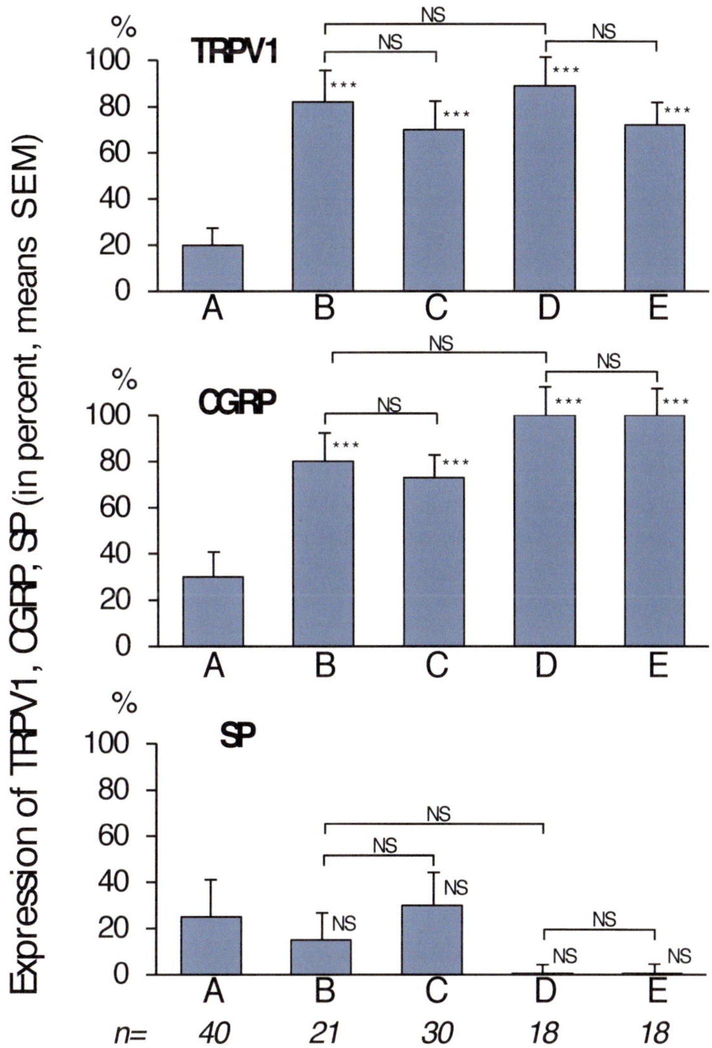

Figure 21. Changes in the expression of capsaicin receptor (TRPV1), calcitonin gene-related peptide (CGRP) and substance P (SP) in the human gastric mucosa of healthy voluntaries (histologically intact) (A), *H. pylori* positive (B), *H. pylori* negative (C) and *H. pylori* positive before (D) and after (E) eradication (pantoprazole 40, amoxicillin 1000 and clarithromycin 500 mg, all two times per day, for seven days) (n=number of patients). (After Mózsik et al., 2014).

4. Discussion

The vagal nerve plays a key role in the gastrointestinal physiology, pathology and pharmacology. The nerve fibres of vagus can be divided into afferent (about 90%) and efferent fibres (10 %) based on animal observations. About 9 per cent of afferent fibres are capsaicin sensitive afferent fibres (Gabella and Pease, 1973; Grijalva and Novin, 1990).

Many observations on the field of Gastroenterology were based on the modification of efferent fibres of vagal nerve, except the classical surgical vagotomy (both in the animal experiments and in human observations with peptic ulcer disease). This standpoint was emphasized during the research period performed by the application of different anticholinergic compounds acting at the level of muscarinic receptor.

Since histamine also plays an essential role in the gastric acid secretion and in many other immunological processes, various H_2 receptor antagonist compounds were developed like cimetidine, ranitidine, famotidine and nizatidine.

After recognition of the H^+-K^+-ATPase as biochemical structure of gastric acid secretion, the so-called proton pump inhibitors (H^+-K^+-ATPase inhibitors) were developed and studied in clinical practice with great efforts (Mózsik, 2006).

The principle problems for clinicians were that the research had not offered any possibilities for studying capsaicin sensitive afferent fibres of vagal nerve in the human physiology, pathology, pharmacology and in human medical therapy. The observations of Jancsó et al. (1967; 1968; 1970) opened a new gate for evaluation of the potential roles of capsaicin sensitive afferent fibres independently from other afferent nerves in various physiological, pharmacological and pathological processes.

Szolcsányi and Barthó (1981) clearly demonstrated the dual actions of capsaicin in peptic ulceration of rat: capsaicin – given in small doses – prevented; meanwhile this compound given in higher doses aggravated peptic ulcer disease in rats. Following them Holzer studied the details of capsaicin actions in the GI tract (see the reviews of Holzer 1998; 1999, 2013; Szolcsányi, 2014).

Our experimental studies with capsaicin have been carried out together with professor Szolcsányi (Department of Pharmacology and Pharmacotherapy, Medical and Health Centre, University of Pécs, Hungary) from 1980, understanding the actions of capsaicin in gastric mucosal damage and protection have been our main focus (Mózsik et al., 1997).

My work team started with the human clinical pharmacological studies from the years of 1960 in patients with peptic ulcer disease (Mózsik et al., 1965; 1967; 1969a; 1969b). These studied tried to reveal the details of absorption, metabolization and excretion of various anticholinergic agents in patients with peptic ulcer before the starting of chronic treatment, after the regular chronic treatment and after cessation of these drugs. The application of anticholinergic agents to patients was used to approach the cholinergic mediated processes both in the development and treatment of peptic ulcer diseases.

After the years of 1970, the H_2R blocking compounds became deeply studied in human GI physiology, pathology and pharmacology. Many clinical pharmacological studies with H_2R blockers have been carried out in patients with peptic ulcer disease (Mózsik et al., 1994; Patty et al., 1984; Tárnok et al., 1979; 1983). In the last two decades the proton pump inhibitors were deeply studied.

The problems, results and difficulties of our clinical pharmacology practice put down the bases of a very clear research line for the observations of capsaicin. The results of the different animal observations offered a new possibility for evaluation of capsaicin sensitive afferent nerves (by the application of capsaicin) during physiological, pathological, pharmacological and therapeutic events of the GI tract (Mózsik et al., 2014).

The results from animal experiments with capsaicin which is widely used in the every-day culinary practice, clearly indicated us that the stimulatory doses of capsaicin acting on capsaicin-sensitive fibres produce gastric mucosal defensive actions and they are able to prevent the NSAID-induced gastric mucosal damage. These scientifically carried out studies with capsaicin in animals also offered a new tool to approach the capsaicin sensitive afferent nerves in the healthy human beings, and to some extent in patients with different GI disorders.

Our studies with capsaicin in human healthy subjects and in patients with different gastrointestinal disorders have been stated from 1997. These studies were permitted by the Regional Ethical Committee of University of Pécs, Hungary, and these observations were carried out according to Good Clinical Practice respecting the Helsinki Declaration.

The human observations were carried out according to the basic laws of human clinical pharmacology (inclusion and exclusion criteria, randomization, prospective studies, generally self-controlled group of healthy human subjects, etc).

We had five aims in these studies with the capsaicin:

1. To understand the main mechanisms of capsaicin sensitive afferent nerves in the gastric functions;

2. To try to understand the potential role(s) of capsaicin sensitive afferent nerves in the development of human physiological, pathological and pharmacological events;

3. To identify the dose range of capsaicin which stimulates only the capsaicin-sensitive afferent nerves and to identify the classical molecular pharmacological parameters (affinity and intrinsic activity curves, ED_{50} and pA_2 values) in comparison the same parameters obtained in cases of every day used drugs;

4. To exclude clearly the existence of desensitation of capsaicin-sensitive afferent nerves to capsaicin (under different observation circumstances, namely in acute administration, before and after two weeks capsaicin treatment, given in dose of 3 x 400 μg /day) to capsaicin;

5. To process and even to produce a new capsaicin containing drug or drug combinations to modify the capsaicin-sensitive afferentation in human healthy subjects and to treat patients with GI mucosal damage against NSAIDs and H. pylori infection.

These aims determined us to use a significant number of the methodologies applied in the human studies. However, we had to use classical molecular pharmacological methods to compare and to understand some details of capsaicin-induced changes in the human physiological, pathological parameters.

The following main trends were applied in the capsaicin research:

1. To determine the dose-response curves for the various drugs and capsaicin.

2. To introduce the classical molecular pharmacological methods for understanding the capsaicin-induced action in comparison to others produced by anticholinergic drugs, H_2R antagonists or proton pump inhibitors.
3. The specific immunohistochemistry (for obtained morphological evidence) was incorporated into the research.
4. Different parameters were simultaneously measured (e.g. plasma glucose, insulin, C-peptide and glucagon were detected during the sugar loading test in the healthy human subjects).
5. Capsaicin studies were carried out not only in acute administration and after a chronic capsaicin administration.
6. The immunohistochemical studies were carried out in the GI mucosa of patients with different GI disorders (acute gastric mucosal damage, chronic inflammation, precancerous state and cancers in the stomach and in the large bowel);
7. The human pathological diagnosis was given by an independent pathologist.
8. The ED_{50} (necessary doses of drugs to produce 50% inhibition) values were determined and expressed in [-] molar values (pD_2).
9. To evaluate the possible role of capsaicin afferentation in the prevention or treatment of gastric mucosal damage produced by NSAIDs in healthy subjects and in patients who are treated with these drugs (as pain killers, platelet aggregation, anti-inflammatory compounds, etc).

4.1. Capsaicin-sensitive efferent nerves vs. gastric secretion in healthy human subjects

The capsaicin dose-dependent manner decreased the gastric basal secretion (BAO) (Mózsik et al., 1999; 2004a; 2005). The capsaicin was applied in very small doses (200 to 800 μg orally), which stimulate the capsaicin-sensitive afferent nerves.

When we applied the molecular pharmacological approach the actions of capsaicin, anticholinergic agents, H_2R antagonists or proton pump inhibitors, we were surprised that capsaicin was able to inhibit gastric acid secretion in smaller molar concentration than other clinically widely used drugs (Figures 3 and 4). Analyzing the intrinsic activity of these drugs and capsaicin by the molecular pharmacological methods (intrinsic activity of atropine was taken to be 1.00), we found capsaicin's action to be lesser than atropine's (Figure 3).

The affinity curves of different drugs and capsaicin were molecular pharmacologically determined and given as pD_2 (the necessary doses of drugs and capsaicin to produce 50% inhibition of gastric acid secretion (basal acid output), which expressed in [-] molar value) and as intrinsic activity (pA_2) (the necessary doses of drugs and capsaicin to produce 50% inhibition, also expressed in [-] molar) values (Table 1).

The results of these molecular pharmacological studies clearly indicated the sensitivity of the various regulatory targets of different drugs and capsaicin in comparison to possible physio-

http://dx.doi.org/10.5772/58360

logical roles of the target organs and the drug actions influence their functional activities and states. There is no question that the stimulation of capsaicin-induced afferent sensitive nerves plays a very significant effect in regulatory processes important for the maintenance of gastric mucosal integrity in human beings (including in healthy subjects and patients with different GI disorders or treated with different drugs, especially with NSAIDs).

The decrease of gastric acid secretion was explained by the increased H^+back diffusion after capsaicin application via the increased vasodilatator processes induced by the release of the CGRP and SP in animal observations or by the increase of somatostatin secretion. The CGRP and SP together with capsaicin receptor (TRVP1) can be detected by inmunohistological methods in the gastric mucosa around nerves, vascular spaces, parietal cells and in epithelial layer.

The increased gastric secretory responses are present along with increased gastric mucosal blood flow. On the other hand, the increased gastric acid (H^+) secretion is closely associated with the increase of K^+, Mg^{2+}, $Ca^+$and albumin in gastric juice. However, the decrease of gastric acid secretion produced by antisecretory agents is associated with the decrease of H^+, K^+, Mg^{2+}, $Ca^{2+}$and albumin (Myren, 1968).

Human observations with capsaicin do suggest presence of increased H^+back diffusion during capsaicin action (except when capsaicin was given in high doses):

1. The increased H^+back diffusion suggests the decreased level of albumin in the gastric juice. Our results cannot prove the existence of gastric H^+back diffusion in human healthy subjects during the capsaicin action:

2. We calculated the "parietal" and "non-parietal "components of gastric juice after Hollander's original observation (Hollander 1934). Our results clearly indicate that the decrease of gastric H^+concentration (and output) is closely associated with the increased extent of "non-parietal component" during the capsaicin action in the healthy human subjects. The "non-parietal component" of the gastric juice is a buffering part, which cannot be obtained in circumstance of passive metabolic processes. Earlier, the significant increase of buffering ("non-parietal component") secretion was obtained in 2-10 days after cessation of a prolonged atropine treatment in patients with peptic ulcer disease (Antal et al., 1966).

3. There are other arguments also exist against the existence of the passive H^+back diffusion in the stomach during capsaicin action in the healthy human subjects. When the capsaicin was directly given to gastric mucosa (using gastroscope), then GTPD increased in a dose dependent manner (Mózsik et al., 2005).

If ethanol was intragastrically given (using the biopsy channel), then GTPD immediately decreased, which could be reversed by the topical application of capsaicin. This action is also dose-dependent from capsaicin after ethanol application in the healthy human subjects (Mózsik et al., 2005).

The capsaicin action on the gastric secretory responses can be explained by different ways:

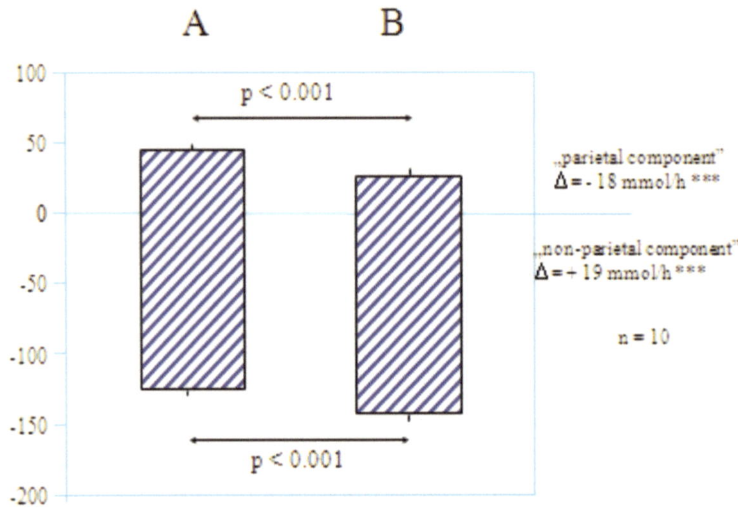

Figure 22. Changes of parietal and non-parietal components of gastric juice before (A) and after (B) capsaicin (400 μg orally, ED_{50} value) administration.

CAPSAICIN-INDUCED CHANGES IN THE "PARIETAL" AND "NON-PARIETAL" COMPONENTS OF GASTRIC JUICE

without capsaicin

	H^+	K^+	Na^+	Ca^{2+}	Mg^{2+}	chloride⁻ proteins (albumin)
H^+↑	↑	↑	↓	↑	↑	↑ ↑
H^+↓	↓	↓	↑	↓	↓	↓ ↓

after capsaicin treatment (ED_{50})

↓	↓	↑	↓	↓	unchanged increased
Typical changes to decrease of inhibition of BAO in human healthy subjects					CAPSAICIN-INDUCED CHANGES

Figure 23. Changes in the contents of electrolytes of gastric juice with increase and decrease of H^+output, without (upper part) and with (below part) capsaicin application.

1. direct cellular action of capsaicin on the parietal cells;
2. direct stimulatory action of capsaicin on the "non-parietal component" of gastric secretory responses;

3. the capsaicin (given in doses producing the stimulation of capsaicin-sensitive afferent nerves) results directly neural (or hormonal) influences on the gastric mucosa;

4. other yet not known mechanism(s) existing in the regulation of the human gastric secretion.

The capsaicin given in ED_{50} increased the gastric emptying (Debreceni et al, 1999; Mózsik et al., 2004a, 2004b). This action of capsaicin on the gastric emptying can be explained at least by two pathways:

1. decrease of gastric acid secretion;

2. direct action on muscular function of the stomach (pylorus).

Up to now, the acute action of capsaicin was evaluated dominantly by the measuring one or two parameters.

4.2. Capsaicin action of glucose absorption from small intestine in human healthy subjects and its hormonal and metabolic backgrounds

The sugar loading test was applied for measuring absolutely different physiological events, e.g. glucose absorption from the proximal part of the small intestine and consequently the produced hormonal regulations during the glucose loading test.

The response to glucose loading in healthy human subject can be divided into three different periods on basis of physiological events after orally applied glucose in human healthy persons:

1. absorption (first period, from 30 to 90 min);

2. insulin (and other hormones) release (second period, from 60 to 150 min);

3. glycogen mobilization by the liver (third period, from 150 to 180 min) under adrenergic neural influences.

The glucose can be absorbed from the proximal part of the small intestine by active transport mechanism (in presence of Mg^{2+}, mitochondrial ATP breakdown into ADP) (Dömötör et al., 2006b). The monitoring of the glucose level was used as biological marker for the equilibrium of the different physiological events. In the first period the plasma glucose level depends only on the glucose absorption; in the second period the plasma level of glucose represents the equilibrium between the absorption and hormone release; and in the third the glucose level represents the mobilization of glucose by the liver in healthy human subjects. It is also important that the insulin and glucagon act contra regulatory on glucose utilization in the serum.

By studying the time sequence of changes in plasma levels of glucose, insulin, C-peptide and glucagon after glucose loading in healthy human subjects without and with capsaicin (400 μg orally), we found the followings:

1. The plasma level of glucose (from 30 to 150 min) and the glucagon (from 90 to 180 min) increased significantly after glucose plus capsaicin administration.

2. The plasma levels of insulin and C-peptide were increased from 90 to 165 min, however, no significant changes were observed between subjects without and with capsaicin.

3. No significance in timing of insulin and glucagon release was observed, which clearly excludes the existence of antagonism between insulin and glucagon release (short time).

4. The plasma level of glucagon was high for longer period than it was in case of insulin. It should be noted that capsaicin increased the glucagon level.

The results clearly indicate that capsaicin sensitive afferent nerves have a key-role in the regulation of glucose absorption from the small intestine (due to a local increase of blood flow), glucose utilization, and release of neuropeptide (presently the glucagon release). This human observation proved clear-cut the active participation of capsaicin sensitive afferent nerves in the carbohydrate metabolism (by the ways of modification of sugar absorption, hormone release). Up till now only the somatostatin release induced by capsaicin has been known (Szolcsányi, 2004).

4.3. Capsaicin given orally in small doses prevents with IND-induced gastric microbleedings in human healthy subjects

The IND was used in these studies as NSAID, which is a non-selective COX blocker (the ratio of ED_{50} of IND on COX-1 /COX-2 = 0.30) (Kawai et al., 1998) (Table 5). The extent of gastric microbleeding appears as consequence of COX-1 and COX-2 inhibition.

The results of our observations (Sarlós et al., 2003; Mózsik et al., 2003, 2004a; 2005) the capsaicin (ig. given) dose dependently prevented the IND-induced gastric microbleeding before and after 2 weeks capsaicin treatment.

Under the results of Kawai et al. (1998), we calculated the extents of gastric microbleeding depending on COX-1 and COX-2 enzyme activity (Table 6). It was found that the capsaicin-induced gastric mucosal protection remained unchanged – before and after 2 weeks capsaicin treatment – after both COX-1 and COX-2 enzyme inhibition.

NSAID	Ratio COX-1 : COX-2
Aspirin	0.12
Diclofenac	38.00
Etodolac	179.00
Ibuprofen	0.86
Indomethacin	**0.30**
Loxoprofen-SRS	3.20
NS-398	1263.00
Oxaprozin	0.061
Zaltoprofen	3.80

Table 5. Comparison of inhibitory effects (IC_{50}) of NSAIDs on COX-1 and COX-2 enzymes in human platelet synovial cell (After Kawai et al.: Eur. J. Pharmacol. 347; 87-94, 1998).*

http://dx.doi.org/10.5772/58360

- **IC_{50} VALUE OF INDOMETHACIN TO RATIO OF COX-1/COX-2 = 0,30 (1: 3,25)**
- **MICROBLEEDING IN THE STOMACH**

	← 2 weeks capsaicin treatment →	
	Before	**After**
Baseline	**2,1 ± 0,1 mL/day**	**2,0 ± 0,1 mL/day**
After IND	**8,25 ± 0,25 mL/day**	**7,8 ± 0,3 mL/day**
Δ IND-induced	**6,15 ± 0,2 mL/day**	**5,8 ± 0,3 mL/day**
	(= inhibition on COX-1 + COX-2) (= 100%)	
COX-1:	**1.447±0.1 mL/day**	**1.364±0.1 mL/day**
COX-2:	**4.70±0.2 mL/day**	**4.44±0.2 mL/day**

- **400 μg CAPSAICIN (IG GIVEN) INDUCED DECREASE OF IND-GASTRIC MICROBLEEDING**

6±0.2 mL/day	**5.9±0.2 mL/day**

* means±SEM in 14 human healthy subjects.

Table 6. Correlation between the capsaicin actions, COX-1 and COX-2 systems and gastric microbleedings produced by indomethacin (IND) in human healthy subjects before and after 2-week capsaicin (3x400μg orally) treatment. (After Mózsik et al.: Inflammmopharmacology 15: 232-45, 2007)*

The orally given 200, 400 and 800 μg capsaicin dose dependently reduced the IND-induced gastric microbleeding. All of the healthy persons included in this study received all the mentioned doses of capsaicin in random allocation.

4.5. Questions of desensibilization in capsaicin receptor to capsaicin

4.5.1. Facts to exclude the presence of the desensibilization of capsaicin receptor to applied doses of capsaicin in acute observation circumstances

When we applied the capsaicin twice in doses of 800 μg ig. after 5 min interval, then we received the same extents of increase in difference of GTPD, indicating a very active metabolic action under these observation circumstances.

The same extent gastric mucosal protection was obtained in the IND-induced gastric mucosal damage in human healthy subjects. The actions of gastric mucosal prevention was dose-dependent on the IND-induced gastric microbleedings (please note that these human observations were carried out in prospective, randomized and multiclinical studies) (Figures 18 and 19).

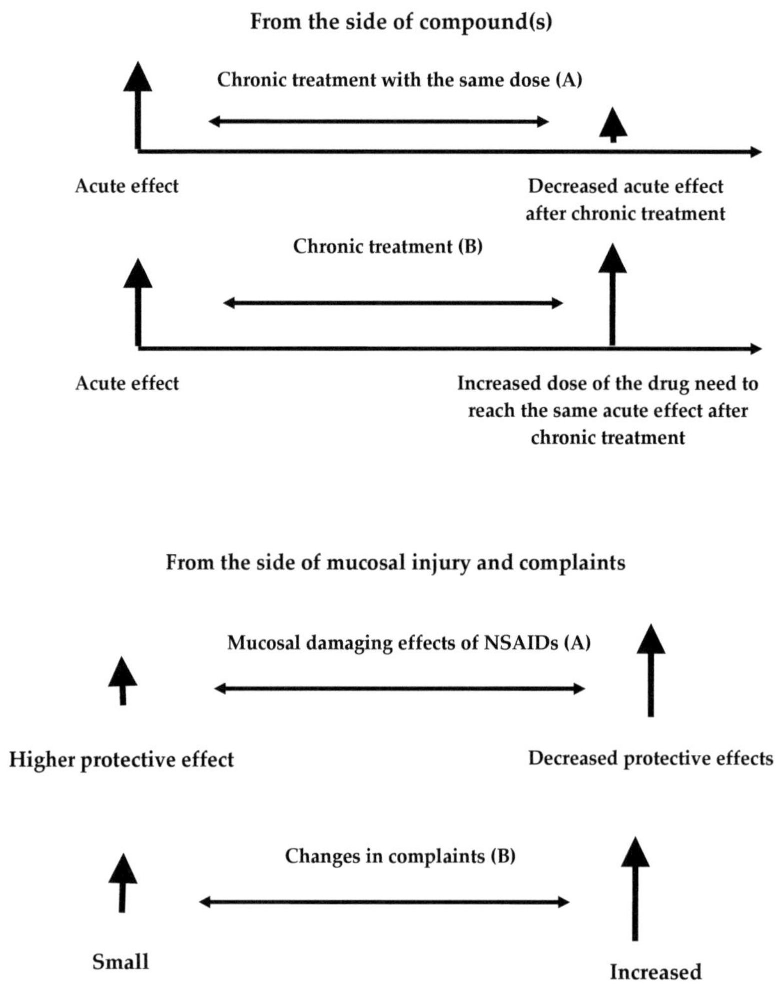

Figure 24. Schematic demonstration the possible pathways in changes of chronic capsaicin treatment from the side of the compound (upper part) and from the side of mucosal injury and complaints (lower part) in human healthy subjects and in patients with different (including gastrointestinal) disorders.

The results of these mentioned observations clearly indicated that the doses of capsaicin in our studies could not produce desensibilization of capsaicin receptors (these doses of capsaicin only were able to stimulate the capsaicin-sensitive afferent nerve).

4.5.2. Facts to exclude the presence of desensibilization to capsaicin receptor by applied doses of capsaicin during 2 weeks capsaicin treatments

The capsaicin exerts gastroprotective effect remained unchanged on IND-induced gastric mucosal microbleeding before and after 2-week capsaicin (3x 400μg orally given) treatment (Figures 19 and 24.

http://dx.doi.org/10.5772/58360

By other words, the gastric baseline microbleeding remained unchanged after the application of different doses of capsaicin (200, 400 and 800 μg orally) induced gastric mucosal prevention.

The registration of these facts are very important, since a very wide scale of capsaicin doses applied in human observations resulted very contradictory data (capsaicin were applied in stimulatory doses to capsaicin sensitive afferent nerve and much higher doses producing reversible and irreversible inhibitory actions in various animal experiments).

The capsaicin acts at the level of capsaicin receptor, which has been cloned (Caterina et al., 1997). It is true that the capsaicin action depends on its doses proved by animal experiments (Szolcsányi, 1984; Mózsik et al., 2001). The small dose (400 μg=ED_{50}) was applied for two weeks (in dose of 400 μg x 3 orally) in healthy subjects. The gastric mucosal microbleeding was produced by orally given IND (Figure 19 and Table 6.

The following results were obtained:

1. The extent of baseline gastric microbleeding before and after 2 weeks capsaicin (without application of any drug) remained unchanged.
2. The extent of acutely given IND-induced gastric microbleeding was also unchanged.
3. The extent of capsaicin-induced gastric mucosal protection was also found to be the same (and dose dependent) before and after 2 weeks capsaicin treatment.

It has been concluded from these observations that the sensitivity of capsaicin receptor (TRVP1) unchanged, and on the other hand, the orally applied capsaicin is capable to exert gastric mucosal protection against IND.

Probably the applied small dose of capsaicin – used in our present studies – could not modify the TRVP1 receptor sensitivity. We have no knowledge in this field by using higher dose(s) of capsaicin in human healthy subjects.

These facts are very important from the point of selection of capsaicin containing drug, because these dosages of capsaicin could exert beneficial effect (given orally in small doses), meanwhile the capsaicin can produce reversible or irreversible damage on the human gastric mucosa.

Earlier similar types of observations were carried out with atropine and other parasympatholytics (Mózsik et al., 1965; 1967; 1969 a,b) and cimetidine (Wildersmith et al., 1990). Tolerance developed to the drugs applied chronically in patients with peptic ulcer disease, and the "pharmacological denervation hypersensibility" occurred with a clinically detectable tolerance (Mózsik et al., 1966; 1967; 1969). These clinical pharmacological examinations modified the periodicity and dosage of applicable drugs (used in chronic treatment).

The careful analysis of the results with capsaicin actions, COX-1 and COX-2 systems and gastric microbleedings produced by IND in human healthy subjects before and after two weeks capsaicin (3 x 400 μg orally) treatment offered an excellent possibility to approach the capsaicin actions on the COX-1 and COX-2 enzyme system (Table 6).

4.5.3. Gastric (gastrointestinal) cytoprotection vs. capsaicin actions (given in stimulatory doses of capsaicin-sensitive afferent nerves)

Observations with different chemical agents (drugs, mediators, nutritive agents like retinoids, prostaglandins and others) indicated a special gastric mucosal protection, which did not depend on the gastric acid inhibition (see the reviews Mózsik et al. 2010, 2011). Later on, many observations indicated that the so-called gastric cytoprotective agents are able to prevent the development of injuries of numerous organs (produced by different actions) and they can accelerate healing processes.

The existence of gastric cytoprotection was earlier proved in patients with peptic ulcer (Mózsik et al., 1965, 2010, 2011) as it was nominated by André Robert (1979).

Only few points are interesting in our present position, namely: 1. the capsaicin-induced gastric mucosal protection in human healthy subjects is accompanied by the decrease of gastric acid secretion (that was one of the criteria differed from "classic" gastric cytoprotection); 2.both "classical cytopotective effects" as well as capsaicin-produced gastric mucosal protection disappear after surgical vagotomy (but not after chemical vagotomy); 3. gastric cytoprotective effect produced by different agents remained to be the same besides application of capsaicin (given in doses to produce stimulation of capsaicin-sensitive afferent nerves) (Mózsik et al., 1997). These results offer us to suggest that: 1. some part a gastric mucosal (cyto)protection is very closely associated with the functional activity of capsaicin-sensitive afferent nerves; 2. increased extent of gastric mucosal damage might develop in consequence of surgical ablation of capsaicin-sensitive afferent nerves (Mózsik et al., 1982, 2011).

These lines of capsaicin and cytoprotection protection in some meaning are similar and differ from each other (Szabó et al., 2012; Mózsik et al., 2011).

4.5.4. Distribution of capsaicin receptor, CGRP and SP in the gastric and large bowel mucosa of patients with different gastrointestinal disorders

The use of specific antisera against TRVP1 receptor, CGRP and SP released by the stimulation of capsaicin sensitive afferent nerve can immunohistochemical demonstrate their presence in the GI mucosa. Please note, that mucosal biopsy cannot be performed in healthy human subjects due to ethical regulations. So „healthy subjects"are represented by human subjects with functional disorders having no endoscopic abnormalities and diagnosed by clinicians and independent pathologist. There is another problem, namely the regular biopsy can be offered a small tissue sample for its regular pathological histological evaluation. Our specific immunohistochemical observations could be done only after successful routine histological examination.

We studied 178 patients with different gastrointestinal disorders (complaints), and the persons, who had normal histology based on the opinion of independent pathologist, were used as normal (healthy) human subjects (Dömötör et al., 2007; Mózsik et al., 2007).

The TRVP1 receptor, CGRP and SP neuropeptides released by the stimulation of capsaicin receptor can be shown by immonohistochemistry both in the human gastric and colon mucosa.

http://dx.doi.org/10.5772/58360

The TRVP1 receptors and neuropetides (CGRP and SP) could be demonstrated in the GI mucosa around the nerve endings, vascular elements, parietal cells, and also in epithelial layer.

The capsaicin application and the immunohistochemical demonstration of TRVP1 receptor in the GI tract newly met in the healthy human subjects. We studied the immunohistochemical distribution of TRVP1, CGRP and SP in the GI mucosa of patients with different disorders. The TRVP1 receptor, CGRP and SP could be detected practically in all patients with different acute, chronic diseases (including benignant, precancerous and cancerous diseases) (Dömötör et al., 2005). The results of these observations can be taken only as preliminary results. Their expression differed significantly in the GI mucosa of patients with acute and chronic disorders. Of course, the critical evaluation of these immunohistochemical observations is extremely hard, since we have only very limited information on the origin, stages, time periods of diseases, drug therapies and suggested etiological backgrounds. The studies dealing with the changes of individual patients with chronic GI disorders – in this research respect – are in progress. We have to emphasize two different main points in these studies, namely 1. The changes of the expressions of TRVP1, CGRP and SP are helpful from the point of development of GI mucosal injury and prevention, and 2. probably the participations of TRVP1, CGRP and SP differ in these GI pathological circumstances.

4.6. Immunohistochemical examinations in patients with chronic H. pylori positive and negative gastritis

In model human observations, the possible participation of TRVP1, CGRP and SP were studies in patients with chronic gastritis. The laboratory tests (quick urease test, urea breath test) and specific histological staining widely used in every day medical practice for demonstration of the presence of H. pylori infection were used, which suggested the presence of bacteria as the etiological for chronic gastritis.

Our studies were carried out in patients with H. pylori positive and negative chronic gastritis. The expression of TRVP1, CGRP and SP increased significantly in the gastric mucosa with chronic gastritis; however, no difference was obtained their expression in patients with H. pylori positive and negative chronic gastritis (Dömötör et al., 2006a).

The inflammation of the tissues does not represent a specific tissue reaction to inducing agents. This statement can be concluded from our results obtained in patients with H. pylori positive and negative chronic gastritis due the potential role of capsaicin sensitive afferent nerves. There is no question that the so-called „neurogenic inflammation" participated in the „general inflammatory processes" in patients with different gastrointestinal disorders.

4.7. Capsaicin sensitive afferentation in patients with chronic H. pylori positive gastritis before and after eradication treatment

The last step of our observations indicated that capsaicin-sensitive afferentation did not differ before and 6 weeks after successful eradication treatment in patients with chronic H. pylori positive gastritis (meanwhile the control biopsy was normal in 22 %, in 78% of cases it indicated a moderate improvement of the histological picture of gastritis) (Lakner et al, 2011; Mózsik et al., 2011, Mózsik et al., 2013; Czimmer et al., 2013).

After careful analysis of these results, it can be stated that the capsaicin-sensitive afferentation represents as an essential pathway in the healing of chronic gastritis (probably without and with H. pylori infection). These results suggest an independent mechanism in the healing of chronic gastritis which differs from the eradication treatment. By other words, besides the H. pylori infection other factors might exist. The H. pylori infection can be taken as one (but probably most important) exogenous factor, however, the capsaicin-sensitive afferent fibres of vagal nerve represents an endogenous factor in the injury and protection of gastric mucosa (Mózsik et al., 2013).

Our results with capsaicin (in healthy human subjects and in patients with different gastrointestinal disorders) are summarized in Figure 21. The vagal nerve is able to modify the GI tract by regulatory steps at the central nervous system and at the level of target organ. The peripheral action of capsaicin is a dose dependent action (Szolcsányi, 1984; Mózsik et al., 2001) (Table 5). The capsaicin mobilizes the CGRP and SP (Inui et al., 1991; Dömötör et., 2005), which modifies the vascular reactions in the GI mucosa (Sipos et al. 2006), recently demonstrated that the existence of neuroimmune link between the CGRP, SP and immune cells in the gastric mucosa of patients with chronic gastritis. Dömötör et al. (2006b) demonstrated the increased release of glucagon during a sugar loading test in healthy human subjects, indicated a new step of capsaicin-induced changes taking place between the capsaicin sensitive afferent nerves and neurohormonal regulation. Dömötör et al. (2006b) gave a direct evidence for the role of capsaicin in the carbohydrates metabolism.

There were a few very surprising matters due to capsaicin from the point of human classical clinical pharmacology prior our observations:

1. no permitted orally applicable capsaicin preparation was available for humans;
2. no chronic toxicology was known to capsaicin by animal observations;
3. no direct clinical pharmacological study had been performed to determine germinative function;
4. the capsaicin (Sigma-Aldrich, USA) chemically is not uniform due to its varying content of dihydrocapsaicin, nordihydrocapsaicin and some other capsaicinoids;
5. no classical human clinical pharmacological study (human phase I and phase II) was found in the literature;
6. no correct Drug Master File (DMF) for capsaicin preparation were developed for the commercially obtained capsaicin (exception of a certain capsaicin preparation obtained from India and used by us);
7. no human pharmacokinetic observations were available for capsaicin (please remember that our capsaicin studies in human healthy subjects were started in 1997).

Bernard et al. (2008) were unable to create pharmacokinetic profile of capsaicinoids after administration of 15 and 30 mg of capsaicin/person; meanwhile, the detection limit was 10 ng/

ml. Chaiyasit et al. (2009) after the application of 5 gram of C. frurenscens orally (equivalent to 26.6 mg pure capsaicin) found that the capsaicin could be detected in plasma after 10 min, and the peak concentration (C_{max}) was 2.47 ± 0.13 ng/mL, t_{max} was 47.1 ± 2.0 min and $t_{½}$ was 24.9 ± 5.0 min. After 90 min, capsaicin could not be detected in the plasma. Chaiyasit et al. (2009) explained the results of Bernard et al. (2008) by the time factor of pharmacokinetic behaviors of capsaicin in humans. The results of these observations were mentioned in the review paper by O'Neill et al. (2012).

We also received new information from the chronic toxicological studies in Beagle dogs (2008). These animals were treated with different doses (0.1, 0.3 and 0.9 mg/kg body weight/day orally given) of capsaicin(noids) for one month. No toxic effects were observed in these dogs during the whole treatment periods. We noticed surprisingly that capsaicin and dihydocapsaicin could not be detected in the sera of Beagle dogs by either high pressure chromatography with the detection limit of 20 ng/mL serum or liquid chromatography-mass spectrometry with the detectation was 26 fg/mL in the serum at any time after the oral administration (Mózsik et al., 2008; Boros et al., 2008).

5. Main conclusion from our obervations on capsaicin application in human healthy subjects and in patients with different disorders

1. The capsaicin (as a specific agent to stimulate the capsaicin-sensitive afferent nerves) plays a special role in the regulation the gastric functions (decrease of gastric acid secretion, increase of gastric emptying, increase in "buffering part" of the gastric secretion, increase of GTDP), absorption of glucose (and in its metabolism as well as in increase of glycagon release) in human healthy subjects, when it is applied in stimulatory doses;
2. The capsaicin given orally in stimulatory doses protects against the alcohol-and NSAID-induced gastric mucosal damage in healthy human subjects;.
3. If the capsaicin is given in stimulatory doses to capsaicin-sensitive afferent nerves in human healthy subjects, it will not produce desensibilization of its receptor (neither in acute administrations nor in chronic administrations) in human healthy subjects ;
4. The presence of capsaicin receptor (also CGRP and SP, which are very close in physiological relation) can be shown by specific immuno-histochemical methods under various GI disorders ;
5. The capsaicin-induced gastroprotection differs from the eradication treatment in patients with chronic H. pylori positive gastritis (and probably the roles of capsaicin receptor and CGRP differ from SP);
6. Very important to note that these gastroprotective actions can be obtained only by administration of capsaicin in stimulatory doses to its sensitive afferent nerves.

After looking of this conclusion list, there are clear evidences that the capsaicin is an orally applicable drug either alone or in combinations with different NSAIDs to human healthy subjects and to patients. Its indication is wide from prevention against drug-induced gastric mucosal damage, from patients under long term aspirin treatment (due to cardiovascular disease, thrombophylia, rheumatoid arthritis), pain killer treatment, patients having chronic H. pylori positive gastritis and to patient with different carbohydrate disorders.

We are of the opinion that we scientifically put down the clinical pharmacological bases of the oral capsaicin or drug combination use. We are in need of competent pharmaceutical partners for commercial introduction of these drug candidates into the everyday medical treatment (Mózsik, 2014; Mózsik et al., 2014).

Of course, we are aware that many other observations are need to be carried out in according to the regulations of international drug development, production and marketing for a capsaicin containing drug to licensed for everyday medical treatment.

Acknowledgements

This study was supported by the National Office for Research and Technology, "Pázmány Péter" Programme, RET-II 08/2005 (2005-2008), and by Baross Grant Programme (REG-DG-09-2-2009-0087, CAPSATAB) (2011-2012).

Author details

Gyula Mózsik[1], András Dömötör[1], József Czimmer[1], Imre L. Szabó[1] and János Szolcsányi[2]

*Address all correspondence to: gyula.mozsik@aok.pte.hu; gyula.mozsik@gmail.com

1 First Department of Medicine Medical and Health Centre, University of Pécs, Hungary

2 Department of Pharmacology and Pharmacotherapy, Medical and Health Centre, University of Pécs, Hungary

The authors confirm that this overview content has no conflicts of interest.

References

[1] Abdel-Salam OME, Czimmer J, Debreceni A, Mózsik Gy (2001) Gastric mucosal integrity: Gastric mucosal blood flow and microcirculation. An overview. J Physiol Paris 95: 105-127

[2] Abdel-Salam OME, Debreceni A, Mózsik Gy (1999) Capsaicin-sensitive afferent sensory nerves in modulating gastric mucosal defense against noxious agents. J. Physiol Paris 93 : 443-454

[3] Aijoka H, Matsuura N, Miyake H (2002) High quality of ulcer healing in rats by lafutidine and new-type histamine H_2-receptor antagonist: involvement of capsaicin of sensitive sensory neurons. Inflammopharmacology 10: 483-493

[4] Aijoka H, Miyake H, Matsuura N (2000) Effect of FRG-8813, a new-type histamine H_2-receptor antagonist, on the recurrence of gastric ulcer healing by drug treatment. Pharmacology 61: 83-90

[5] Antal L, Mózsik Gy, Jávor T, Krausz M. (1965) The electrolyte content of gastric juice after prolonged atropine treatment. In: Magyar I (ed) Acta Tertii Conventus Medicinae Internae Hungarici. Gastroenterologia. Akadémiai Kiadó, Budapest, pp 167-169

[6] Bernard BK, Tsubuku S, Kayhara T, Maeda K, Hanada M, Nakamura T, Shirai Y, Nakayaha A, Ueno S, Mihara H (2008) Studies of the toxicological potential of capsaicinoids. X. Safety assessment and pharmacokinetics of capsaicinoids in healthy male vlonteers after single oral ingestion of CH-19 Sweet extract. Int J Toxicol 27 (Suppl 3): 137-147

[7] Boros B, Dornyei Á, Felinger A (2008) Determination of capsaicin and dihydrocapsaicin in dog plasma by Liquid Chromatography- Mass Spectography (analytical method report). PTE TTK Analitikai Kémiai Tanszék, Pécs,Hungary

[8] Buck SH, Burks TF (1986) The neuropharmacology of capsaicin: a review of some recent observation. Pharmacol Rev 38: 179-226

[9] Caterina MJ, Schumacher MA, Tominaga H, Rosen TA., Levine JD, Julius D (1997) The capsaicin receptor: a heat-activated ion channel in the pain pathway. Nature 389: 816-824.

[10] Chaiyasit E, Khovidhunkit W, Wittayertpanya S (2009) Pharmacokinetic and the effect of capsaicin in Capsicum flourescens on decreasing plasma glucose level. J Med Assoc Thai 92:108-113

[11] Czimmer J, Szabó IL, Szolcsányi J, Mózsik Gy (2013) Capsaicin-sensitive afferentation represents a new mucosal defensive neural pathway system in the gastric mucosa in patients with chronic gastritis.In: Mozsik Gy (ed) Current Topics in Gastritis – 2012.INTECH Publishers, Rijeka, Croatia, pp 61-75

[12] Csáky TZ (1969) Introduction to general pharmacology. Appleton–Century-Craft Educational Division, Meredith Corporation, New York. pp 17-34

[13] Debreceni A, Abdel-Salam OME, Figler M, Juricskay I, Szolcsányi J, Mózsik Gy (1999). Capsaicin increases gastric emptying rate in healthy human subjects measured by ^{13}C-labeled octanoid acid breath test. J Physiol Paris 93: 455-460

[14] Dömötör A, Peidl Zs, Vincze Á, Hunyady B, Szolcsányi J, Szekeres Gy, Mózsik Gy. (2005) Immunohistocemical distribution of vanilloid receptor, calcitonin- gene related peptide and substance P in gastrointestinal mucosa of patients with different gastrointestinal disorders. Inflammopharmacology 13: 161-177

[15] Dömötör A, Kereskay L, Szekeres Gy, Hunyady B, Szolcsányi J, Mózsik Gy (2006a) Participation of capsaicin sensitive afferent nerves in the gastric mucosa of patients with Helicobacter pylori-positive or –negative chronic gastritis. Dig Dis Sci 52:411-417

[16] Dömötör A, Szolcsányi J, Mózsik Gy (2006b) Capsaicin and glucose absortion and utilization in healthy human subjects. Eur J Pharmacol 534:280-283

[17] Fisher MA, Hunt JN (1976) A sensitive method for measuring haemoglobin in the gastric juice. Digestion 14:409-414

[18] Gabella G, Pease H (1973) Number of axons in the abdominal vagus of the rat. Brain Res 58: 465-469

[19] Grijalva CV, Novin D (1990) The role of hypothalamus and dorsal vagal complex in gastrointestinal function an pathophysiology. Ann N Y Acad Sci.. 597: 207-221

[20] Hollander F (1934) The component of gastric secretion. Am J Dig Dis Sci 1:319-329

[21] Holzer P (1998) Neural emergency system in the stomachs. Gastroenterology 114: 823-839

[22] Holzer P (1999) Capsaicin cellular targets. Mechanisms of action, as selectivity for thin sensory neurons, Phamacol Rev 43:143-201

[23] Holzer P (2013) Transient receptor potential (TRP) channels as drug targets for diseases of the gastrointestional system. Pharmacol & Ther 131: 142-170

[24] Hossenbocus A, Fitzpatrick P, Colin-Jones DG (1975) Measurement of gastric potential difference at endoscopy. Gut 14: 410-415

[25] Inui T, Kinoshita J, Yamahuchi A, Yamatani T, Chiba T (1991) Linkage between capsaicin-stimulated calcitonin gene-related peptide and somatostatin release in the rat stomach. Am J Physiol. 261: G770-774

[26] Jancsó N, Jancsó- Gábor A, Szolcsányi J (1967) Direct evidence for neurogenic inflammation and its prevention by denervation and by pretreatment with capsaicin. Brit J Pharmacol 31:138-151

[27] Jancsó N.,Jancsó- Gábor A, Szolcsányi J (1968) The role of sensory nerves endings in the neurogen inflammation induced in human skin and in the eye and paw of the rat. Brit J Pharmacol 33: 32-41

[28] Jancsó-Gábor A, Szolcsányi J, Jancsó N. (1970) Irreversible impairment of the irregulation induced by capsaicin and similar pungent substances in rat and guinea-pigs. J Physiol London 206: 495-507

[29] Karádi O, Mózsik Gy (2000) Surgical and Chemical Vagotomy on the Gastrointestinal Mucosal Defense. Akadémiai Kiadó, Budapest

[30] Kawai S, Nishida S, Kato M, Furumaya Y, Okamoto R, Koshino T, Mizushima Y (1998) Comparison of cyclooxygenase-1 and -2 inhibitory activities of various non-steroidal anti-inflammatory drugs using human platelets and synovial cells. Eur J. Pharmacol 347:87-94

[31] Lakner L, Dömötör A, Tóth Cs, Szabo IL, Mecker Á, Hajós R, Kereskay L, Szekeres Gy, Döbrönte Z, Mózsik Gy (2011) Capsaicin-sensitive afferentation represents an indifferent defensive pathway from eradication in patients with Helicobacter pylori positive gastritis. World J Gastrointest Pharmacol Ther 2: 36-41

[32] Marfertheimer P, Megraud F, 0'Morain C, Bazzoli F, El-Omar E, Graham D, Hunt R, Rokkas T, Vakil N, Kuipers EJ (2007) Current concept in the management of Helicobacter pylori infection: the Maastricht III Consensus Report. Gut 56: 772-781

[33] Mózsik Gy (2006) Molecular pharmacology and biochemistry of gastroduodenal mucosal damage and protection. In Mózsik Gy (ed) Discoveries in Gastroenterology: from Basic Research to Clinical Perspectives (1960-2005). Akadémiai Kiadó, Budapest, pp 139-224

[34] Mózsik Gy (2010) Gastric cytoprotection 30 years after its discovery by André Robert: a personal perspective. Inflammopharmacology 18: 209-221

[35] Mózsik Gy (2014). Capsaicin is new orally applicable gastroprotective and therapeutic drug alone or in combination in human healthy subjects and in patients. In: Abdel Salam OME (Ed) Capsaicin as an Therapeutic Molecule. Springer Verlag, Basel, pp. 209-258.

[36] Mózsik Gy, Abdel-Salam OME, Szolcsányi J (1997) Capsaicin-Sensitive Afferent Nerves in Gastric Mucosal Damage and Protection. Akadémiai Kiadó Budapest.

[37] Mózsik Gy, Belágyi J, Szolcsányi J, Pár G, Pár A, Rumi Gy, Rácz I (2004a) Capsaicin-sensitive afferent nerves and gastric mucosal protection on human healthy subjects. A critical overview, in: Takeuchi K, Mozsik Gy (eds) Mediators in Gastrointestinal Protection and Repair. Research Signpost, Kerala, India, pp 43-62

[38] Mózsik Gy, Debreceni A, Abdel-Salam OME, Szabó I, Figler M, Ludány A, Juricskay I, Szolcsányi J (1999) Small doses capsaicin given intragastrically inhibit gastric basal gastric secretion in healthy human subjects. J Physiol Paris 93:433-436.

[39] Mózsik Gy, Berstad A, Myren J, Setekleiv J (1969a) Absorption and urinary excretion oxyphencyclamin HCI in patients before and after a prolonged oxyphencyclimide treatment. Med Exp 19: 10-16

[40] Mózsik Gy, Dömötör A, Past T, Vas V, Perjési P, Kuzma M, Blazics Gy, Szolcsányi J (2009) Capsaicinoids: from the Plant Cultivation to the Production of the Human Medical Therapy. Akadémiai Kiadó, Budapest

[41] Mózsik Gy, Hunyady B, Garamszegi M, Németh A, Pakodi F, Vincze A. (1994) Dynamism of cytoprotective and antisecretory drugs in patients with unhealed gastric and duodenal ulcers. J Gastroenterol Hepatol 9: S88-92

[42] Mózsik Gy, Jávor T (1969b) Development of drug cross-tolerance in patients treated chronically with atropine. Eur J Pharmacol 6:169-174.

[43] Mózsik Gy, Jávor T, Dobi S (1965) Clinical-pharmaological analysis of long term parasympatholytic treatment. In: Magyar I (ed) Acta Tertii Conventus Medicinae Internae Hungarici. Gastroenterologia.Akadémiai Kiadó, Budapest, pp 709-715

[44] Mózsik Gy, Jávor T, Dobi S, Petrássy K, Szabó A. (1966) Development of "pharmacological denervation phenomenon" in patients treated with atropine. Eur J Pharmacol 1: 391-395

[45] Mózsik Gy, Moron F, Jávor T (1982) Cellular mechanisms of the development of gastric mucosal damage and of gastroprotection induced by prostacyclin in rats. A pharmacological study, Prostagland Leukot Med 9: 71-84

[46] Mózsik Gy, Past T, Abdel-Salam OME, Kuzma M, Perjési P (2009) Interdisciplinary review for correlation between the plant origin capsaicinoids , nonsteroidal antiinflammatory drugs, gastrointestinal mucosal damage and prevention in animals and human beings. Inflammopharmacology 17: 113-150

[47] Mózsik Gy, Past T, Dömötör A, Kuzma M, Perjési P (2010) Production of orally applicable new drug or drug combinations from natural origin capsaicinoids for human medical therapy. Curr Pharm Des 16, 1197-1208

[48] Mózsik Gy, Past T, habvon T, Keszthely Zs, Perjési P, Kuzma M, Sándor B, Szolcsányi J, Abdel-Salam OME, Szalai M.(2014) Capsaicin is a new gastrointestinal mucosal protecting drug candidate in humans – pharmaceutical development and production based on clinical pharmacology. In: Mózsik Gy, Abdel-Salam OME, Takeuchi K (Eds) Capsaicin-Sensitive Neural Afferentation and the Gastrointestinal Tract: from Bench to Bedside. INTECH Publishers, Rijeka (in press).

[49] Mózsik Gy, Pár A, Pár G, Juricskay I, Figler M, Szolcsányi J (2004a) Insight into the molecular pharmacology to drugs acting on the afferent and efferent fibres of vagal nerve in the gastric mucosal protection In:: Ulcer Research, Proceedings of the 11th International Conference, Sikirič P., Seiwerth P., Mózsik Gy., Arakawa T., Takeuchi K. (eds) Ulcer Research, Proceedings of the 11th International Conference. Monduzzi, Bologna, pp 163-168.

[50] Mózsik Gy, Sarlos P, Racz I, Szolcsányi J (2003). Evidence for the direct protective effect of capsaicin in human healthy subjects. Gastroenterology 124: Suppl 1, A-454

[51] Mózsik Gy, Past T, Perjési P, Szolcsányi J (2008) Determination of capsaicin and dihydrocapsaicin content of dog's plasma by HPLC-FLD method. In: Mózsik Gy., Past T, Pejési P., Szolcsány J: Original reports on toxicology of capsaicin.VII. 8-day oral tocicity study of test item capsaicin natural USP 37 in Beagle Dogs (Final report). LAB International research Centre Hungary Ltd. Veszprém,Hungary by the date of final repot 13 June 2008.Study Code: 07/496-100K, pp 1-35 text and 190 pages in Appendices (Appendix 2.11) pp 1-37

[52] Mózsik Gy, Rácz I, Szolcsányi J (2005) Gastroprotection induced by capsaicin in human healthy subjects. World J. Gastroenterol 11: 5180-5184

[53] Mózsik Gy, Szabo IL, Czimmer J (2011a) Approaches to gastrointestinal cytoprotection: from isolated cell, via animal experiments to healthy human subjects and patients witg different gastrointestinal disorders. Curr Pharm Des 17: 1556-72

[54] Mózsik Gy, Szabó IL,Dömötör A (2011b) Approach to role of capsaicin-sensitive afferent nerves in the development and healing in patients with chronic gastritis. In: Tonito P (ed) Gastritis and Gastric Cancer. New Insights in Gastroprotection,Diagnosis and Treatments. INTECH Publishers, Rijeka, Croatia, pp 25-46

[55] Mózsik Gy, Szabó I L, Czimmer J (2014) Vulnerable points of the Helicobacter pylori story – based on animal and human observations (1975-2012).In: Buzas Gy (ed) Helicobacter Pylori – a Worldwide Perspective 2013.Bentham Science Publishers, Oak Park, IL, USA, pp. 429-480.

[56] Mózsik Gy, Szolcsányi J, Dömötör A. (2007) Capsaicin research as a new tool to approach of the human gastrointestinal physiology, pathology and pharmacology. Inflammopharmacology 15: 232-45

[57] Mózsik Gy, Vincze Á, Szolcsányi J (2001) Four responses of capsaicin sensitive primary afferent neurons to capsaicin and its analog. Gastric acid secretion, gastric mucosal damage and protection. J. Gastroenterol. Hepatol. 16:193-197

[58] Myren J (1968) Gastric secretion following stimulation with histamine, histology and gastrin in man. In: Semb L, Myren J (eds) The Physiology of gastric Secretion. Universitetforlaget, Oslo, pp 413-428

[59] Nagy L, Mózsik Gy, Feledi É, Ruzsa Cs, Vezekényi Zs, Jávor T (1984) Gastric microbleeding measurements during one day treatment with indomethacin and indomethacin plus sodium salicylate (1:10) in patients. Acta Physiol. Hung 64: 373-377

[60] O'Neill J, Brock C, Olesen E, Andersen T, Nilsson M, Dickenson AH (2012) Unravelling the mystery of capsaicin: a tool to understand and treat pain. Pharmacol Rev 64: 939-97

[61] Onodera S, Shibata M, Tanaka M (1999) Gastroprotective mechanisms of lafutidine, a novel anti-ulcer drug with histamine H_2-receptor antagonist activity, Artneim. Forsch., Drug. Res. 49: 519-526

[62] Onodera, S., Shibata, M., Tanaka M (2002) Gastroprotective activity of FRG-8813, a novel histamine H_2-receptor antagonist, in rats. Jpn J Pharmacol 68: 161-173

[63] Patty I, Tárnok F, Simon L, Jávor T, Deák G, Benedek Sz, Kenéz P, Nagy L, Mózsik Gy (1984) A comporative dynamic study of the effectiveness of gastric cytoprotection by the vitamin A, De-Nol, sucralfate and ulcer healing by pirenzepine in patients with chronic gastric ulcer (A multi-clinical and randomized study). Acta Physiol Hung 64:379-384

[64] Robert A, Nemazis JE, Lancastter C, Hanchar A (1979) Cytoprotection by prostaglandins in rats. Prevention of gastric necrosis by alcohol, HCl, NaOH, hypertonic NaCl and thermal injury. Gastroenterology 77: 4433-443

[65] Sarlós P, Rumi Gy, Szolcsányi J, Mózsik Gy, Vincze Á (2003) Capsaicin prevents the indomethacin-induced gastric mucosal damage in human healthy subject. Gastroenterology 124: Suppl. 1, A-511

[66] Sipos G, Altdorfer K, Pongor É, Chen LP, Fehér E (2006) Neuroimmune link in the mucosa of chronic gastritis with Helicobacter pylori infection. Dig Dis Sci 51: 1810-1017

[67] Szabo IL, Czimmer J, Szolcsányi J, Mózsik Gy (2013). Molecular pharmacological approaches to effects of capsaicinoids and of classical antisecretory drugs on gastric basal acid secretion and on indomethacin-induced gastric mucosal damage in human healthy subjects (mini review). Curr Pharm Des 19: 84-89

[68] Szabo S, Taché Y, Tarnawski A (2012) The "Gastric Cytoprotection" concept of André Robert and the origins of a new series of international symposia. In: Filaretova LP, Takeuchi K (eds) Cell/ Tissue Injury and Cytoprotection/Organoprotection in the Gastrointestinal Tract. Front Gastrointest Res. Basel, Karger. Vol. 30, pp 1-23

[69] Szállasi A, Blumberg M (1999) Vanilloid (capsaicin) receptors and mechanisms. Pharmacol Rev 51:159-211

[70] Szolcsányi J (1984) Capsaicin sensitive chemoprotective neural system with dual sensory-afferent function. In: Chalh LA, Szolcsányi J, Lembeck F (eds) Antidromic Vasodilatation and Neurogenic Inflammation. Budapest, Akadémiai Kiadó, pp. 27-56

[71] Szolcsányi J (1997) A pharmacological approach to elucidation of the role of different nerve fibres and receptor endings inmediation of pain. J Physiol Paris 73: 251-259

[72] Szolcsányi J (2004) Forty years in capsaicin research for sensory pharmacology and physiology. Neuropeptide 38: 377-384.

[73] Szolcsány J.(2014) Discovery and mechanism of gastroprotective action of capsaicin. In: Mózsik Gy., Abdel-Salam OME, Takeuchi K (eds). Capsaicin Sensitive Neural Afferentation and the Gastrointestinal Tract: from Bench to Bedside. INTECH Publishers, Rijeka,Croatia (in pres).

[74] Szolcsányi J, Barthó L (1979) Capsaicin-sensitive innervation of the guinea-pig small intestine and its selective blockade by capsaicin. Naunyn-Schmidede-berg's Arch Pharmacol 305: 83-90

[75] Szolcsányi J, Barthó L (1981) Impaired defense mechanisms to peptic ulcer in the capsaicin-desensitized rat. In: Mózsik Gy, Hänninen O, Jávor T (eds) Advances in Physiological Sciences Vol.29, Gastrointestinal Defense Mechanisms.Pergamon Press, Oxford-Akadémiai Kiadó, Budapest, pp 39-51

[76] Takeuchi K (2006) Unique profile of Lafutidine: a novel histamine H_2-receptor antagonist: mucosal protection throughout GI mucosal mediated by capsaicin-sensitive afferent nerves. Acta Pharmacol. Sinica Suppl.pp 27-35

[77] Tárnok F, Deák G, Jávor T, Mózsik Gy, Nagy L, Patty I (1983) Effect of combination atropine and cyproheptadine and atropine+carbenoxolone in duodenal ulcer therapy. Int J Tiss React 5:315-321

[78] Tárnok F, Jávor T, Mózsik Gy, Nagy L, Patty I, Rumi Gy, Solt I (1979) A prospective multiclinical study comparing the effects of placebo, carbenoxolone, atropine cimetidine in patients with duodenal ulcer. Drugs Exp Clin Res 5 : 157-166

[79] Vincze A, Szekeres Gy, Király Á, Bódis B, Mózsik Gy (2004) The immunohistochemical distribution of capsaicin receptor, CGRP and SP in the human gastric mucosa in patients with different gastric disorders.In: Sikirič , Seiwert S, Mózsik Gy, Arakawa T, Takeuchi K (eds). Ulcer Research.Proceedings of 11th International Congress of Ulcer Resarch. Monduzzi, Bologna, pp 149-153

[80] Wildersmith, CH, Ernst T, Gennoni M, Zeyen B, Halter F, Merki HS (1990) Tolerance to H_2-receptor antagonist. Dig Dis Sci 35: 976-983

Section 6

Development and Industrial Production of Capsaicin(oids)-Containing Drug and Drug Combinations: Preclinical Dossier, Chronic Capsaicin Toxicology, Pathways of Classical Clinical Pharmacology in Human Healthy Subjects and in Patients

Chapter 11

Capsaicin is a New Gastrointestinal Mucosal Protecting Drug Candidate in Humans — Pharmaceutical Development and Production Based on Clinical Pharmacology[1]

Gyula Mózsik, Tibor Past, Tamás Habon,
Zsuzsanna Keszthelyi, Pál Perjési, Mónika Kuzma,
Barbara Sándor, János Szolcsányi,
M.E. Abdel-Salam Omar and Mária Szalai

Additional information is available at the end of the chapter

http://dx.doi.org/10.5772/58359

1. Introduction

Backgrounds. 1. The intact gastrointestinal mucosa is a result of excellently well regulated equilibrium between the aggressive (physical and other stress, xenobiotics, wide scale of drugs, chemicals, bacterial and viral infections) and defensive (bicarbonate secretion, mucus secretion, blood supply, prostaglandins, mucosal energy systems, etc.) factors, which are further controlled by different neural, hormonal and pharmacological mechanisms. 2. The vagal nerve takes an essential place both in the development of gastrointestinal mucosal damage and protection. 3. The physicians have widely been applied the nonsteroidal antiinflammatory drugs (such as aspirin, diclofenac, Naproxen, etc.) as antipyretic, anti-inflammatory, painkiller and platelet aggregation inhibitor agents in healthy humans and in patients with different disorders (such as myocardial infaction, different forms of thrombophylia, rheumatoid arthritis and arthrosis or trauma) in the everyday medical practice. The administration of these drugs produces gastrointestinal complaints (mucosal damages, bleedings, perforations). So in one hand, the applications of these drugs are absolutely indicated, on the other hand, the

1 Important note: The term "capsaicin" is used in the text, however capsaicinoids of natural origin are used for during different studies.Some times the term "capsaicinoids" are used to emphasize their plant origin.

applications of these drugs are contraindicated from the points of gastroenterologist. 4. We earlier proved clearly that the small doses of capsaicin (given orally in doses of nanogram to microgram / kg in animal experiments and 200 to 800 μg in human observations) prevents the aspirin, indomethacin (a mixed COX-1 and COX-2 inhibitor)-induced gastrointestinal mucosal damage.

Aims: 1. The development and pharmaceutically production of the planned production of new gastrointestinal mucosal protective drug (capsaicin alone and/or capsaicin in combination with different nonsteroidal anti-inflammatory drugs) for the use in human healthy beings and in patients. 2. For the development and production of a new drug, we had to respect the following aspects: **a**. the knowledge of the chemical composition of natural origin capsaicin(oids); **b**. problems of the analytical measurements of capsaicin(oids) in the biological samples (in animals and humans); **c**. correct and complete preclinical dossier; **d**. correct dossier of acute and chronic toxicological studies with capsaicin (including the different tests) in two speciments of animal experiments; **e**. existence of a complete drug master file (DMF); **f**. the exclusion of pesticides, fusariums, aflatoxin and other toxicological agents (which are used during the plant cultivation in the different countries) from the capsaicin(oids) preparations used for drug production; **g**. to collect the necessary permissions from the different international and national authrorities before starting of pharmaceutical production of drug alone or in combinations; **h**. different pharmaceutical controlling measurements and other pharmaceutical aspects of planned drug or drug combinations (such as stability, drug preparation, different pharmaceutical technologies, etc.); **i**. preparation of different protocols for human human phase examinations (especially for human phase I.); **j**. to receive the permissions from the the different national authorities to carried out the prepared protocols before starting of the classical pharmacological studies; **k**. to gather the necessary numbers of experts from the very different scientific fields, who are able to solve all of above mentioned scientific, pharmaceutical, research problems (in animal experiments and in human observations); l. to find accredited institutes to perform human clinical pharmacological (phase) examinations. 2. When we solved all of above scientific problems, the human phase I. examinations with capsaicin alone and with combination+aspirin and capsaicin+diclofenac, the human phase I. examinations were in the Clinical Pharmacological Units of First Department of Medicine and of Institute of Cardiology, Medical and Health Centre, University of Pécs, Hungary, meanwhile the pharmacokinetic measurements were done in the Laboratories of PannonPharma Pharmaceutical Ltd., Pécsvárad, Hungary. 3. The aims of these human phase I. examinations were: **a**. to measure of capsaicin in the plasma of male human healthy subjects, when the capsaicin was given orally (in doses of 400 and 800 μg) alone or in combination with aspirin (500 mg orally) and with diclofenac (100 mg orally); **b**. to measure the pharmacokinetic parameters (C_{max}, T_{max}, $AUC_{0\text{-}tlast}$, $AUC_{0\text{-}\infty}$, $t_{½}$, MRT, mean residence time) of ASA and diclofenac given alone and after in combinations with different doses (400 and 800 μg) of capsaicin; **c**. to study extents of inhibitory effect on platelet aggregation of ASA and diclofenac on the epinephrine-induced platelet aggregation.

The observations were carried out on volunteers of healthy male human subjects. The volunteers were selected by special experts of human clinical pharmacology based on the strict criteria of inclusion and exclusion. The time period of phase I. examinations was maximally 8 weeks, from which two weeks for randomisation of the volunteers (15 in each study), the clinical pharmacological study was done in five sequences during 5 weeks, and the post-study procedure took one week after the closing the clinical pharmacological studies. The observations were carried out in random allocation, and the human phase I. examinations covered hospitalization (two days) and outpatients (4 days) periods. The observations were carried out according to the written and permitted protocols ("Human phase I. single-blind study comparing the pharmacokinetic properties of ASA after single administration alone and co-administration with two different doses of capsaicin (400 and 800 μg) and evaluating their safety in healthy male subjects". Protocol number: 1.4.1; EudraCT number: 2008-007048-32 and " Human phase I. single-blind study comparing the pharmacokinetic properties of diclofenac after single administration alone and co-administration with two different doses of capsaicin (400 and 800 μg) and evaluating their safety in healthy male subjects". Protocol number: 1.4.2; EudraCT number: 2008-007050-36).

Our observations were to produce clinically and pharmaceutically a new capsaicin containing drug and drug combinations started from 2005 as an "innovative drug research", meanwhile the human phase I. examinations started from March 10, 2011 and finished by December 31, 2013 (including the examinations, pharmacokinetic measurements, mathematical analysis of obtained results, closing of written reports).

Main results and conclusions: 1. The presence of capsaicin and dihydrocapsaicin (after orally given capsaicinoids of 400 and 800 μg) was not able to detect in the plasma of the healthy male volunteers, who were treated with capsaicin(oids); 2. The capsaicin(oids) does (do) not modify the absorption, metabolism and excretion of orally given ASA and diclofenac; 3. The capsaicin(oids) does(do) not modify the epinephrine-induced platelet aggregation by ASA and diclofenac, meanwhile the different doses of capsaicin(oids) alone has (have) no direct action on the epinephrine-induced platelet aggregation; 4. We have learned a lot of new research, juristic, patent, pharmaceutical and other clinical pharmacological problems (from basic research problems, requisted animal toxicological examinations by the different authorities,

preparation of preclinical dossier, the different pathways for obtaining official permission from the different authorities to carried out the human clinical phase examinations, chemical qualification of capsaicin(oids) in the plasma in treated animals and human healthy subjects);

5. We were able to start with the development and production of pharmaceutical production of gastroprotective capsacin(oids) containing drug alone and in combinations with ASA and diclofenac based on the internationally accepted laws of human clinical pharmacology; 6.

We established the scientific basis of the capsaicin-sensitive afferentation vs. gastric mucosal protection against the different noxious agents (including the nonsteroidal anti-inflammatory drugs) in human healthy subjects and in patients treated with different anti-inflammatory drugs.

2. Historic backgrounds

The biological regulation of living organ is very complex process, including the efferent nerves as well as afferent nerves as recently discovered. These regulatory processes influence main cellular physiological mechanisms. Of course, for the understanding these mechanisms we have to learn the principal physiological laws at the level of cells (including the classical physiology, biochemistry and in different pathological circumstances) (Mozsik, 2006).

The primary aim of pharmacology is to give different biological or chemical substances, which are able to modify cell functions under normal and pathological conditions (Mózsik et al., 1997; Mózsik, 2006). The field of pharmacology changed significantly nowdays by the application of various research trends (chemical synthesis of new drugs, drugs of plant origin, molecular biology plus immunology, etc).

We deal briefly in this paper with the interdisciplinary challenges in new drug (and drug combinations) production of plant origin capsaicin (alone or in combination with NSAIDs) modulating (used in doses, which have stimulatory actions on the capsaicin-sensitive afferent nerves) pharmacologically the afferent nerves in the gastrointestinal (GI) tract. From that point of views we carefully and critically evaluated the correlations between the plant origin capsaicinoids, NSAIDs with GI mucosal damage and preventions in animals and human healthy beings (Abdel Salam et al., 1994; 1995a,b,c,e,f,g; 1996a,b; 1997a,b,c,d; 1999; 2001; 2006 ; Mózsik et al., 1999; 2006 a,b; 2005; 2007).

3. Main problems of pharmacological treatment in patient with different diseases

The patients with myocardial infarction, thromboembolic episodes, stroke of central nervous system, cancers and persons who have to be treat as preventions of different diseases (reinfarction after myocardial infarction, prevention of thromboembolic episodes produced by atrial fibrillation, cancers, after different surgical intervention and immobilization) and in healthy subjects treated with NSAIDs in order to prevent the development of colorectal cancers. The number of these groups of patients reaches to 50-60 per cent of total population in Hungary.

The majority of patients who underwent cardiac and other surgeries are treated permanently with aspirin (in dose of 100 mg/day/person). This is a basic stand-point of the different consensus meetings of Europe and of the World (Megettigan et al., 2006; Patrono et al., 2004; Todd and Clisson, 1990).

The administration of aspirin in absolutely indicated from medical points of view in patients mentioned above, accepting the opinion of cardiologists; however, we have to emphasize that the aspirin very frequently produces GI bleeding (which do not favour gastroenterologists). Really, there is a great and principal question from the general medical practice (and of research), namely whether all patient can be taken as the same, in whom the medical science should offer medical treatment from the point of cardiology, which produces severe GI disorders (bleedings, peptic ulcer). Consequently there is a contradictory medical (and evidence-based proved) standpoint between the cardiologists vs. gastroenterologists (during the treatment of one patient, and as well as in the treatment of populations of patients mentioned above).

Another big population of patients suffers from different degenerative joint diseases, trauma or from acute and chronic pain. These patients have to receive permanent treatment with NSAIDs. The NSAIDs are not GI protective agents neither in healthy person and nor in patients with these disorders. Large portion of patients appearing on gastrointestinal wards suffer from the drug-induced side effects.

Patients with NSAIDs-induced gastrointestinal disorders (blood losing, bleeding, peptic ulcer) represent a significant number of populations. Furthermore, these patients have to treat permanently by different NSAIDs.

The actions of NSAIDs are associated with the selective and non-selective inhibitory properties on cyclooxygenase system (emphasizing the key role of COX-1 and COX-2). Aspirin is a specific COX-1 inhibitor; meanwhile other NSAIDs applied in the clinical practice represent the compounds acting as non-selective COX-1 and COX-2 inhibitors. Recently, the specifically acting compounds, inhibiting COX-2 enzyme, have been produced to reduce gastric mucosal damage, however, the number of myocardial infarction was increase in such patients (Megettigan et al., 2006; Patrono et al., 2004; Tood and Clissold, 1990; Couzin 2004a,b; Lenzer, 2004).

We have to emphasize clearly, that the small doses of capsaicin are able to prevent gastric mucosal bleeding induced by NSAIDs (both COX-1, COX-2 inhibitors). It is true that COX-2 inhibitors produce smaller side effects in GI tract of patients; however these compounds have no inhibitory properties on the thrombocyte aggregation. When the patient with angina pectoris and degenerative joint disease received only COX 2 inhibitors, than the number of patients with myocardial infarctions and of cardiac origin death increased significantly ("Vioxx story") (Couzin, 2004a,b ; Lenzer, 2004; Green, 2005; Lawler, 2005; Tanne, 2006a,b,c). Recently, the European and American Consensus Meetings uniformly accepted the salicylate application in about dose of 100 mg/day and of 300 mg/day in cumarine resistant patient (Megettigan et al., 2006; Patrono et al., 2004).

Our aim was to product a capsaicin containing drug or drug combinations with a NSAID for the treatment of above mentioned groups of patients hoping that application of these compounds will be able to prevent the NSAIDs induced GI side effects in patients (Mózsik et al., 2009a,b, 2010; Szabo et al., 2013).

4. Experts' opinion up to 2008

We successfully applied funding for innovative academic pharmacological and pharmaceutical industrial research to the National Office for Research and Technology (Hungary) in 2005 (Regional University Science Centre Pécs, Hungary, MEDIPOLISZ, Pázmány Péter Programme RET-II, 08/2005) for time period of 2006-2008, and later on BAROS GÁBOR Programme, Hungary (REG_DKI_O,CAPSATAB) for time period of 2010-2011.

The aims of these research programmes (in these time periods) were to produce new capsaicin(oids) drug alone and in different combinations for patients with different gastrointestinal disorders, for patients with myocardial infarctions (orally applicable combinations of capsaicin(oids) with aspirin) and for those with chronic degenerative locomotive diseases (orally applicable capsaicin(oids) with diclofenac and Naproxen).

Twenty-one researchers (chemist, pharmaceutical chemist, physicians, clinical pharmacologists, pharmaceutics, laboratory experts, biologists, engineers and agricultural engineers) have participated in this innovative pharmacological and pharmaceutical research.

The capsaicin(oids) are well-known species, which are able to modify the action of capsacin-sensitive afferent nerves. Their actions are dose-depependent, and they are capable to modify the neurogenic inflammantion, pain, and the defence of the various target organs against different noxious agents.

The research of capsaicin is a traditional and internationally well accepted research line at Pécs University, Hungary (Department of Pharmacology and Pharmacotherapy, First Department of Medicine in a well successful cooperation) in the 50 years period. We arrived to the production of orally given capsaicin(oids) new drug and capsaicin(oids) plus nonsteroidal anti-inflammatory drugs in the time of our innovative pharmacological and pharmaceutical research in the 2005.

The production of new drug or different drug combinations represented an interdisciplinary challenge for all of us (which significantly differed from the traditional basic and clinical research).

The first step of our common work was to write an interdisciplinary experts' opinion based on the most important research data from the capsaicin research to be used for the new drug production, for receiving different permissions from the different authoritities to start with the classical clinical pharmacological studies.

The experts's opinion was prepared (Mózsik et al., 2007b), and this material was published in Inflammopharmacology (Mózsik et al., 17:113-150, 2009a). This part of book chapter deals with these experts' opinion (subchapter of 3). The authors summarized their obtained significantly different results in these studies from the years of 2005 to 2008 (Mózsik et al., 2009b).

4.1. Brief introduction

Capsaicin is an active ingredient of red pepper and paprika. These plants have been well known in about 9500 years, and these have been applying in the every day of the culinary practice.

It was an important discovery that the capsaicin (capsaicin, dihydrocapsaicin, nordihydrocapsaicin and other capsaicinoids) specifically modify the function of capsaicin sensitive afferent nerves (Jancsó et al., 1967; 1968; 1970).

The action of capsaicin on the capsaicin sensitive afferent nerves is dose dependent (Szolcsányi and Barthó, 1981; Szolcsányi, 1984, 1997, 2004; Abdel-Salam et al., 1999; 2001; Mózsik et al., 2001). Szolcsányi indicated four different stages of capsaicin action (depending on the dose and duration of the exposure of the compound): a. excitation (stage 1); b. sensory blocking effect (stage 2); c. long-term selective neurotoxin impairment (stage 3) and d. irreversible cell destruction (stage 4) (Szolcsányi, 1984). The stages 1 and 2 are reversible; meanwhile the stages 3 and 4 are irreversible compound-induced actions on the capsaicin sensitive afferent nerve. These stages of capsaicin actions can be detected in the gastrointestinal tract (Mózsik et al., 2001).

Capsaicin activates the capsaicin (vanilloid) receptor expressed by a subgroup of primary afferent nociceptive neurons (Szolcsányi, 2004). The capsaicin receptor had been cloned (Caterina et al., 1997) and turned out to be a cation channel. It is gated besides capsaicin and other capsaicinoids (some vanilloids) by low pH, noxius heat and various pain-producing endogenous and exogenous chemicals. Thus, these sensory nerve endings equipped with these ion channels are prone to be stimulated in gastric mucosa.

The vagal nerve has a key role in the development of gastrointestinal mucosal damage and prevention (Mózsik et al., 1982). The key role of vagal nerve has been emphasized dominantly in the aggressive processes to gastrointestinal mucosa (such as peptic ulcer disease, gastric mucosal damage, etc.) both in the GI research of animal models and as well as in human clinical practice. The "chemical" and " surgical" vagotomy widely used in the treatment of patients with peptic ulcer disease in the years up to middle of 1970s (Karádi, Mózsik, 2000). By the other words, the primary aims of this therapy were to decrease the activity of vagal nerve at the level of efferent vagal nerve.

The application of capsaicin in the animals experiments was used as a specific tool to approach to the group of primary afferent nociceptive neurones (Szolcsányi, 2004; Buck and Burks, 1986; Holzer, 1998; 1991; Szállasi and Blumberg, 1999) involved in the different physiological and pathological processes.

Szolcsányi and Barthó (1981) were the firsts, who clearly indicated the beneficial and harmful effect of capsaicin in the peptic ulcer disease in rats, on dependence of applied doses of capsaicin. Later on, Holzer started with a very extensive research work with capsaicin in the field of Gastroenterology (Holzer, 1998; 1999; Buck and Burks, 1986; Szállasi and Blumberg, 1999). We also participated in the GI capsaicin research in animals experiments from 1980 (Mózsik et al., 1997). Recently, the new drug, Lafutidine, was processed in the medical treatment of GI mucosal damage (Ajioka et al., 2000; 2002; Onodera et al., 1999; 2002; Takeuchi, 2006). The Lafutidine is a H_2R blocking compound together with typical capsaicin actions at the target organ.

The new and interesting results obtained with capsaicin application in animal experiments offered an excellent tool to approach the different events of human GI physiology, pathology and pharmacology. Our clinical studies with capsaicin have been started from 1997 (Mózsik et al., 1999; Debreceni et al., 1999; Mózsik et al., 2004a; 2004b; 2005).

The aim of this paper is given a short summary on the possibility of capsaicin application as a new tool to understand the various steps of human physiology, pathology and pharmacology.

4.2. Physiological and pharmacological research tool by capsaicin

4.2.1. The chemistry of capsaicinoids

4.2.1.1. Chemical composition of Natural Capsaicin

The degree of pungency (heat or bite) of the Capsicum fruits is determined by the amount of compounds called capsaicinoids. These substances are responsible to produce the characteristic sensations associated with injestion of spicy cuisine as well as responsible for causing severe irritation, inflammation, erythema, and transient hypo-and hyperalgesia at sites exposed to capsaicinoids.

All capsaicinoids posses a 3-hydroxy-4-methoxy-benzylamide (vanilloid) pharmacophore, but differ in their hydrophobic alkyl side chain. Differences in the side chain moiety include saturation of the carbon carbon double bond, deletion of a methyl group and changes in the lenght of the hydrocarbon chain (Figure 1). Previous structure-activity studies using models for the study of acut pain and altered pain sensitivity in mice have demonstrated a strict structural requiremenet for both the vanilloid pharmacophore and a hydrophobic alkyl chain that may be saturted or unsaturated, branched or unbranched, and consisting of 8 to 12 carbon atoms for optimal binding and activation of the capsaicin receptor, TRPV1 (Bevan and Szolcsányi, 1990; Walpole et al., 1993a,b,c).

It is worth mentioning that there are some contradictions in meaning of the term "capsaicin" in different sources of literature. On one hand, the term capsaicin refers to one chemical entity: (*E*)-8-Methyl-N-vanillyl-6-nonenamide (CAS-number: 404-86-4). On the other hand, the term capsaicin is frequently used for Capsicum extracts containing capsaicin and related capsaicinoids (e.g., see Capsaicin USP 29). These latter preparations are frequently referred to as Natural Capsaicin. In addition to the natural capsaicin preparations, capsaicin can be obtained by synthesis as well. The synthesized capsaicin is frequently referred to as *trans*-capsaicin, since during the syntheses not only the natural *trans* but the *cis* isomer can also be obtained.

The two main components of Natural Capsaicin (a mixture of capsaicinoids of Capsicum origin) are capsaicin and dihydrocapsaicin. There are, however, other structurally related alkyl vanillylamides (capsaicinoids) generally found in smaller amounts in Capsicum extracts. The names and structures of the main components of Natural Capsaicin are shown below (Figure 1).

Separation and quantitation of the components can be performed by gas chromatography (GC) or liquid chromatography (HPLC). The GC and HPLC chromatograms of Natural Capsaicin (Capsaicin USP 29) are shown on Figures 2 and 3, respectively.

http://dx.doi.org/10.5772/58359

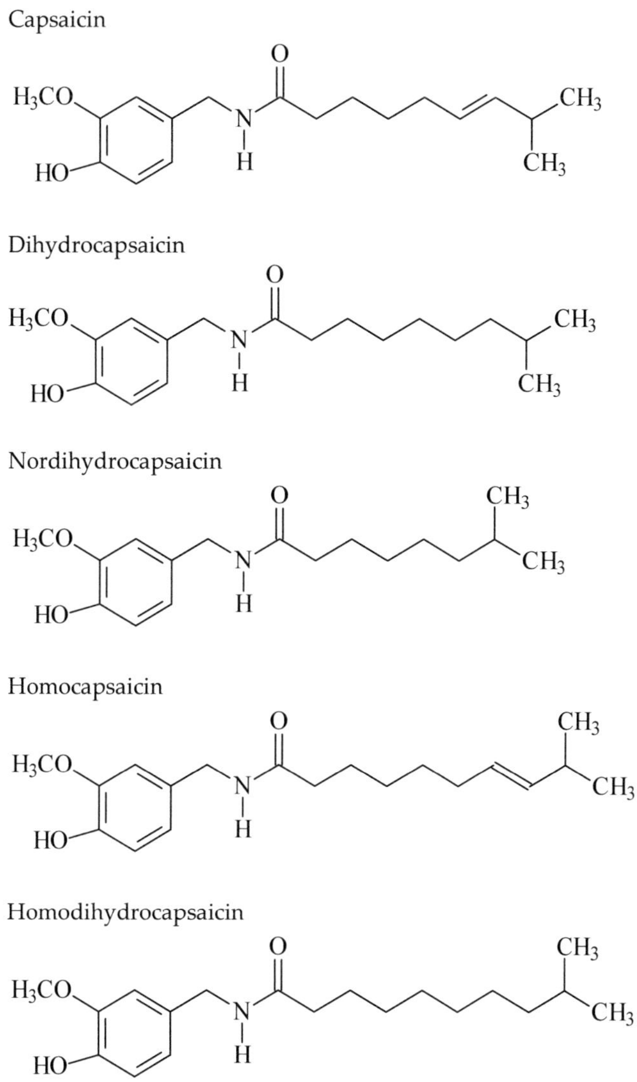

Figure 1. Names and chemical structures of the main components of the Natural Capsaicin preparations

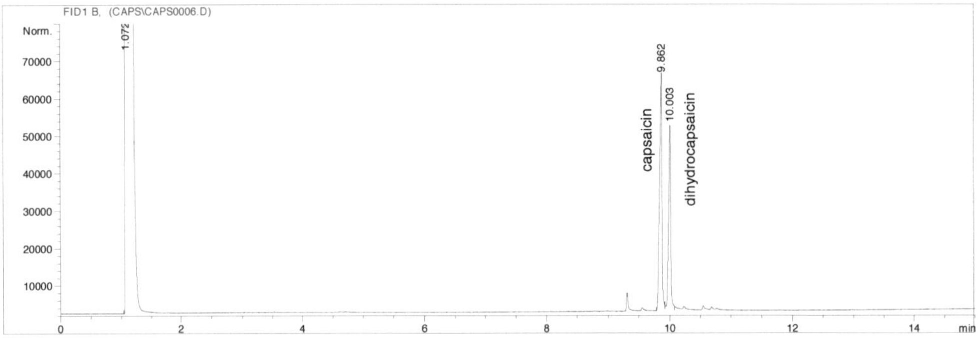

Figure 2. Gas-Chromatographic (GC-FID) analysis of capsaicin and dihydrocapsaicin of a Natural Capsaicin sample. (Identification of the components was performed by GC-MS method.) (Kuzma M. et al., unpublished results)

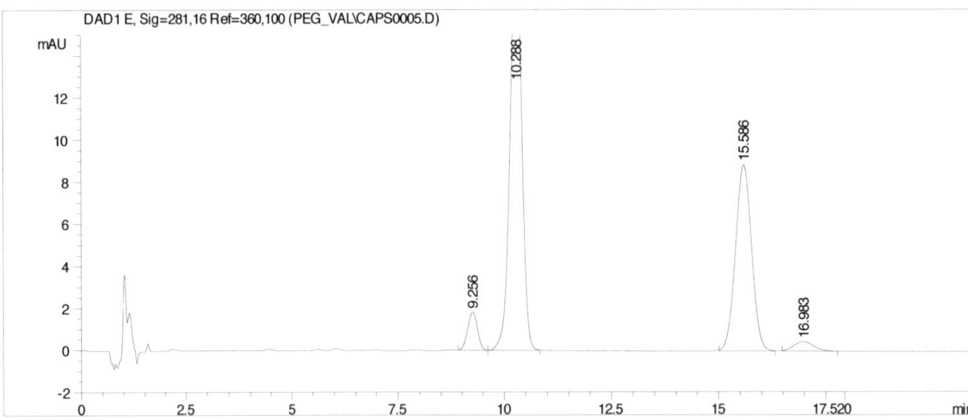

Figure 3. High Pressure Liquid Chromatography (HPLC-DAD) chromatogram of a Natural Capsaicin sample. (Retention times: Capsaicin $t_{R=}$10.29 min, Dihydrocapsaicint_R=15.59 min. Identification of the components was performed by means of the respective USP standards.) (Kuzma M. et al., unpublished results)

4.2.1.2. Capsaicin USP 29

Chemical name: 6-Nonenamide, (*E*)-N-[(4-Hydroxy-3-methoxy-phenyl)methyl]-8-methyl

Formula: $C_{18}H_{27}NO_3$

Molecular weight: 305.41

(*E*)-8-Methyl-N-vanillyl-6-nonenamide CAS-number: 404-86-4

Capsaicin contains not less than 90.0 percent and not more than 110.0 percent of the labeled percentage of total capsaicinoids. The content of capsaicin (C18H27NO3) is not less than 55 percent, and the sum of the contents of capsaicin and dihydrocapsaicin ($C_{18}H_{29}NO_3$) is not less than 75 percent, and the content of other capsaicinoids is not more than 15 percent, all calculated on the dried basis.

http://dx.doi.org/10.5772/58359

Packaging and storage: Preserve in tight containers, protected from light, and store in a cool place.

Caution: Handle Capsaicin with care. Prevent inhalation of particles of it and prevent its contact with any part of the body.

Solubility: It does not dissolve in water. It well dissolves in alcohols (methanol, ethanol 96%), ethylacetate and acetonitrile.

Identification: Prepare a test solution of Capsaicin in methanol containing 1 mg/mL. Prepare a Standard solution of *USP Capsaicin RS* in methanol containing 1 mg/mL. Separately apply 10-µL portions of the test solution and the Standard solution to a thin-layer chromatographic plate coated with a 0.25-mm layer of chromatographic silica gel mixture.

Develop the chromatograms in a solvent system consisting of a mixture of ether and methanol (19:1) until the solvent front has moved about three-fourths of the length of the plate. Remove the plate from the chamber, and allow it to air-dry. Spray the plate with a 0.5% solution of 2,6-dibromoquinone-chlorimide in methanol, allow to stand in a chamber containing ammonia fumes, and examine the chromatograms: the blue color and the *Rf* value of the principal spot obtained from the test solution correspond to those properties of the principal spot obtained from the Standard solution.

Melting range: between 57° and 66°, but the range between beginning and end of melting does not exceed 5°.

Loss on drying: Dry it in vacuum over phosphorus pentoxide at 40° for 5 hours: it loses not more than 1.0% of its weight.

Residue on ignition: not more than 1.0%.

4.2.1.3. Stability of capsaicinoids

Stability of capsaicin and dihydrocapsaicin are different according to the respective MDSD documents: The recommended storage temperature of capsaicin and dihydrocapsaicin are 2-8 °C and-20 °C, respectively. According to the MDSD sheet, the Sigma-Aldrich Capsaicin natural (pruduct number 21750, CAS number: 404-86-4) ((~65 % capsaicin) should be stored at 2-8 °C.

Literature data only to capsaicin chemistry:

Kopec et al. tested the stability of 100 % ethanol solution of capsaicin of different concentrations. It was found that the solutions of 4 mM or more concentrated solutions protected from light and stored at 4 ºC have been proved to be stable for a period of 12 months (Kopec et al., 2002).

While investigating stability of a capsaicin containing ointment Jaiarj et al. found the preparation to show higher stability stored at 4 °C other than at ambient temperature (Jaiarj et al., 2000).

Schweiggert et al. investigated stability of chilli powder. They found that the capsaicin, dihydrocapsaicin and nordihydrocapsaicin content of the samples dropped by 6-11 %. Based on their experience it was recommended that paprika (pepper) samples should be heat-treated before processing, in order to reduce the number of microorganisms producing enzymes with peroxidase activity (Schweiggert et al., 2006).

Conclusions: The presence of phenolic hydroxyl gruop and that of the carbon carbon double bond makes capsaicinoids sensitive to oxidation. Accordingly, natural capsaicin should be protected from exposure to light, heat, moisture, and oxidizing agents, wich initiate and/or catalyse the decomposition processes.

4.2.2. Capsaicin as a pharmacological tool in research

The term Capsicum refers to the fruit of numerous species of the solanaceous genus Capsicum. The genus name Capsicum is either derived from Greek "Kapso" meaning to bite, referring to its purgency or from the Latin "Capso" or box referring to the fruit pod. Members of the genus vary widely in size, shape, flavor, and much more importantly in purgency. Red hot peppers, also called chilies, paprika, and sweet non-purgent peppers are consumed widely by humans (Maga, 1975; Rozin, 1990, Mózsik et al., 2007). Capsaicin (8-methyl-N-vanillyl-6-nonenamide) is the major purgent ingredient of hot peppers.

4.2.3. Selective sensory effects of capsaicin

Apart from being used as a food additive, the compound has wide important pharmacological actions. Capsaicin uniquely selective for mammalian small afferent neurons of dorsal root ganglia C and Aδ fibers, a property which led to its use to investigate the role of these afferent fibres in a number of physiological processes (Jancsó and Jancsó-Gábor, 1959; Szolcsányi, 1982; 1984). In the skin the polymodal sensory receptors, chemoreceptors and warm receptors are affected by capsaicin (Szolcsanyi, 1977; 1982; 1993; 1996; Szolcsányi et al., 1994; Bevan and Szolcsányi, 1990; Holzer, 1990; 1991a, 1992 a; 1992 b). Most of these afferents contain substance P (SP) and /or calcitonin gene-related peptide (CGRP) (Holzer, 1991a; 1991 b; Maggi, 1995).

The action of capsaicin expresses itself as an initial short-lasting stimulation that can be followed by desensibilization to capsaicin itself and to other stimuli of afferent sensory neurons. Capsaicin in ng – μg/kg doses applied to the peripheral or central endings or cell bodies of sensory neurons induces transient excitation of these sensory neurons. In response to stimulation peptide mediators are released from the central and peripheral nerve endings (Szolcsányi, 1984; 1996; Holzer, 1998; 1991a; Maggi, 1995).

In the periphery neuropeptide release exerts local neuroregulatory tissue responses (Szolcsányi, 1984; 1991; 1996). Neuropeptides are stored in sensory vehicles (Gulbekian et al., 1986; Merighi et al., 1988) and are released on stimulation with capsaicin by a Ca^{2+}-dependent manner (Maggi et al., 1989). In this way the peripheral terminals of capsaicin sensitive nerves are not only sensory receptors for conveying impulses in the afferent direction but also effector sites from where mediators are released for neurotransmission (Szolcsányi, 1984; 1996). With large doses (mg /kg) there is an initial stimulation, the duration of which is not yet defined, followed by sensory desensitization (Szolcsányi, 1984; 1993).

http://dx.doi.org/10.5772/58359

Four response stages of the capsaicin-sensitive primary afferents to capsaicin have been introduced by Szolcsányi (Szolcsányi, 1984; 1985) depending on the dose and duration of exposure to the drug. These are excitation, sensory blocking effect, long-term selective neurotoxic impairment and irreversible cell destruction.

4.2.4. Mechanism of action of capsaicin on sensory receptors

To explain the mechanism of these sensory effects of capsaicin it has been hypothetized that in the polymodal nociceptive primary afferent neurons a capsaicin-gated cation channel exists which operates at the peripheral receptive terminals as at the level cell body. Capsaicin exerts its excitatory effect by activation of this cation channel which is permeable to a wide range of cations as Na^{+}, $K^{+}$and Ca^{2+}, but not to anions as Cl^{-}(Winter, 1987; Wood et al., 1988). The influx of $Na^{+}$and Ca^{2+}induces membrane depolarization which at a certain level, opens tetrotodotox-in-sensitive fast sodium channels at the regenerative region of the sensory receptor and in this way triggers nerve terminal spike and direct stimulation of transmitter release by Ca^{2+}.

Opening of the capsaicin-gated cation channel for shorter or longer periods of time triggers a chain of intracellular events (Bevan and Szolcsányi, 1990). Functional blockage with reversible intracellular molecular changes (stage 2) or neurotoxic degeneration (stages 3 and 4) develop depending on the concentration and the contact time at the site of action on different parts (receptor, axon, cell body, central terminal) of the capsaicin-sensitive primary afferent neurones (Mózsik et al., 2001). Prolonged stimulation and consequently prolonged opening of this cation channel results in osmotic swelling due to intracellular NaCl accumulation together with intracellular accumulation of Ca^{2+}at the exposed sites of the nerve terminal which will activates Ca^{2+}-dependent enzymes and impairs mitochondrial functions (Bevan and Szolcsányi, 1990; Chard et al., 1995). Prolonged activation of $Ca^{2+}$is therefore the first step in sequence of events ultimately leading to cell death.

In mammals, the long-lasting sensory blocking or neurotoxic effects of capsaicin on primary afferent neurones have been described following topical, perioxonal, or systemic pretreatment in adults or neonates. Autonomic efferent neural mechanisms are not affected by drug (Maggi and Meli, 1988; Szolcsányi, 1982; Holzer, 1991a). This selective sensory blocking effect of capsaicin has been used as an experimental tool for the elimination of the capsaicin-sensitive subset of primary afferent neurones and consequently for identifying those tissue responses that are mediated by capsaicin-sensitive afferent (Szolcsányi, 1996; Mózsik et al. 1997c). The later tissue responses being absent in sensory desensitized animals.

4.2.5. Capsaicin actions of the gastrointestinal tract in animals

In their experiments, Makara et al. (1965) found that intragastric capsaicin (1 mg/0.5 ml volume/ rat) enhanced the development of Shay ulcer at 12 hours. After four consecutive daily doses of reserpine (1.0 mg/kg, sc.), the above dose of capsaicin given simultaneously enhanced gastric ulceration by the latter. On the other hand, daily administration of paprika oil containing 1.0 mg/kg of capsaicin tended to accelerate rather than retard the healing process of reserpine-induced gastric ulcer in rats.

This was attributed by the authors to the capsaicin-induced local hyperaemia or the carotenoids and other pigments present in paprika oil. When Lee (1963) kept rabbits for 12 months on various diets (high fat,high carbohydrate or high protein) supplemented with large doses of ground hot pepper, ulcers developed in the stomach of all animals and cirrhosis of the liver occurred in animals fed with either high fat or high carbohydrate supplemented with capsaicin.

In the study of Nopanitaya (1974), the effect of capsaicin (1.0 mg/kg) and its combination with various diets on the morphology of duodenal mucosa of young rats was investigated for period of 28 and 56 days. The author reported ultrastructural alterations in the mitochondria of the absorptive cells of rats fed with low protein diet and also those supplemented with capsaicin. The changes, however, were less pronounced at the 56th day than at 28th day, indicating some sort of adaptation to capsaicin.

It was not known until 1981, that Szolcsányi and Barthó proved, namely that capsaicin protects against experimental gastric ulcer. Introduction of capsaicin into the stomach of pylorus-ligated rats (Shay)-rats in small doses (5 to 50 μg) and low concentration (10 μg/ mL) markedly reduced the ulcer formation at 18 hours later. On the other hand, acute gastric ulceration induced by pylorus-ligation (Shay-ulcer) or acid distension was aggravated in rats desensitized 2 weeks earlier with systematic capsaicin in high doses which selectively impairs capsaicin sensitive sensory nerves.

In capsaicin desensitized rats the aggressive side of the balance remained apparently unchanged since hypersecretion of the pylorus-ligated rats did not differ from that of the controls with respect to volume, $H^+$and pepsin concentration. This suggested that it is the gastric defense mechanism which was impaired in capsaicin desensitized rats. As a result of these data a role of capsaicin sensitive afferents in modulating gastric mucosal defenses was forwarded by the authors. In explaining the nature of this novel gastroprotective action of low dose capsaicin, it was postulated that intragastric capsaicin exerts opposite effects on gastric ulcer formation depending on the concentration in which it is introduced into the gastric lumen. Low concentrations trend to inhibit the development of ulceration and high concentrations promote ulcer formation. Release of vasodilator mediators from capsaicin-sensitive sensory nerve endings with the consequent enhancement of the microcirculation was proposed as the mechanism responsible for the mucosal protective effects on intragastrically administered capsaicin in low concentrations.

These mechanisms suggested a resistance or defense mechanism against ulcer formation working under physiological conditions. In capsaicin desensitized rats, mucosal sensory receptors will be unresponsive to stimuli, and consequently no release of vascular dilator mediators will take place upon challenge with noxious agents. As a result gastric ulcer will be aggravated (Szolcsányi and Barthó, 1981).

These observations and the drawn conclusions were confirmed by other investigators. Intragastric application of capsaicin in small doses has been shown to protect rat gastric mucosa against experimental ulcerations induced by ethanol (Holzer and Lippe, 1988; Esplugues and Whittle, 1989), acidified aspirin (Holzer et al., 1989) and indomethacin (Gray

http://dx.doi.org/10.5772/58359

et al., 1994). Furthermore, after desensitization rats exhibited more severe gastric mucosal damage than their sensory intact controls in response to chemical challenge with ethanol (Holzer and Lippe, 1988; Lippe et al., 1989; Esplugues and Whittle, 1990; Esplugues et al., 1992; Pabes et al., 1993), cysteamine (Holzer and Samettz, 1986; Gray et al., 1994), platelet activating factor (Esplugues et al., 1989; Pique et al., 1990) and endothelin-1 (Whittle and Lopez-Belmonte, 1991).

Capsaicin desensitation performed 6 days prior to cold restraint stress, however, was reported to have a little effect on gastric ulcer formation. Only the number of lesions was higher in capsaicin treated rats restrained for 3 hours (Dugani and Glavin, 1986). Acute intragastric capsaicin (40 mg/kg) followed immediately by stress resulted in significantly more frequent and more severe ulceration (Dugani and Glavin, 1985). Cysteamine-induced duodenal ulcers (Holzer and Sametz, 1986) and gastric mucosal damage evoked by 0.6 M HCl (Takeuchi et al., 1994) were not changed after capsaicin desensitization.

Studies have shown that gastric mucosal barrier disruption is accompanied with an increase of gastric mucosal blood flow (GMBF), which appears to be triggered by H^+rediffused through the breached mucosal defenses (Bruggeman et al., 1979; Starlinger et al., 1981a). Such an increase in GMBF is through to be a defense mechanism, whereby the increased blood flow prevents the accumulation of injurious concentration of H^+in the submucosa. Capsaicin-sensitive nerves which are unduly sensitive to H^+(Bevan and Yeats, 1991) have been shown to respond to H^+back-diffused through breached mucosal defenses and to signal for an increase in gastric mucosal blood flow (Holzer et al., 1991b). This further strengthened the role of these nerves in maintaining mucosal integrity. Holzer el al. (1991a, b) postulated that the acid-induced mucosal hyperaemia results from local axon reflex between collaterals of afferent nerve fibres within the gastric wall. Li et al. (1992) found that gastric mucosal hyperaemia in response to perfusion of the rat stomach with 0.15 M HCl in 15 v/v ethanol to be completely blocked by close arterial infusion of a hCGRP receptor antagonist.

Lippe and Holzer (1992) reported in rats that, N-nitro-L-arginine methyl ester (L-NANE) (an inhibitor of endothelium derived nitric oxide formation) depressed the increase in GMBF produced by gastric perfusion with ethanol diluted in 0.15 M HCl The loss of $H^+$from the lumen under these circumstances was also markedly enhanced by L-NAME. Considerable controversy still exists in the literature in regards to the mediators of the hyperaemic response to back-diffusion of acid (Whittle, 1977; Ritchie, 1991; Gislason et al., 1995).

The involvement of capsaicin-sensitive sensory nerves in repair mechanisms of the injured mucosa have also been investigated. In anaesthetized rats, 180 min after exposure to 50 v/v ethanol, rapid repair of the injured mucosa (assessed by reduction of deep mucosal damage and partial reepitheliazition of the denuted surface) was reported to be similar in sensory denervated and sensory intact groups. This suggested that nociceptive neurones control mechanisms of defense against acute gastric mucosal injury, but they are not required for the rapid repair of the injured mucosa (Pabst et al., 1993). On contrary, sensory differention delayed healing of gastric ulcers provoked in rats by 0.6 M HCl.

In addition capsaicin-desensitized not sensory intact animals showed no hyperaemic responses in response to intragastric instillation of 50 mM HCl. The conclusion was that capsaicin-sensitive sensory nerves contribute to healing of gastric ulcer (lesions) by mediating the hyperaemic responses associated with acid back-diffusion following injury (Takeuchi et al., 1994). Similarly sensory denervated rats showed marked increased area of acetic acid-induced ulceration at 1 and 2 weeks following the acetic acid injection indicating that the sensory function adversely affected the healing of gastric ulcer (Tramontana et al., 1994).

Capsaicin exerts protective effects on the chemical-induced mucosal injury not only in the stomach, but also in the colon. Evangelista and Meli (1989) found that systemic capsaicin neonatal pretreatment enhanced trinitrobenzene sulfonic acid-induced colitis (one week) in rats. This pretreatment, however, had no acute affect (24 hours) on colitis caused by trinitrobenzene sulfonic acid, ethanol or acetic acid.

Reinshagen et al. (1994) employed systemic capsaicin pretreatment as a tool to investigate the role of sensory nerves in an immune-complex model of colitis in rabbits. They found that capsaicin pretreatment per se caused no histological inflammation. Meanwhile, colitis was more severe in sensory denervated state than in sensory intact rabbits. The increase in ulcer index and neutrophyl infiltration was more marked in the capsaicin pretreated control group at both 48 and 96 hours.

The difference in neutrophyl infiltration between the two groups was, however, more marked at 48 than at 96 hours (Reinshagen et al., 1994). Endoh and Leung (1990) reported that topical capsaicin application protected against acetic acid-induced colitis. In the trinitrobenzene sulfonic acid-induced colitis rat model, however, only partial and transient protective effect was seen by Goso et al. (1993) after topical capsaicin administration. Co-administration of 640 μM capsaicin reduced the ulcerative area from 91% to 64% only when colon was examined 1 hour later. An approximatically 8 fold higher dose of capsaicin (5000 μM) yielded similar protection, while 100 μM had no protective effect. No protection by capsaicin was however seen when the colon was examined 24 hours after noxious challenge.

4.2.6. Capsaicin-sensitive sensory nerves and gastric acid secretion

Several studies in rats have indicated the involvement of capsaicin-sensitive sensory nerves in the regulation of gastric acid secretion; however, contradictory data were reported. In most studies, the indirect approach through functional ablation of capsaicin-sensitive afferent nerves with systemic neonatal (Evangelista et al., 1989; Esplugues et al., 1990), adult (Alföldi et al., 1986; 1987; Dugani and Glavin, 1986; Robert et al., 1991) or peripheral capsaicin (Raybould and Taché, 1989) treatment was used as a tool to investigate the role of capsaicin-sensitive afferent nerves in the regulation of gastric acid secretion.

Adult rats treated with systemic capsaicin (60 mg/kg, sc.) showed depressed pentagastrin-stimulated gastric acid secretion (Dugani and Glavin, 1986). On the contrary, adult systemic capsaicin pretreatment with 300 mg/kg sc. did not modify gastric acid secretion elicited by pentagastrin, carbachol or by small dose of histamine (0.1 mg/kg). However, the gastric acid secretory response to 0.5 and 5.0 mg/kg histamine was greatly reduced in capsaicin desensitized rats. It was suggested that the histamine-induced increase in gastric acid secretion involves a capsaicin-sensitive mechanism, while these mechanisms are not required for pentagastrin or cholinergic stimulation of gastric acid secretion (Alföldi et al., 1986; 1987).

Similar data were reported by Raybould and Taché (1989) using topical capsaicin application into the cervical vagus. The gastric acid secretory response to distension (5 ml for 6 min) was reduced in capsaicin-treated rats. This mechanism by which capsaicin-sensitive vagal afferent fibres play a role in the secretory response to histamine was explained by histamine acting in part by increasing vagal C-fibres discharge resulting in a vago-vagal reflex increase in gastric acid secretion or by that histamine stimulates vagal afferent C-fibres resulting the release of peptides from sensory nerves terminals.

A peptide increasing gastric acid secretion and would be localized in vagal afferent nerves has not been identified. In contrast that adult rats treated with systemic capsaicin (300 mg/kg, sc.) at neonate age did not show any reduction in their gastric acid secretory to histamine, pentagastrin or carbachol, while acid secretion in response to distension was abolished. On the other hand, capsaicin desensitation (neonatal treatment) substantially reduced the gastric acid secretion to 2-deoxy-D-glucose (Evangelista et al., 1989), while it did not modify when stimulated by insulin (Esplugues et al., 1990).

The conflicting observations regarding the effect of capsaicin continue to be seen when it was given into the stomach. It was reported that intraduodenal (but not intragastric) instillation of capsaicin (1.0 mg in 2 ml saline solution) in pylorus-ligated rats induced a significant rise in total acidity 12 hours later (Makara et al.,1965). The results with capsaicin indicated in some meaning contradictory results in the gastrointestinal tract mentioned above. Relatively same attention was played to the applied doses of capsaicin. Szolcsányi and Barthó (1981), however, emphasized well that capsaicin protects against the chemical induced gastric ulcer formation, when the capsaicin was given in 5 and 50 μg doses (10 μg/mL concentration) intragastrically, meanwhile capsaicin in high dose aggravated the ulcer formation by the induction of desensitazion.

Very systematic observations were carried out by us with capsaicin on dependence of its concentration (or pretreatment produced desensitization of capsaicin sensitive afferent nerves) on different experimental models (aspirin, HCl, indomethacin, ethanol, cysteamine). The changes of gastric acid secretion, gastric mucosal damage, gastric H^+back-diffusion, gastric mucosal blood flow were measured and calculated, when the capsaicin was applied in small doses and in high doses producing desensitization (Mózsik et al., 1997c). The results of these observations clearly demonstrated that: 1. capsaicin, given in small doses, dose-dependently inhibited all of the parameters in all experimental models; 2.the gastric mucosal protective effects of capsaicin remained at the level of other drugs (acting on efferent nerves, eg. atropine, and cimetidine or at topically such as sucralfate, retinoids). Consequently, the capsaicin enhanced the other drug-induced gastric mucosal protective effects (Mózsik et al., 1997c); 3. after denervated states of capsaicin-sensitive afferent nerves (produced by pretreatment of high dose of capsaicin) the gastric mucosal lesion formation was enhanced. These results offered to conclude that the gastric mucosal protective effects can be obtained only capsaicin, when it is given in small doses, however this gastric mucosal protective effect of capsaicin can not be obtained by the application of higher doses (Abdel-Salam et al., 1994, 1995a, 1995b, 1995c, 1995d, 1995e, 1995f, 1995g, 1996a, 1996b, 1997a, 1997b, 1997c, 1997d; Mózsik et al.,1993, 1996a, 1996b, 1997a, 1997b, 1997)

4.2.7. Molecular-pharmacological studies

The molecular pharmacological observations were carried out (and calculated based on the dose-response curves of drugs) with capsaicin, atropine, cimetidine, omeprazole, PGI_2, vitamin A, β-carotene, studying their effects on the gastric acid secretion in 2 and 4 hours pylorus-ligated rats alone, or in combination of betanechol (7.6 and 15.4 nmol/kg), histamine (2.7 and 13.6 μmol/kg) and pentagastrin (65.1 and 325.6 nmol/kg) and on the gastric mucosal damage produced by intragastrically applied ethanol, HCl, acidified aspirin and subcutaneously applied indomethacin (alone and in combinated with application of 7.6 and 15.2 μmol/ kg betanechol, 13.6 and 54.3 μmol/kg histamine and 6.51 and 325.6 nmol/kg pentagastrin) (calculated the number and severity of gastric mucosal damage) in rats (Figures 4-7, Tables 1-7).

The doses of the necessary for the producing 50% inhibition on the gastric acid secretion and gastric mucosal damage were calculated in molar values/kg body weight (ED_{50}).

The values for affinity (pD) and intrinsic (α-values) were calculated according to standard procedures employed in molecular pharmacology (Csáky, 1969). The values of the pD_2 (necessary dose to inhibit the gastric acid secretion and gastric mucosal damage in 50%) and pA_2 (necessary dose to produce 50% in gastric acid secretion and on gastric mucosal damage) were calculated from the affinity and intrinsic activity curves.

The doses of drugs (compounds) were calculated as molar values for the determination of their biological effects. The affinity (pD_2 values) and intrinsic activity (α-values) are shown as molar values. The intrinsic activity of atropine (α) was taken as 1.00 for comparing the effects of agents on gastric acid secretion and gastric mucosal damage (Figures 4-7, Tables 1-7) (Mózsik et al., 2006).

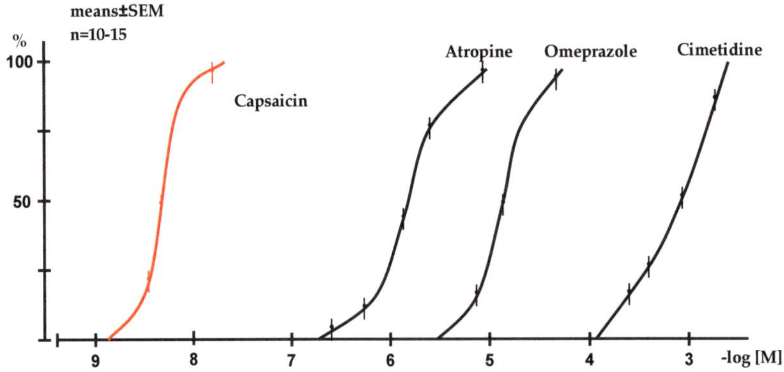

Figure 4. Affinity curves for different drugs, compounds inhibiting the gastric acid secretion of 4 h pylorus-ligated rats (Mózsik et al., 2006b). For further details of the observations see the cited paper.

http://dx.doi.org/10.5772/58359

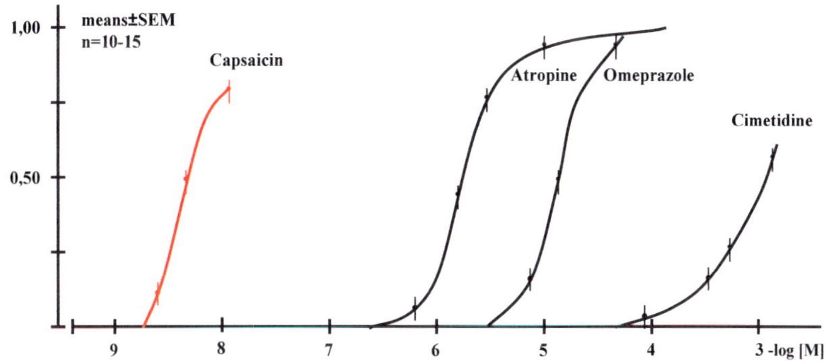

Figure 5. Intrinsic affinity curves for different drugs, compounds inhibiting the gastric acid secretion of 4 h pylorus-ligated rats, which were expressed in relation to that of atropine (1,00)($\alpha_{atropine}$) (Mózsik et al., 2006b). For further details of the observations see the cited paper.

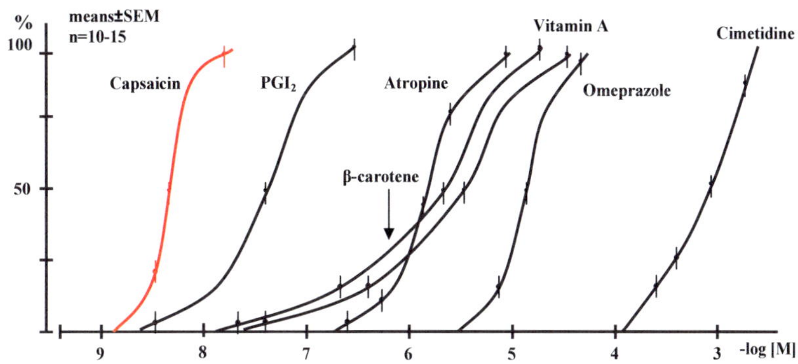

Figure 6. Affinity curves for different drugs, compounds inhibiting the gastric mucosal damage produced by various chemical agents in rats (Mózsik et al., 2006b). For further details of the observations see the cited paper.

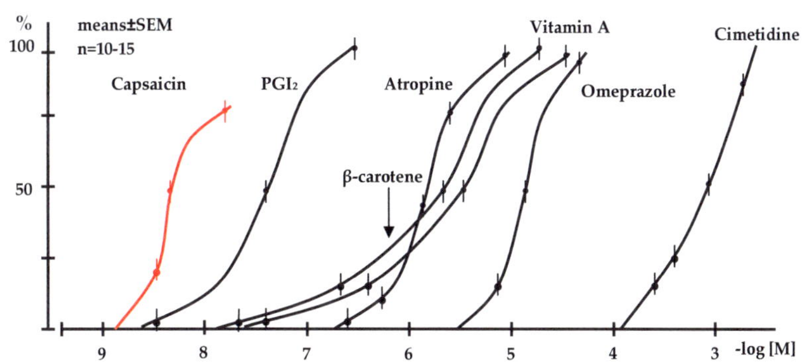

Figure 7. Intrinsic activity curves for different drugs, compounds inhibiting the gastric mucosal damage produced by chemical agents which were expressed relative to that of atropine ($\alpha_{atropine}$=1,00) in rats (Mózsik et al., 2006b). For further details of the observations see the cited paper.

Compounds	Models	ED_{50} values
Capsaicin	2 h pylorus ligated rats	**3.27 nmol/kg**
Capsaicin	4 h pylorus ligated rats	**3.27 nmol/kg**
RTX	4 h pylorus ligated rats	**0.954 nmol/kg**

*(Mózsik et al., 2006b)

Table 1. Inhibitory effects of capsaicin and resiniferatoxin on basal gastric acid secretion in rats.*

Compounds	Models	ED_{50} values
Capsaicin	1 h pylorus ligated rats + betanechol (7.6 μmol/kg)	0.954 nmol/kg
Capsaicin	1 h pylorus ligated rats + betanechol (15.2 μmol/kg)	0.954 nmol/kg
Capsaicin	1 h pylorus ligated rats+ histamine (13.6 μmol/kg)	0.954 nmol/kg
Capsaicin	1 h pylorus ligated rats + histamine (54.3 μmol/kg)	0.954 nmol/kg
Capsaicin	1 h pylorus ligated rats + pentagastrin (65.1 nmol/kg)	0.954 nmol/kg
Capsaicin	1 h pylorus ligated rats pentagastrin (325.6 nmol/kg)	0.954 nmol/kg
RTX	4 h pylorus ligated rats + betanechol (7.6 nmol/kg)	0.954 nmol/kg
RTX	4 h pylorus ligated rats+ betanechol (15.2 nmol/kg)	0.954 nmol/kg
RTX	4 h pylorus ligated rats + histamine (2.7 μmol/kg)	0.954 nmol/kg
RTX	4 h pylorus ligated rats + histamine (13.6 μmol/kg)	0.954 nmol/kg
RTX	4 h pylorus ligated rats + pentagastrin (65.1 nmol/kg)	0.954 nmol/kg
RTX	4 h pylorus ligated rats pentagastrin (325.6 nmol/kg)	0.954 nmol/kg

* (Mózsik et al., 2006b)

Table 2. Inhibitory effects of resiniferatoxin on stimulated gastric acid secretion in rats.*

Compounds	Models	ED_{50} values
Capsaicin	0.6 M HCl (2 ml) (4 h)	0.135 μmol/kg
Capsaicin	aspirin (200 mg/kg) + 0.15 M HCl (4 h)	0.13 μmol/kg
Capsaicin	ethanol (96% in 1 ml) (1 h)	0.13 μmol/kg
Capsaicin	4 h pylorus ligated rats+ IND (20 mg/kg)	1.98 nmol/kg
RTX	4 h pylorus ligated rats + IND (20 mg/kg)	0.95 nmol/kg
Capsaicin	4 h pylorus ligated rats +IND (20 mg/kg) + 0.15 N HCl (2 ml)	0.25 μmol/kg
RTX	4 h pylorus ligated rats + IND (20 mg/kg)+ 0.15 N HCl (2 ml)	0.95 nmol/kg
Capsaicin	4 h pylorus ligated rats+ IND (20 mg/kg) 0.3 N HCl (2 ml)	2.78 μmol/kg
RTX	4 h pylorus ligated rats + IND (20 mg/kg) 0.3 N HCl (2 ml)	0.15 μmol/kg

*(Mózsik et al., 2006b)

Table 3. Protective effects of capsaicin and resiniferatoxin on gastric mucosal damage caused by exogenous agents in rats.*

Compounds	Models	ED_{50} values
RTX	4 h pylorus ligated rats+ bethanechol (7.6 µmol/kg) + IND (20 mg/kg)	0.20 µmol/kg
RTX	4 h pylorus ligated rats+ bethanechol (15.2 µmol/kg) + IND (20 mg/kg)	0.20 µmol/kg
RTX	4 h pylorus ligated rats+ histamine (13.6 µmol/kg) + IND (20 mg/kg)	0.13 µmol/kg
RTX	4 h pylorus ligatedrats + histamine (54.3 µmol/kg) + IND (20 mg/kg)	0.13 µmol/kg
RTX	4 h pylorus ligated rats+ pentagastrin (6.51 nmol/kg)+ IND (20 mg/kg)	0.13 µmol/kg
RTX	4 h pylorus ligated rats+ pentagastrin (325.6 nmol/kg) + IND (20 mg/kg)	0.13 µmol/kg

*(Mózsik et al., 2006b)

Table 4. Protective effects of resiniferatoxin on gastric mucosal damage caused by exo-, and endogenous agents in rats.*

Compounds	pD_2	Intrinsic activity	pA_2
Capsaicin	8.48	0.76	8.50
Atropine	5.75	1.00	5.80
Cimetidine	3.00	0.64	3.20
Omeprazole	4.88	1.00	4.90

* For further information, see Figures 1 and 2 (Mózsik et al., 2006b)

Table 5. The pD_2, intrinsic activity ($\alpha_{atropine}$=1.00) and pA_2 values for different drugs (compound) inhibiting the gastric acid outputs in 4 h pylorus-ligated rats.*

Vitamin A:	3.49 x 10-8 – 3.49 x 10-5 (0.01-10.0 mg/kg): no inhibitory action on the gastric acid secretion
β-carotene:	1.86 x 10-8 – 1.86 x 10-5 (0.01-10.0 mg/kg): no inhibitory action on the gastric acid secretion
PGI_2 :	2.8 x 10-9 – 1.42 x 10-8 (1.0-5.0 µg/kg): no inhibitory action on the gastric acid secretion
PGE_2 :	1.33-1.99 x 10-7 (50.0-150.0 µg/kg): no inhibitory action on the gastric acid secretion

*(Mózsik et al., 2006b)

Table 6. Dose ranges of the tested nutritional compounds (vitamin A and β-carotene), PGI_2 and PGE_2 on the gastric acid secretion of 4 h pylorus-ligated rats, without presence any inhibitory actions.*

Compounds	pD_2	Intrinsic activity	pA_2
Capsaicin	8.48	0.76	8.50
PGI_2	7.45	1.00	7.44
Atropine	5.75	1.00	5.80
Cimetidine	3.00	0.64	3.20
Omeprazole	4.88	1.00	4.90
Vitamin A	5.45	1.00	5.44
β-carotene	5.73	1.00	5.73

* For further information, see Figures 4-7. (Mózsik et al., 2006b)

Table 7. The pD_2, intrinsic activity ($\alpha_{atropine}$=1.00) and pA_2 values for different drugs, compounds inhibiting the gastric mucosal damage produced by chemical agents in rats.*

The results obtained demonstrated the following conclusions:

1. Only the values of pD_2 and pA_2 (expressed in [-] molar doses) can be used for the evaluation of physiological and pharmacological regulations of the target organ(s) in animal-experiment(s) (Mózsik et al., 2006).
2. The following pD_2 (ED_{50}%) values were obtained for the different drugs (compounds) for actions in inhibiting gastric acid secretion: atropine 5.75; omeprazole 4.88; cimetidine 3.00; capsaicin 8.50,whereas no effects were observed with PGI_2, vitamin A and β-carotene.
3. The intrinsic activity values ($\alpha_{atropine}$=1.00) obtained in relation to atropine were 0.64 for cimetidine, 0.75 for capsaicin, 1.00 for omeprazole; no effects were observed for PGI_2, vitamin A and β-carotene.
4. The following pD_2 (ED_{50}) values were obtained for he different drugs or compounds inhibiting the gastric mucosal damage produced by chemicals: capsaicin 8.48, PGI_2 7.45, atropine 5.75, cimetidine 3.00, omeprazole 4.88, vitamin A 5.45 and β-carotene 5.73.
5. The intrinsic activity values ($\alpha_{atropine}$=1.00) were obtained: capsaicin 0.76, cimetidine 0.64, of other components were 1.00 on the gastric mucosal damage.
6. The values of pA_2 values were obtained as follows: capsaicin 8.50, PGI_2 7.44, atropine 5.80, cimetidine 3.00, omeprazole 4.90, vitamin A 5.44 and β-carotene 5.70.

The results of these molecular pharmacological observations clearly indicated (proved) that the capsaicin-sensitive afferent nerves have essential role both in the regulation of gastric acid secretion and in the defense of the gastric mucosal damage produced by the different chemical agents. It has been emphasizing that the capsaicin exerts the gastric acid inhibitory and the

http://dx.doi.org/10.5772/58359

gastric mucosal protective effect in smaller molar concentrations than other compounds (atropine, cimetidine, omeprazole and other compounds without any gastric acid inhibitory effects). That is a clear explanation for why the essential role of capsaicin-sensitive afferent nerves is deeply emphasized in the physiological and pharmacological regulation of gastro-intestinal tract.

4.2.8. Capsaicin actions in human healthy subjects and in patients with different gastrointestinal disorders

Early work regarding the effect of peppers on the human stomach has yielded conflicting results. In peptic ulcer patients, Schneider et al., (1956) studied the influence of a variety of spices on sensation of pain and healing peptic ulcer. Ulcer patients placed on established treatment with anticholinergics and diet were given different purgent species in capsules that contained the average quantity habitually consumed by Americans with three of their daily meals for six weeks. With the exception of black pepper, which resulted in distressing pain after one or two days, none of the tested spices have modified pain sensation or delayed healing of ulcers.

In other study, instillation of red chilli powder was reported to be associated with significant increase of DNA from gastric aspirates (Desai et al., 1973). Viranuvatti et al. (1972) studies the local effect of capsicum in twenty human subjects by instillation a 3% capsicum solution through an intragastric tube or via the lumen of gastrofiberscope. There was no change in 13 cases, oedema and/or hyperaemia developed in three cases, haemorrhagic spots occurred in another three cases and bleeding occurred in one case.

Capsaicin was reported to increase the gastric acidity in human subjects receiving intragastrically aqueous suspensions from hot peppers (Berkessy, 1934; Varga, 1936; Ketusinh et al., 1966; Solanke, 1973). Solanke (1973) studied the effect of red pepper suspension (200 ml of 4% solution) instilled through a nasogastric tube on gastric acid secretion in patients with duodenal ulcer and non-duodenal ulcer. Patients were allocated into two treatments: fresh red pepper suspension and a red pepper suspension with pH adjusted to 7.4 with 0.01 N sodium hydroxyde. They found a significant increase in gastric acid secretion after treatment with either form of the red pepper suspension. Many other observations were carried out in human beings with different extractions of chilli, paprika. Consequently we have no scientifically well controlled human studies on the applied doses of capsaicin. On the other hand, these studies were carried out in sporadic pathways.

The Good Clinical Practice (GCP) was introduced in the clinical research of human beings and patients.

From the years of 1997, the clinical studies with capsaicin were carried out in prospective and randomized, multiclinical conditions as those had been officially accepted in the multiclinical pharmacological studies in all over the World.

The following observation facts were accepted in these human observations:

1. The pure capsaicin (Sigma, USA, later on Sigma-Aldrich, USA) was used in the studies with healthy human subjects and in patients with different diseases (instead of different extractions of different capsaicin containing plants),
2. The clinical observations were carried out according to the medical laws of clinical pharmacology (in random allocation and in prospective and randomized studies),
3. The clinical observations were carried out according to the criteria of GCP,
4. All of the persons participating received all doses of capsaicin in random allocation.

We have to emphasize that the classical pharmacological studies were carried out with capsaicin obtained from the firm of Sigma (USA), or later from Sigma-Aldrich (USA).

The main results of the human multiclinical pharmacological studies with capsaicin:

1. The capsaicin (in range of 100 to 800 μg dose orally given to each person) dose-dependently inhibited the gastric basal acid output (BAO) in healthy human subjects (Fig. 8.) (Mózsik et al., 1999; Mózsik et al., 2005).
2. The capsaicin dose-dependently enhanched the the gastric transmucosal potential difference (GTPD) in healthy human subjects (Fig. 9) (Mózsik et al., 2005).
3. The ethanol-induced decrease of GTPD can be dose-dependently reversed by topical application of capsaicin (given it in doses of 100, 200,400 and 800 μg orally) (Fig. 10) (Mózsik et al., 2005).
4. The indomethacin (3x 25 mg/day given orally,plus 25 mg given immediately before measuring of gastric blood losing) produced a significant increase of gastric microbleeding in comparison to control (untreated) conditions (Fig. 11) (Mózsik et al., 2005; Mózsik et al., 2006).
5. The extent basal and indomethacin-induced gastric microbleeding unchanged before and after weeks treatment with capsaicin (3x 400 μg/ person/day) (Mózsik et al., 2005; Mózsik et al., 2007).
6. The dose-dependent gastroprotective effect of capsaicin on the indomethacin-induced gastric microbleeding remained the same after two weeks (3 x 400 μg given orally /day/ person) of capsaicin treatment (Mózsik et al., 2005; Mózsik et al., 2006).

These observations proved that the capsaicin (dose-dependently) prevents the ethanol- and indomethacin-induced gastric mucosal damage in healthy human subjects (Mózsik et al., 2005; Mózsik et al., 2007) before and after two weeks treatment with capsaicin (3x 400 μg orally /day/ person) (Mózsik et al., 2005; Mózsik et al., 2006), however, we have to emphasize that the indomethacin (3x25 mg given orally, plus 25 mg given immediately before the measuring of gastric microbleeding) produced the same extent of gastric microbleeding. We also have to emphasize that the extent of baseline of gastric microbleeding remained the same before and after two week treatment with capsaicin (Mózsik et al., 2005; Mózsik et al., 2007).

http://dx.doi.org/10.5772/58359

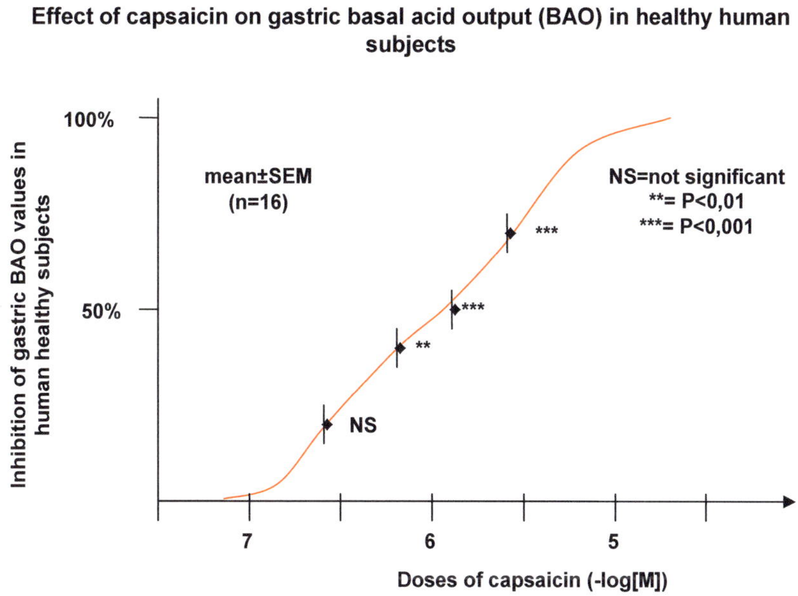

Figure 8. Dose-response curve of capsaicin on the gastric basal acid output (BAO) in healthy human subjects (Mózsik Gy. et al., 2005). The determination was carried out at one hour after the beginning of the human observations.

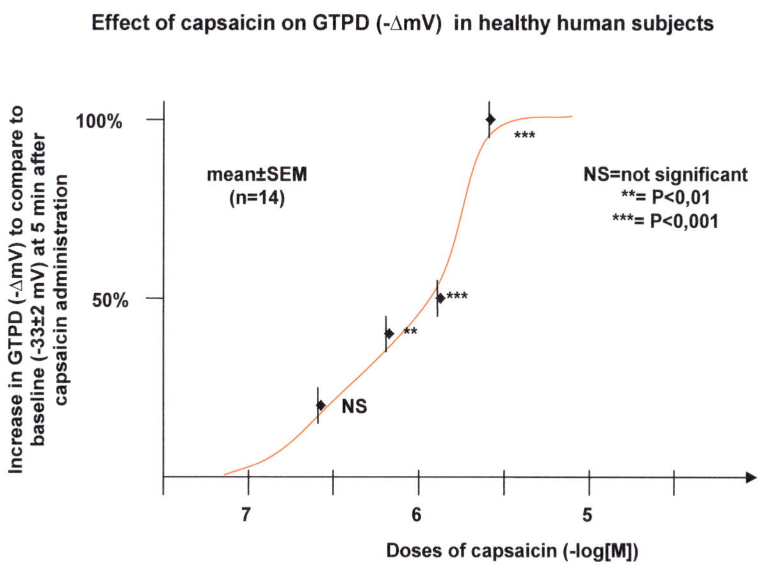

Figure 9. Dose-response curve of capsaicin on the gastric transmucosal potential difference (GTPD) in healthy human subjects (Mózsik Gy. et al., 2005), when the different doses were directly intragastrically via endoscopic chanel. The GTPD measurements were carried out at 1, 2, 3, 4, and 5 minutes. The results are expressed at 5 min after capsaicin intragastric application.

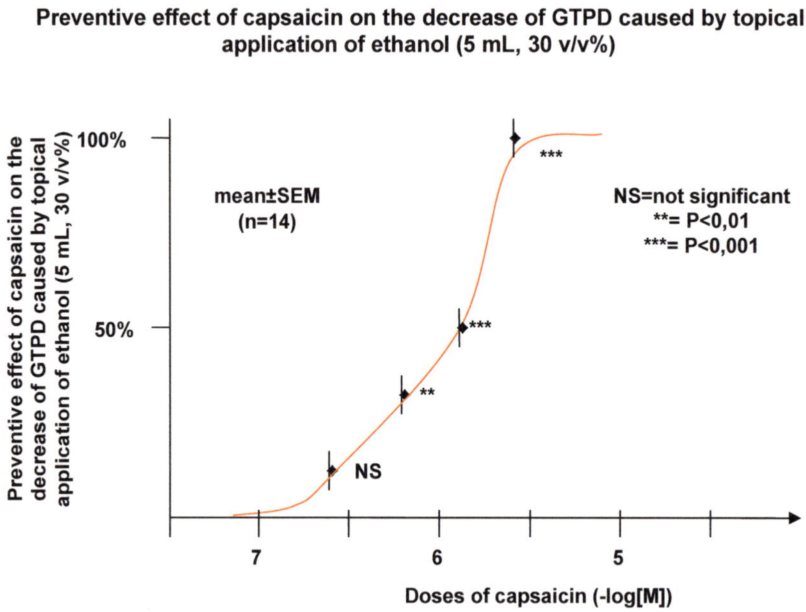

Figure 10. Dose-response curve of capsaicin on the gastric transmucosal potential difference after intragastric administration of ethanol in healthy human subjects (Mózsik Gy. et al., 2005). Intragastrically applied (via endoscopic chanel) ethanol (5 mL of 30 v/v) decreased GTPD with 30 mV which reversed with intragastric application of capsaicin at 1-2 min after capsaicin intragastric application.

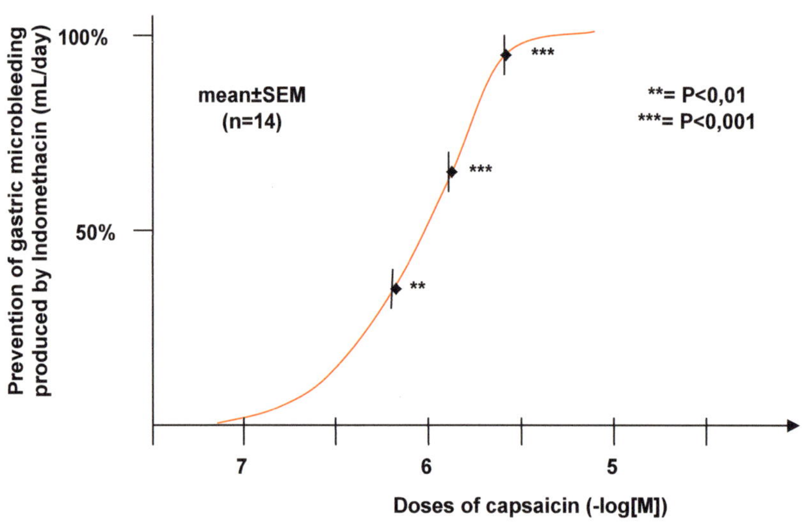

Figure 11. Dose-response curve of capsaicin on the Indomethacin (3x25+25mg given orally in pills) induced gastric microbleeding in healthy human subjects. The different doses 200, 400, 800 μg capsaicin was intragastrically applied in gelatin capsule (Mózsik Gy., et al., 2005).

4.2.8.1. Results of the comparative molecular-pharmacological studies of capsaicin, atropine, Omeprazole, Famotidine, Ranitidine and Cimetidine on the gastric basal acid output (BAO) in human subjects

The affinity (pD values) and intrinsic activity (pA values) curves of capsaicin, atropine, Omeprazole, Famitidine, ranitidine and cimetidine (used in their physiological and human therapeutic doses) were determined in patients with gastrointestinal disorders, according to the method of Csáky (1969) (Figures 12 and 13, Table 8).

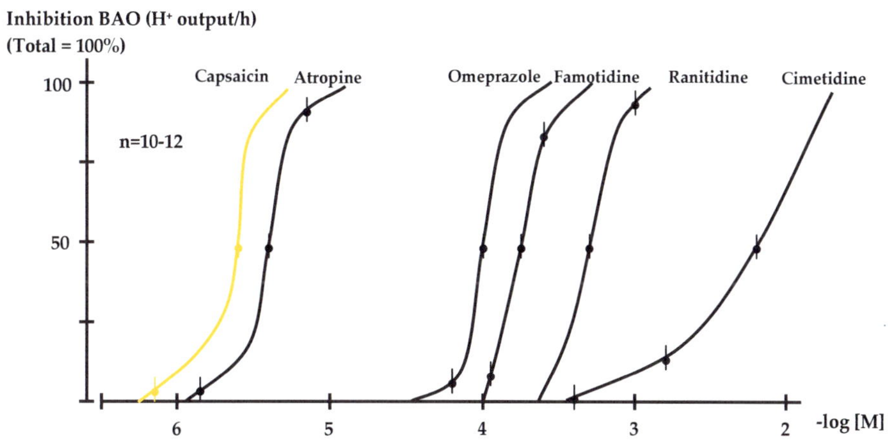

Figure 12. Affinity curves for the inhibitory actions of different drugs on the gastric basal acid output (H^+output/h) in healthy human subjects (Mózsik et al. 2007c). For further explanation see the cited paper.

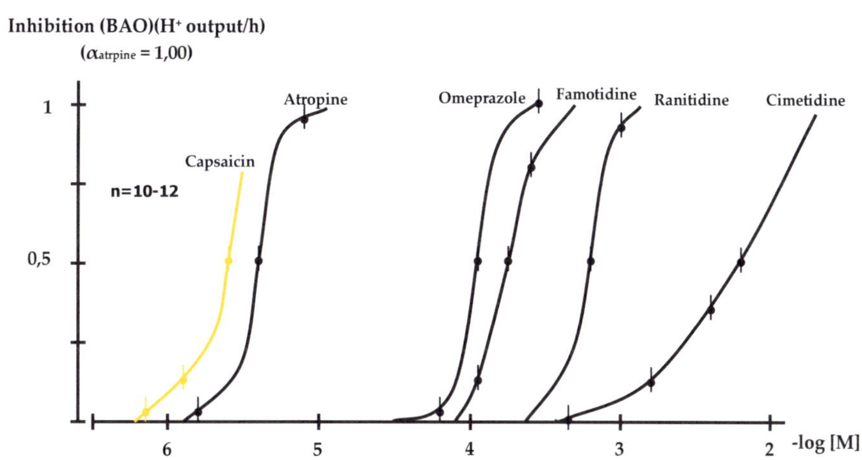

Figure 13. Intrinsic activity curves for the inhibitory effects of different drugs on the gastric basal acid output (H^+output/h) in healthy human subjects, which were expressed to action of atropine (1,00)($\alpha_{atropine}$) (Mózsik et al. 2007c). For further explanation see the cited paper.

Compounds	M.W.	pD_2	Intrinsic activity	pA_2
Capsaicin	305,4	5,88	0,76	5,87
Atropine	289,38	5,40	1,00	5,40
Pirenzepine	424,34	3,93	0,89	3,93
Cimetidine	252,34	2,23	1,00	2,23
Ranitidine	314,41	3,33	1,00	3,33
Famotidine	337,43	3,77	1,00	3,77
Nizatidine	331,47	3,34	1,00	3,34
Omeprazole	345,42	3,97	1,00	3,97
Esomeprazole	345,42	3,97	1,00	3,97

Table 8. Summary of the affinity (pD_2) and intrinsic activity (expressed in value of $\alpha_{atropine}$=1,00)(pA_2) values of capsaicin, atropine, Pirenzepine, cimetidine, ranitidine, famotidine, Omerazole and Esomeprazole on the gastric basal acid output (BAO) in healthy human subjects

4.2.9. Side effects of aspirin and other nonsteroidal anti-inflammatory drugs (NSAIDs) in the gastrointestinal tract of patients

The patients with myocardial infarction, thromboembolic episodes, stroke of central nervous system, cancers and persons who have to be under secondary preventional terapy (against reinfarction after myocardial infarction, prevention of thromboembolic episodes produced by atrial fibrillation, cancers, after different surgical intervention and immobilization) and in healthy subject treated with NSAIDs in order to prevent the development of colorectal cancers were randomized for further study.

The number of these groups of patients reaches to 50-60 per cent of total population in Hungary; however, an extremely big number of patients with these diseases is included in the different countries of the World.

The patients who underwent cardiac and other surgeries we have to treat permanently with aspirin (in dose around 100 mg / day / person). This is a basic staind-point of the different consensus meetings of Europe and of the World (Mcgettigan and Henry, 2006; Expert Consensus Document on the Use of Antiplatelet Agents 2004; Todd, and Clissold, 1990).

The administration of aspirin is absolutely indicated from medical points of view in patients with mentioned disorders, accepting the opinion of cardiologists we have to emphasize that the aspirin very frequently produces harmful gastrointestinal bleeding (which is not accepted by gastroenterologists). Really, there is a great and principal question from the general medical practice (and of research), namely wheather all patients can be taken uniformally, in whom the medical science offers such medical treatment from the point of cardiology, which produces severe gastrointestinal disorders (bleedings, peptic ulcer). Consequently, there is a contradiction medically (and evidence-based proved) in standpoint of cardiologists and gastroenterologists (during the treatment only one patient, and as well as in the treatment of populations of patients mentioned above).

Another big population of patients suffers from different degenerative joint diseases, trauma, acute and chronic pain producing states.These patients have to receive permanently treatment with NSAIDs. The NSAIDs are not gastrointestinal protective agents neither in healthy person and nor in patients with these diseases. The patients appearing at ambulance of Gastrointestinal Units are suffered from the drug-induced side effects in gastrointestinal tract

The number of patients with NSAIDs-induced gastrointestinal disorders (blood losing, bleeding, peptic ulcer) also represents a significant number of populations. Furthermore, these patients have to be treated permanenly by different NSAIDs.

The actions of NSAIDs are associated with the selective and non-selective inhibitory properties on cycloxygene system (emphasizing the key role of COX-1 and COX-2). Aspirin represents as a specific COX-1 inhibitor; meanwhile the other NSAIDs applied in the clinical practice represent the compounds acting as non selective COX-1 and COX-2 inhibitors. Recently, the specifically acting compounds, inhibiting COX-2 enzyme, have been produced, however, it was also observed that during the treatment an extremely big number of patients received myocardial infraction (Couzin, 2004a, 2004b; Lenzer, 2004; McGettigan, and Henry, 2006).

We have to emphasize clearly, that the small doses of capsaicin are able to prevent gastric mucosal bleeding in humans, which are able to inhibit both the COX-1 and COX-2 enzymes. This discovery opened a new pathway in the physiological and pharmacological regulation of different tissues (see later).

4.3. Animal observations

4.3.1. Acute toxicology studies of capsaicin in animal experiments

During acute toxicity study with capsaicin eight of 17 rats died in which capsaicin was administered in four increasing s.c. doses to a cumulative amount of 21.0 – 66.0 mg/ rat (Cabanac et al., 1976). Additionally, Molnár (1965), Molnár and György (1967) reported that capsaicin administered i.v. at a dose higher than 10 μg/ kg to cats caused a rapid fall in the mean arterial pressure which was followed by either a pressor phase or death.These results called our attention to methods of administration of capsaicin (intravenously or orally in animal observations.

The LD_{50} dose of capsaicin (given i.p.) was calculated as 7.65 mg/kg in adult female and male mice (please to note that capsaicin was not given in as pure agents, however as extracts) (Glinsukon et al., 1980). The toxicity of capsaicin present in the capsicum extract was approximately four fold higher than that of pure capsaicin given intraperitoneally to mice. Capsaicin had a sligtly LD_{50} in weanking female rats administred in propylene glycol of those observed when administered intraperitoneally in dimethylsulfoxyde (DMSO) (*$P < 0.05$*) (Glinsukon et al., 1980). Guinea pigs are the most susceptible species to capsaicin toxicity with LD_{50} of 1.10 mg/mg, whereas hamsters and rabbits are less susceptible (Glinsukon et al., 1980).

The main results of these toxicological observations were as follows: LD_{50} values were 7.65 (5.28 – 11.09) for male and 6.50 (4.33-9.75) mg /kg for female mice; 10.40 (9.71 – 18.12) mg/ kg for rats; 1.10 (0.79 – 1, 52) mg /kg for guinea pig; > 50 mg/kg for rabbits and > 120 mg/kg for hamsters (Glinsukon et al., 1980).

The relative lethality of capsaicin administered by various routes in the mouse:

- 0.56 (0.36 – 0.87) mg/ kg intravenously,
- 1.60 (1.03-2.48) mg/kg intratracheally,
- 7.65 (5.28 – 11.09) mg/ kg intraperitoneally,
- 7.80 (5.53 – 10.99) mg/kg subcutaneusly,
- 60 to 190 mg/kg intragastrically,
- > 218 mg/kg intrarectally and
- > 512 mg/kg dermally (Glinsukon et al., 1980).

At the autopsy, only hyperemia without hemorrhage was observed in the visceral organs and the muscular wall of the peritoneal cavity with a slight increase in the amount of peritoneal fluid in the rats treated intraperitotoenally treated with capsaicin. A similar observation was also found in mice treated intraperitoneally with capsaicin. Histopathologic changes seen in the gastric mucosa of mice treated intragastrically with capsaicin was desquamatic necrosis with increase mucus material (PAS's Schiff stain). Some of the chief and parietal cells showed an appearance of pale basophylic cytoplasm and vacuolization. No significant histopathological changes were observed in other organs.

The pattern of the electrocardiogram and heart rate did not change for 5 min after capsaicin adminsitration. Respiratory rates were slightly increased during the first min, whereas a small increase of the tidal volume was also observed. The tidal volume then decreased to 10 to 20 per cent of the control whithin 3-4 min and the respiration stopped. During this time, heart rate gradually decreased and electrocardiograph signals disappeared much later (in about 6-14 min). Mean arterial pressure was variable in the rats treated with capsaicin. At the beginning, capsaicin causes a transient hypotension and followed by hypertensive period. Mean arterial pressure gradually decreased along with the decrease in the tidal volume. Convulsions were not observed in these anesthetized with a lethal dose of capsaicin. This finding was confirnmed in mice anesthetized with sodium barbital and subsequently given a single lethal dose of capsaicin.

The LD_{50} values indicate a high susceptibility, in guinea pigs, rats and mice, whereas hamsters and rabbits are less susceptible to capsaicin. Capsaicin is a highly toxic compound when administered by all routes except gastric, rectal and dermal. Cabanac et al. (1976) published a report on the acute toxicity of capsaicin in which adult male rats were given four increasing subcutaneosly doses of capsaicin (cumulative amount of 21.0 to 66.0 mg/kg).

The letality of capsaicin administered gastrically to the mouse is much more less than that of the intraperitoneal adminsitration route. The minimum lethal dose of capsaicin per kg was 100 mg, which would be contained in 32.4 g dry weigth of fruits. For a 60 kg person, this toxic level would be comparable to the consumption of about 1.94 kg of dry weet of capsinum fruits, this prevents the over consumption of this spice (Molnar, 1965).

4.3.2. Acute toxicity studies with pure trans-capsaicin derivated to dogs after intravenous administration

The *trans*-geometric isomer of capsaicin, or *trans*-8-methyl-N-vanillyl-6-nonenamide, is the most abundant pungent molecule in chilli peppers and thus represents the most important ingredient in spicy foods. Although there are two geometric isomers of capsaicin (*trans* and *cis*), only *trans*-capsaicin occurs naturally (Cordell and Araujo, 1993). The capsaicin content of chilli peppers ranges from 0.1 to 1.0 % w/w (Govindajarajan and Sathyanarayna, 1991). Furthermore, this food addidive has been widely used to evaluate the different physiological or pathological regulatory mechanisms in the human observation in the form of non-prescription (in USA) or prescribtion (in the Europe) topical analgetics, and self-defense products (e.g. pepper spray).

The *trans*-geometric isomer of capsaicin is a highly selective agonist for the transient receptor potential vanilloid receptor 1 (TRVP1 or also known as VR1 according to older nomenclature) (Caterina et al., 1997).

TRVP1 is a ligand-gated, non-selective, cation channel preferentially expressed in small-diameter in primary afferent neurones (C-fibres and Aδ-fibres), especially nociceptive sensory nerves. TRPV1 responds to noxious stimuli including capsaicin, heat and extracellular acidification, and integrates simultaneous exposures to these stimuli (Tominaga et al., 1998). Based on the highly selective agonistic property of capsaicin toward TRVP1 receptors, drug products containing pure synthetic trans-capsaicin are under evaluation as topical and injectable therapies (Bley, 2004).

Formal studies of the toxicological potential of capsaicin *in vivo* began in 1935, when De Lille and Ramirez (1935) reported that administration of a capsaicin extract into dogs produces a fall in blood pressure accompanied by variable effect on the respiration, an increase is salivary secretion, and a relatively small increase in gastric secretion. The capsaicin can really be increased the buffering ("non-periatal component" of the gastric secretion, in association with the decrease of "parietal component" of gastric secretion by the application of pure capsaicin (Sigma, USA) in the human healthy subjects (Mózsik et al., 2007).

The capsaicin materials tested in the studies cited above were generally natural extracts and may not exhibit the same toxicological profile as pure synthetic *trans*-capsaicin. Although the extract content and nature of impurities in the test articles used in these studies are often not explicitly stated, a typical capsaicin extract is a mixture of *trans*-capsaicin (*cis*-capsaicin does not occur naturally) and other capsaicinoids (including capsaicin, nordyhydrocapsaicin, dihydrocapsaicin, homocapsaicin and homodihydrocapsaicin). Earlier Burk et al. (1986) clearly proved that there is no physiological difference of between the application of capsaicin or dihydrocapsaicin in animal experiments.

The actual percent of capsaicin and other capsaicinoids will vary depending on the peppers used and method of extraction. In fact, **the United States Pharmacopoeia definies capsaicin**

as a product which contains >55% capsaicin and in combination of capsaicin and dihydrocapsaicin to be >75%; total capsainoid content may be as little as 90% (United States Pharmacopoeica, 2005). Additionally, each extracts are expected to contain chemical entities other than vanilloid compounds.

Chanda et al. (2005) performed observation with pure *trans*-capsaicin in dogs. The objectives of their study were to evaluate the possible cardivascular and respiratory effects of the pure capsaicin, and to evaluate the potential of any target organ toxicity and that might occur as a result of introduction of the pure trans-capsaicin given into the systemic circulation in dogs.

These studies were carried out in approximatively 10-17 months old dogs weighed between 19 and 21.8 kg at the time of observations. Capsaicin for this study was dissolved in 10 % w/v hydroxypropyl-β-cyclodextrin (Aldrich Chemical Gillingham, UK). Doses of capsaicin used in the main study were 0.03, 0.1 and 0.3 mg/kg given intravenously. The studies were carried out in acute observations and after two weeks of capsaicin (in doses of 0.03, 0.1 and 0.3 given intravenously) treatment as well. Different biochemical parameters (glucose, urea nitrogen, creatinine, total protein, albumin, albumin/globulin ratio, cholesterol, alanine aminotransferase, alkaline phosphatae, calcium, gamma glutamyltransferase, inorganic phosphorus, sodium, potassium, chloride, total bilirubin), hematological parameters (red blood count, hemoglobin, hematocrit, mean corpuscular volume, mean corpuscular hemoglobin, mean corpuscular hemoglobin concentration, platelet count, leucocyte count, different blood cell count, blood smear, prothombin time, activated partial thromboplastin time). Urine sapmles were tested for appearance/color, volume, specific gravidity, pH, protein, glucose, ketones, bilirubin, blood, microscopic examination of urine sediments, and urobilinogen. At the necropsy, the macroscopic observations were recorded, the organs were weighed, and selected tissues were collected and preserved. Microscopic examinations were carried out from all the tissue samples.

The capsaicin concentration of the plasma samples was determined by high performance liquid chromatography (HPLC).

- All of these observations were carried out in acute and after two weeks capsaicin treatment.
- The studies reported were conducted according to the priciples of Good Laboratory Practice (GLP). The *trans*-capsaicin (CAS 404-86-4) used in both the studies decribed was manufactured under the Current Good Manufacturing Practice (CGMP) conditions. The two batches of *trans*-capsaicin used for the studies had > 99%.
- The main results of these observations with *trans*-capsaicin in acute administration (before a chronic capsaicin treatment) are the followings:

4.3.2.1.Acute effects on cardiovascular and respiratory parameters

Administration of capsaicin (given in vehicle, 0.03 and 0.1 mg/kg) had no detectable effect on the cardiac and respiratory systems. However, after administration of 0.3 mg/kg trans-capsaicin elicited a rise in mean arterial blood pressure from a baseline of 96±7 to 138±21 mmHg whithin 2 min of starting the infusion. This effect peaked at 146±17 mmHg at the end of infusion

(15 min). The administration of the vehicle, capsaicin from 0.03 mg/kg to 0.1 mg/kg had no measurable effectc on arterial blood pressure, change in force of ventricular contraction (dP/dt_{max}), heart rate ECG waveform, and femoral blood flow. However, administration of 0.3 mg/kg capsaicin elicited a rise in mean arterial blood pressure from a base line of 96±7 to 138±21 mmHg within 2min of starting the infusion. The hypertensive effect was accompanied by increases in heart rate (from 71±3 at baseline to 119±25 bpm), dP/dt_{max} (from 4050±91 at baseline to 6679±1027 mmHg/s) and femoral blood flow (from 117±27 at baseline to 174±34 mL/min). These changes were statistically significant (*P*) in comparison with the results obtained after application of vehicle, 0.03 or 0.1 mg/kg capsaicin injection.

The change in heart rate was also associated with decreases in the RR and QT intervals of the ECG. However the corrected QT intervals (both QT_{CF} and QT_{CB}) were unchanged.

The administration of the vehicle elicited a decrease in deep of respiration. This was reflected as decreases at 30 min post-infusion in tidal volume (TV) (from 143±19 to 118±20 mL), peak inspiratory flow (PIF) (from 253 ±12 to 198±10 mLs) and peak expiratory flow (PEF) (from 297±47 to 246±24 mL/s). The rate of respiration was unaffected. After administration of 0.03 and 0.1 mg/kg *trans*-capsaicin did not elicit any further changes in respiration. After administration of high (0.3 mg/kg) dose of *trans*-capsaicin (given intravenously) elicited increases in PIF, PEF and TV. The increase of in PIF and PEF following 0.3 mg/kg *trans*-capsaicin is significantly different from the decrease in these parameters following the vehicle treatment ($P<0.05$). However, these increases were transients, lasting for only 5 to 10 min following the infusion.

4.3.2.2. Plasma levels of capsaicin

No detectable levels of capsaicin were found 5 min after administration of 0.05 mg/kg capsaicin. Following the administration of the intermediate dose (0.1 mg/kg i.v.), two and four dogs showed detectable levels of capsacinin (in ranges approximatively 17 and 11 ng/mL). The high dose (0.3 mg/kg) produced an increase in the plasma levels in all dogs (ranging 32.2 to 65.6 ng/mL, mean of 47.9±6.4 ng/mL).

4.3.3. Results of subacute toxicology of capsaicin in dogs

4.3.3.1. Two weeks treatment with trans-capsaicin

All dogs survived until scheduled termination on Day 15. Only capsaicin solution-related clinical sign observed during the study was vacualization during dosing, which was noted in all dogs.

In general, the observation was noted more frequently in male dogs than in female dogs. Clear nasal discharge was seen across all groups, and the daily incidence was slighly higher in male than in females given 0.3 mg/kg *trans*-capsaicin (intravenously), althought the daily incidence in males given 0.1 or 0.3 mg/kg/day of *trans*-capsaicin and in females given 0.3 mg/kg/day was slightly higher than controls. Slight tremors (head, limbs and/or body) were seen across all groups during this study. The majority of these observations were noted during the study.

As the study progressed, dogs given 0.3 mg/kg *trans*-capsaicin demonstrated an apparent tolerance to the general anesthetic and analgesic, as indicated by a general vacualization during the dosing period.

There were no statistically significant differences in the body weights and food consumption values, among the groups of dogs treated with capsaicin chronically. The body weights, however, were slightly lower (in about 7 %) in males treated with 0.3 mg/kg *trans*-capsaicin for 14 days. Over the duration of the study, males lost approximately 0.4 kg, whereas the control gained 0.1 kg. Through this value statistically was not significant, the food consumption of males and females given 0.3 mg/kg/ day was sligthly lower than that of controls (approximately 11 and 12 per cent, respectively).

4.3.3.2. Clinical chemistry and hematology

The only the difference considered related to test article was minimally higher ALT for males and females given 0.3 mg/kg/day *trans*-capsaicin intravenously after 14-day treatment. Other statistically significant differences for clinical chemistry test results were considered incidental, because they did not exhibit dose relatioship and they were present before the initiation of treatment. In hematology, WBC was statistically significant ($P < 0.05$) lower in female dogs in the 0.3 mg/kg/day treated group. A few animals, including controls, had notably high neutrophil counts, which were likely secondary to inflammated lesions at injection sites.

4.3.3.3. Organ weights, macroscopic and microscopic observations

There were no capsaicin solution-related organ weight changes, macroscopic or microscopic observations.

The statistically significant differences with respect to controls of prostate, brain and adrenal weight values were considered incidental because there were no correlating macroscopic and microscopic findings. Thrombosis, due to administration of vehicle, was noted at the intravenous injection sites in all groups. Other lesions observed with the thrombosis induced inflammmation, fibrosis, edema and hemorrhage.

4.3.3.4. Pharmacokinetic data after 14-day treatment with trans-capsaicin in dogs

After intravenous administration, peak of the plasma concentration (C_{max}) was obtained in all cases immediately at the end of infusion. Capsaicin was rapidly eliminated and measurable values were only obtained immediately after the end of infusion (0.25 h) in 0.03, 0.1 and 0.3 mg/kg/day dose groups. In the 0.3 mg/kg/day group, measurable values were obtained at 0.5 h in all dogs on Day 1, but they were very close to the limit of quantitation (10 ng/mL). On Day 15, only one dog still had a measurable value at this timepoint.

Females generally had higher or similar mean C_{max} values compared to males, but the largest difference did not exceed 44%. The increases in mean C_{max} for males and females were throughly proportional to the increase of dose level from 0.03 to 0.3 mg/kg/day.

4.3.4. Absorption and metabolism of oral application of the capsaicinoids in animal experiments

Due to the increasing experimental use and planned drug production in humans of capsaicin in a very wide field of medical research and medical treatment, we have to know correct facts on the absorption, metabolism and excretion of capsaicinoids.

It is known that capsaicin given directly into the stomach of rats has only minimal excitatory effects on immediate blood pressure responses (Lippe et al., 1989) in contrast to intravascular or subcutaneous administration (Donnerer and Lembeck, 1983). On the other hand it has been shown that capsaicin disappears from the intestinal lumen whithin a rather short time (Kawada et al., 1984) and should therefore reach the circulation.

Since biotransformed products of capsaicin are difficult to detect, the use of [^{3}H]-labelled dihydrocapsaicin ([^{3}H]-DHC) allowed us to determine the percentage of unchanged compound in the total ectracted radioactivity. Dihydrocapsaicin (DHC) has been shown to display pharmacodynamic and pharmacokinetic properties compared with those of capsaicin (Burk et al., 1982; Kawada et al., 1984).

[^{3}H]-dihydrocapsacin ([^{3}H]-DHC) and unlabelled capsaicin were readily absorbed from the gastrointestinal tract but were almost completely metabolized before reaching the general circulation. A certain degree of biotransformation already took place in the intestinal lumen. Unchanged compounds (identified by chromatography) were present in the portal vein blood. These seem to be result of a saturable absorption and degradation process in the gastrointestinal tract and a very effective metabolism limit of the liver (Donnerer et al., 1990).

Less than 5% of the total amount of extracted radioactivity consisted of unchanged [^{3}H]-DHC in truck blood and brain 15 min after gastrointestinal application. On the other hand, approximatively 50% unchanged [^{3}H]-DHC was detected in these tissues in 3 min after intravenously application or 90 min after subcutaneously application of capsaicinoids (Donnerer et al., 1990). Dihydrocapsaicin (DHC) or [^{3}H]-DHC were metabolized when incubated *in vitro* with liver tissue but not with brain tissue (Donnerer et al., 1990). The metabolic product(s) did not show capsaicin-like biological activity (Donnerer et al., 1990). These results clearly indicate that the rapid hepatic metabolization limits systemic pharmacological effects of enterally absorbed capsaicin in rats (Donnerer et al., 1990)

4.3.5. Toxicological studies with pure trans-capsaicin derivated to dogs after intravenous administration in acute and after subacute experimental circumstances

4.3.5.1. Chemistry of capsaicin

Trans-capsaicin, or *trans*-8-methyl-N-vanillyl-6-nonenamide, is the most abundant pungent molecule in chilli peppers and thus represents the most important ingredient in spicy foods. Although there are two geometric isomers of capsaicin, only the *trans*-isomer occurs in natural sources (Cordell and Araujo, 1993). The capsaicin content of chilli peppers ranges from 0.1 to 1.0 % w/w (Govindajarajan and Sathyanarayna, 1991). Furthermore, this food addidive has been widely used to evaluate the different physiological or pathological regulatory mechanisms in the human observation in the form of non-prescription (in the USA) or prescribtion (in Europe) topical analgetics, and self-defense products (e.g. pepper spray).

The *trans*-geometric isomer of capsaicin is a highly selective agonist for the transient receptor potential vanilloid receptor 1 (TRVP1 or as known VR1 according to older nomenclature) (Caterina et al., 1997).

TRVP1 is a ligand-gated, non-selective, cation channel preferentially expressed in small-diameter, primary afferent neurones (C-fibres and Aδ-fibres), especially nociceptive sensory nerves. TRPV1 responds to noxious stimuli including capsaicin, heat and extracellular acidification, and integrates simultaneous exposures to these stimuli (Tominaga et al., 1998). Based on the highly selective agonistic property of capsaicin toward TRVP1 receptors, drug products containing pure synthetic *trans*-capsaicin are under evaluation as topical and injectable therapies (Bley, 2004).

Formal studies of the toxicological potential of capsaicin *in vivo* began in 1935, when De Lille and Ramirez (1935) reported that administration of a capsaicin extract into dogs produced a fall in blood pressure accompanied by variable effect on the respiration, an increase is salivary secretion, and a relatively small increase in gastric secretion. The capsaicin really can increase the buffering ("non-perietal component" of the gastric secretion, in association with the decrease of "parietal component" of gastric secretion by the application of pure capsaicin (Sigma, USA) in human healthy subjects (Mózsik et al., 2007a).

The capsaicin materials tested in the studies cited above were either natural extracts or racemic mixtures, and may not exhibit the same toxicological profile as pure *trans*-capsaicin. Although the extract content and nature of impurities in the test articles used in these studies are often not explicitly stated, a typical capsaicin extract is a mixture of *trans*-capsaicin (*cis*-capsaicin does not occur naturally) and other capsaicinoids (including capsaicin, nordyhydrocapsaicin, dihydrocapsaicin, homocapsaicin and homodihydrocapsaicin). Earlier Burk et al. (1986) clearly proved that there is no physiological difference between the applications of capsaicin and dihydrocapsaicin in animal experiments).

4.3.5.2. Observations in acute experiments in the dogs

The actual percent of capsaicin and other capsaicinoids will vary depending on the peppers used and method of extraction: In fact, the United States Pharmacopocia definies capsaicin as a product which contains >55% capsaicin and in combination of capsaicin and dihydrocapsaicin to be >75%; total capsainoid content may be as little as 90% (United States Pharmacopoeica, 2005). Additionally, per extracts are expected to contain chemical entities other than vanilloid compounds.

Chanda et al. (2005) did observation with pure *trans*-capsaicin in dogs.The objectives of this study were to evaluate the possible cardiovascular and respiratory effects of the pure capsaicin, and to evaluate the potential of any target organ toxicity and that might occur as a result of introduction of the pure *trans*-capsaicin given into the systemic circulation in dogs.

These studies were carried out in dogs, approximatively 10-17 months old and weighed between 19 and 21.8 kg at the time of observations. Capsaicin for this study was dissolved in 10 % w/v hydroxypropyl-β-cyclodextrin (Aldrich Chemical, Gillingham, UK). Doses of capsaicin used in the main study were 0.03, 0.1 and 0.3 mg/kg given intravenously. The studies were carried out in acute observations, and after two weeks capsaicin (in doses of 0.03, 0,1 0nd 0,3 mg/ kg given intravenously) treatment. Different biochemical parameters (glucose,urea nitrogen, creatinine, total protein, albumin, albumin / globulin ratio, cholesterol, alanine aminotransferase, alkaline phosphatae, calcium, gamma glutamyltransferase, inorganic phosphorus, sodium, potassium, chloride, total bilirubin), hematological parameters (red blood count, hemoglobin, hematocrit, mean corpuscular volume, mean corpuscular hemoglobin, mean corpuscular hemoglobin concentration, platelet count, leucocyte count, differenrt blood cell count, blood smear, prothombin time, activated partial thromboplastin time). Urine samples were tested for appearance/color parameters, volume, specific gravidity, pH, protein, glucose, ketones, bilirubin, blood, microscopic examination of urine sediments, and urobilinogen. At the necropsy, the macroscopic observations were recorded, the organs were weighted, and selected tissues were colected ans presenved. Microscopic examinations were carried out from all the tissue samples.

The capsaicin concentration of the plasma samples was determined by high performance liquid chromatography (HPLC).

All of these observations were carried out in acute and after two weeks capsaicin treatment.

The studies reported were conducted according to the priciples of Good Laboratory Practice (GLP). The *trans*-capsaicin (CAS 404-86-4) used in both the studies decribed was manufactured under the Current Good Manufacturing Practice (CGMP) conditions. The two batches of trans-capsaicin used for the studies had > 99%.

The main results of these observations with *trans*-capsaicin in acute administration (before a chronic capsaicin treatments) are as follows:

Administration of capsaicin (given in vehicle, 0.03 and 0.1 mg/kg) had no detectable effect on the cardiac and respiratory systems. However, after administration of 0.3 mg/kg *trans*-capsaicin elicited a rise in mean arterial blood pressure from a baseline of 96±7 to 138±21 mm Hg whithin 2 min of starting the infusion. This effect peaked at 146±17 mmHg at the end of infusion (15 min). The hypertensive effect was accompanied by increases in heart rate (from 71±3 at baseline to 119±25 bpm) left ventricular pressure and derivitave (dP/dt_{max}) (from 4050±91 at baseline to 6679± 1079 mmHgs), and femoral blood flow (from 117±27 at baseline to 174±35 mL/min). These changes were statistically significant in comparison with the results obtained after vehicle, 0.03 or 0.1 mg/ kg capsaicin injection

Administration of the vehicle elicited a decrease in deep of respiration. This was reflected as decreases at 30 min post-infusion in tidal volume (TV) (from 143±19 to 118±20 mL), peak inspiratory flow (PIF) (from 253 ±12 to 198±10 mLs) and peak expiratory flow (PEF) (from 297±47 to 246±24 mL/s).The rate of respiration was unaffected. After administration of 0.0.3 and 0.1 mg / kg trans-capsaicin did not elicit any further changes in respiration. After administration of high (0.3 mg/kg) dose of *trans*-capsaicin (given intravenously) elicited increases in

PIF, PEF and TV. The increase of in PIF and PEF folloowing 0.3 mg/kg *trans*-capsaicin is significantly different from the decrease in these parameters following the vehicle treatment (*P<0.05*). However, these increases were transients, lasting only 5 to 10 min after the end of infusion.

No detectable levels of capsaicin were found in the plasma level at 5 min after administration of 0.05 mg/kg capsaicin. Following the administration of the intermediate dose (0.1 mg/kg i.v.), two and four dogs showed detectable levels of capsacinin (in ranges approximatively 17 and 11 ng/mL). The high dose (0.3 mg/kg) produced an increase in the plasma levels in all dogs (ranging 32.2 to 65.6 ng/mL, mean of 47.9±6.4 ng /mL).

4.3.5.3. Results of the subacute and chronic toxicology of capsaicinoid in dogs

All dogs survived until the scheduled termination on day 15. Only capsaicin solution-related clinical sign observed during the study was vacualization during dosing, which was noted in all dogs.

In general, the observation was noted more frequently in male dogs than in female dogs. Clear nasal discharge was seen across all groups, and the daily incidence was slighly higher in male than in females given 0.3 mg/kg *trans*-capsaicin (intravenously), althought the daily incidence in males given 0.1 or 0.3 mg/kg/ day of *trans*-capsaicin and in females 0.3 mg/kg/day was slightly higher than controls. Slight tremors (head,l imbs, and/or body) were seen across all groups during this study. The majority of these observations were noted during the study.

As the study progressed, dogs given 0.3 mg/kg *trans*-capsaicin demonstrated an apparent tolerance to the general anesthetic and analgesic, as indicated by a general vacualization during the dosing period.

There were no statistically significant differences in the body weights and food consumption values, among the groups of dogs treated chronically. The body weights, however, were slightly lower (in about 7 %) in males treated with 0.3 mg/kg *trans*-capsaicin for 14 days. Over the duration of the study, males in this group lost approximately 0.4 kg, whereas the control gained 0.1 kg. Altough it was statistically not significant, the food consumption of males and females given 0.3 mg/kg/day was sligthly lower than that of controls (approximately 11 and 12 per cent, respectively) (Changa et al., 2005).

4.3.5.4. Clinical chemistry and hematology

The results of the clinical chemistry [aminotransferase (ALT), aspartate aminotransferase (AST) and alkaline phosphatase], and hematology (RBC, count of MCV, MCV, platelet count,WBC) tests from days – 1 and 15 only are measured. There were few statistically significant or otherwise notable differences for clinical chemistry test results between the control and treated animals.

The only the difference considered related to test article was minimally higher ALT for males and females given 0.3 mg/kg/day *trans*-capsaicin intravenously after 14 days treatment. Other significant differences for clinical chemistry test results were considered incidental because they exhibited no dose relationship or were present before initiation of the treatment. In hematology, female dogs in the 0.3 mg/kg/day treated group the WBC was statistically significant ($P < 0.05$) lower. A few animals, including controls, had notably high neutrophil counts, which were like secondary to inflammated lesions at injection sites.

4.3.5.5. Organ weights, macroscopic and microscopic observations

There were no capsaicin solution-related organ weight changes in macroscopic or microscopic observations.

The statistically significant differences with respect to controls of prostate, brain and adrenal weight values were considered incidental because there were no correlating macroscopic and microscopic findings.

Thrombosis, due to administration of vehicle, was noted at the intravenous injection sites in all groups. Other lesions observed with the thrombosis induced inflammation, fibrosis, edema and hemorrhage.

4.3.5.6. Pharmacokinetic data after 14 days treatment with trans-capsaicin in dogs

After intravenous administration, peak plasma concentration (C_{max}) was attained in all cases immediately after the end of infusion. Capsaicin was rapidly eliminated and measurable values were only obtained immediately after the end of infusion (0.25 hour) in 0.03, 0.1 and 0.3 mg/kg/day dosage groups. In the 0.3 mg/kg/day group, measurable values were obtained out to 0.5 hour in all dogs on day 1, but they were very close to the limit of quantitation (10 ng/mL). On day 15, only one dog still had a measurable value at this timepoint.

Females generally had higher or similar mean C_{max} values compared to males, but the largest difference did not exceed 44%. The increases in mean C_{max} for males and females were throughly proportional to the increase of dose level from 0.03 to 0.3 mg/kg/day. Mean C_{max} values for males increased 1: 3.3: 10-fold on Day 1 and 1: 2.9: 9.2 fold on Day 14. These results clearly indicate that no acumulation exists to capsaicin after multiple dosing by this route of its administration (Chanda et al., 2005).

4.3.5.7. Summary and conclusions of the administration of trans-capsaicin in its acute and subacute experiments in dogs (on dependence of different doses of trans-capsaicin)

In the acute study, surface lead II ECG was monitored to determine the QTc intevals and the duration of cardiac repolarization. However, there were no observable changes in the QT_{CF} (Fridericia's correlation QT_{CF}, $QT_{CF}=QT/^{3}\sqrt{}$ (RR intervall)). Such a change would have been theoretically possible, as capsaicin has been reported to block voltage-activated potassium channels in rat ventricular myocytes (Castle, 1992). Because many drugs are able to block voltage-activated channels actuallly shorten the duration of cardiac action potentials, there are limited correlations between the potassium channel blocking activity and QT interval prolongation (Martin et al., 2004). The lack of measurable effects on the cardiac action potential make it likely that the hemodynamic effects of capsaicin measured during the acute study with 0.3

mg/kg/kay capsaicin due to agonistic activity on TRVP1 receptors. This is probably due to the reported potency of capsaicin being severalfold higher than for either calcium and potassium ion channels (Castle, 1992); Cheng et al., 2003). Thus, it is likely that capsaicin receptors expressed on pericardiac sensory nerves induced the transient increases in the heart rate observed during the acute dosing study, in the course of performing their role to sense cardiac ischemia (Pan and Chem, 2004). For longer administration of capsaicin, it is possible that the putative antihypertensive actions of capsaicin result from either prolonged desensitation of pericardiac sensory fibres, or including the release of vasoactive peptides (CGRP and SP) from the perivascular C-fibres, or activating and endogenous system with counterbalances hypertension caused by sodium salt loading (Vaishnava and Wang, 2003).

Other than cardiac effects, capsaicin has also been studied in animals for other possible target organ toxicity. Almost all of these studies used pepper plant extracts, which are likely to display varying degrees of capsaicinoids content and possible diverse impurity profiles. These impurities may be the contributing factor in some of toxicities observed. Chanda et al. (2004) observed that pure capsaicin displays a different genotocity profil than that described in some previous literature. Additionally, in contrast to the high dose levels used in toxicological studies, human exposure to dietary capsaicinoids (a mixture of capsaicin, dihydrocapsaicin, nordihydrocapsaicin, homocapsaicin and homodihydrocapsaicin) in the USA and in European countries is about 1.5 mg/ day, which translates into 0.025 mg/ day/ day dose (Chanda et al., 2005).

When capsaicin was dissolved in diethylene gycol monoethyl eher and Dulbecco's phosphate-buffered saline and administered intravenous infusion for14 days (in a 15 min time period to anesthetized dogs), the vehicle itself caused marked vascular irritation at the administration sites. There were no deaths, no test article-related organ weight changes, and no macroscopic and microscopic observations. The only test article-related clinical sign observed in the study was vacualization by the dogs treated with 0.3 mg/kg /day dose. The only test article-related clinical pathology finding was maximal higher in ALT for male and female dogs receiving 0.3 mg/kg/day capsaicin. This may indicate the liver as a possible target organ when capsaicin is delivered at high doses directly into the systemic circulation. When the capsaicin was given in dose of 0.1 mg/kg/day for 14 days, capsaicin was rapidly eliminated in dogs.

Capsaicin dissolved in dimethyl sulfoxide (DMSO) has been studied by Glinsukon et al. (1980) for determination of LD_{50} values using several administration routes in mice. The authors also determined the LD_{50} values of capsaicin for one administration route (intraperitoneal) in different species. The oreder of sensitivity (LD_{50} values) for species, from at least to most, by the intraperitoneal route using DMSO as the delivery vehicle was repoted to be: hamsters (>120 mg/kg), rabbit (>50 mg/kg), rat (9.5 mg/kg), mouse (6.5 to 7.65 mg/kg) and guinea pig (1.1 mg/kg). This study and those described above were mixed with respect to gender. Electrocardiograms (ECGs), mean arterial presure and resporiratory rates were also measured by Glinsukon et al. (1980) in anesthetized rats after treatment with a lethal intraperitoneal dose of capsaicin. Saito and Yamamoto (1996) reported the oral LD_{50} values for capsaicin extract for both genders in mice and rats from experiment, where propylene glycol was used as vehicle. They did not found any significance in the LD_{50} values in both genders. The major toxic signs in mice and rats included salivation, straggering gait, bradypnoe and cyanosis. Tremor, clonic convulsion, dyspnoe and lateral or prone position were observed, and then the animals died in time period of 4 to 26 min after oral dosing by gavage.

The cause of death was proposed to be due to hypotension and respiratory paralysis in rats and mice although the authors noted that the pathophsiology of these deaths was not clearly understood.

In a study with Monsereenusorn (1983), 50 mg /kg capsaicin was given orally by gavage to rats for up to 60 days. The effects of capsaicin on body weight, rectal temperature, food and water consumption, hematological parameters, plasma biochemistry, urine concentration and dilution tests were evaluated at 10, 20, 30, 40, 50 and 60 days. The major finding was decreased body weight gain starting at 40 days, despite an increase in food cosumption. Minor changes in the clinical chemistry (reduced plasma urea nitrogen, glucose, phospholipids, triglycerides, total cholesterol, free fatty acids, glutaminic piruvic transaminase and alkalic phosphatase) were noted after one month treatment, however, these differences were not biologically significant,

The results of observations done by Chanda et al. (2005) indicate that *trans*-capsaicin given into the sytemic circulation, induces transient increases in heart rate and blood pressure without the alterations in cardiac repolarization.

4.3.6. Metabolism of capsaicin

Early studies by Lee and Kumar (1980) showed that phenobarbital-induced rat liver microsomes converted the capsaicin and dihydrocapsaicin to corresponsing catechol metabolites, N-(4,5-dihydroxyl-3-methoxybenzyl)-acetamides via hydroxylation on the vanillyl moiety. This finding was further confirmed by Miller et al. (1983) who demonstrated the covalent binding of [3H]-dihydrocapsaicin to hepatic microsomal proteins following *in vitro* incubation or administration to rats. Based on these results, it has been postulated that capsaicin is activated by the liver mixed-function oxidase system to an electrophilic intermediate, most likely a ring epoxide, capable of covalently interactiving with nucleophilic sites of hepatic protein (Figure 14).

This irreversible interaction of capsaicin with liver microsomal protein may account for its impact binding of capsaicin observed in spinal cord or brain, and it was concluded that capsaicin-induced neuropathy in rodents might be mediated by mechanisms other than covalent intercation (Miller et al.,1983). The alkyl side chain of capsaicin is also considered to be susceptible to enzymatic oxidation. Thus, when capsaicin was incubated with NADPH and the liver S9 fraction from phenobarbital pretreated rats, it was hydroxylated at the terminal carbon of the side chain (Surh et al., 1995).

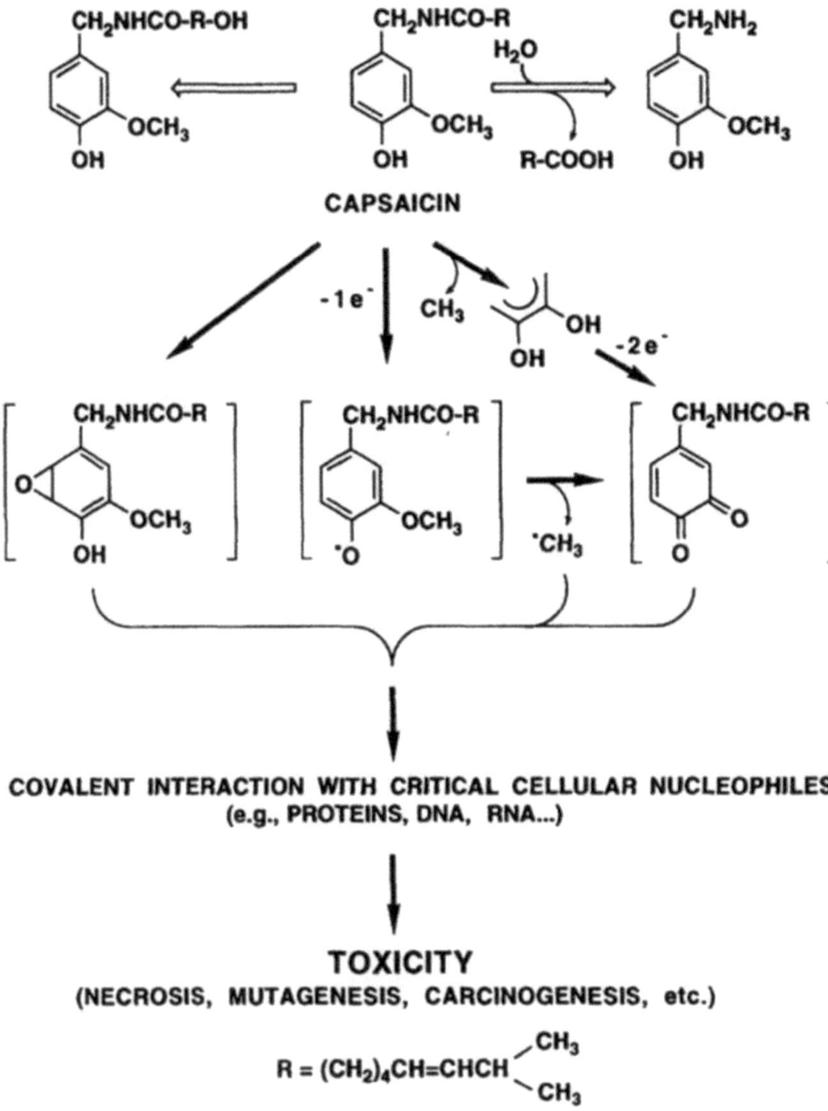

Figure 14. Metabolism of natural capsaicin in the experimental animals. After Surh and Lee, 1995 with modification.

4.3.6.1. The potential routes of metabolism in capsaicin

4.3.6.1.1. Enzymatic oxidatic metabolism of capsaicin

One-electron oxidation of capsaicin has been investigated by means of electrochemical, enzymatic and chemical procedures (Lawson and Gannett, 1989; Boersch et al., 1991). Lawson and Gannett (1989) reported that incubation of capsaicin with microsomes or non-enzymatic reaction with potassium ferricyanide resulted in the formation of a dimer, 5,5′-bis-capsaicin.

A phenoxy radical was proposed to be involved in the mutagenesis by capsaicin. Formation of phenoxy radical has often been observed with certain plant phenolics (Newmark, 1984; 1987), which plays a critical role of in lignin biosynthesis in the process of wood formation (Freudenberg, 1960). Formation of dimetric tyrosine by oxidation of tyrosine with horseradish peroxidase-catalized coupling reaction has been proposed as a mechanism for the dimerization of two diiodotyrosyl residues in thyroglobin to form the thyroid hormone, thyroxine (Taurog et al., 1994). Boersch et al. (1991) have demonstrated that incubation of capsaicin with peroxidase and hydrogen peroxide produced a flouescent dimer analogue similar to that previously reported by Lawson and Gannett (1989). The formation of this flourescent oxidation product was also observed by chemical or electrochemical oxidation of capsaicin (Lawson and Gunnett, 1989). Gunnett et al. (1990) has shown that the liver cytochrome P450 2E1 (CYP2E1) activity is responsible for conversion to the reactive phenoxy radical which, in turn, dimerizes or covalently binds to CYP2E1, thereby interacting the enzyme (Figure 14).

4.3.6.1.2. Non-oxidative metabolism of capsaicin

Cell-free extracts of various tissues of rats contained enzyme activity for hydrolyzing capsaicin or its dihydro analoque at the acid-amide bond to produce vanillylamine and the corresponding fatty acyl moieties (Kawada and Iwai, 1985; Tawada et al., 1992; Oi et al., 1992) (Table 1). The highest enzyme activity was found in the liver followed by such extrahepatic tissues as kidney, lung and small intestine (Kawada and Iwai, 1985). It is of oral administration of capsaicin (Oi et al., 1992). The splitting of the side chain of dihydrocapsaicin also occurred *in vivo* (Kawada and Iwai, 1985), which is considered to be rate-limiting step in the overall metabolism of this compound. Hydrolysis of the amide linkage of capsaicinoids will thus lead to the formation of vanillylamine as a common metabolite regardless of the fatty acid type in their side chain. Indeed, the systhemic vanilloid, olvanil [N-(3-methoxy-4-hydroxybenzyl)oleamide] having longer side chain than capsaicin, has been found to be susceptible to hydrolysis of the amide bond as determined in various metabolic model systems including cell-free extracts of liver and intestine, isolated hepatocytes, enterocytes, and perfused isolated intestine, and also in whole animal studies (Wehmeyer et al., 1990). Oxydative deamination of the resulting vanillylamine produces the aromatic alcohol for excretion as a free form or a glucoronic conjugate (Kawada and Iwai, 1985; Wehmeyer et al., 1990). Capsaicin hydrolyzing enzymes have been purified from the rat hepatic microsomes (Park and Lee, 1994), and identified as previously known isoenzymes of carbylesterase based on such biochemical and biophysical parameters as Mr, pI value, pH-dependency, mode of inhibition and subcellular toxicity. The enzymes are likely to be present either free in the lumen of endoplasmatic reticulum or loosely bound to the terminal surface of the membrane (Park and Lee, 1994). Capsaicinoids administered to rats intragastrically were readily absorbed from the gastrointestinal tract, and further metabolized to a great extent in the liver before reaching the general circulation (Park and Lee, 1994). As a result, gastrointestinally absorbed capsaicinoids are expected to reach the central nervous system or other extrahepatic organs almost exclusively as degradation products (Donnerer et al., 1990).

4.3.6.2. Role of metabolic activation in capsaicin-induced toxicity

There is no clear-cut mechanism which can solely explain the toxicity exerted by capsaicin. Bioactivation to an electrophylic intermediate with subsequent covalent modification of critical cellular macromolecules such as DNA, RNA and proteins has been thought to play a role in cell death (Miller et al., 1983; Anonymous, 1986), fueling interest in towards the role of these observed metabolic processes. Based on the results of previous metabolic studies, the following activation pathways can be postulated which may account for the capsaicin-induced cellular damage (Figure 15):

a. cytochrome P450-catalyzed epoxidation of the vanillyl moiety to produce an arene oxide;

b. one-electron oxidation of the hydroxyl group to form a phenoxy radical;

c. O-demethylation at the aromatic ring and subsequent oxidation of the resulting catechol to the semiquinone and quinone derivates.

The possible involvement of an electrophilic epoxide by others (Miller et al., 1983), but the presumed oxirane epoxidation of capsaicin is expected to occur since the formation of arene oxide. Nonetheless, ring epoxidation of capsaicin is expected to occur since the formation of arene oxide intermediates is a best general phenomenon in the monooxigenase-catalized metabolism of aromatic compounds. The best evidence for the epoxidation of capsaicin might be the actual isolation of the presumed arene oxide, but the chemical reactivity of such species precludes its direct isolation from incubation mixtures or from the biological fluids or tissues of treated animals. The advances in the development of novel mild oxidating agents such as dimethyl dioxirane have made it possible to prepare the extremely reactive epoxides of certain chemical carcinogens including alflatoxin B1-8,9 oxide (Baertschi et al., 1988). A similar synthetic approach could be applied to synthesis of the benzoepoxide derivate of capsaicin for testing its biological activity as well as chemical reactivity. The covalent binding of tritium-labeled capsaicin to hepatic microsomal protein was significantly inhibited by reduced glutathione, which implies the formation of a reactive intermediate (epoxide) during metabolism of capsaicin (Miller et al., 1983). Since glutathione is relatively nonspecific in terms of interacting with reactive intermediates including not only oxiranes but also of capsaicin does not necessarily suggest the aforementioned arene oxide as a sole electrophilic epoxide hydrolase being more sensitive approach in exploring the possible involvement of an epoxi metabolite in the toxification processes induced by capsaicin.

The intermediacy of the phenoxy radical of capsaicin has been investigated by using the electrochemical or chemical methods (Lawson and Gannett, 1989; Boiesch et al., 1991; Gannett et al., 1990). Furthermore, horseradish peroxidase plus the phenoxy radical intermediate (Boesch et al., 1991; Gunnett et al., 1990). Likewise, hepatic microsomal cytochrom P450 (particularly CYP2E1) might generate the same reactive radical species that is capable of attacking the nucleophilic sites of the enzyme or the target cell protein (Gunnett et al., 1990) leading to the loss of catalytic activity in other crutial biological functions.

A quinone type intermediate also represents a potential ultimate electrophilic metabolite of capsaicin. The formation of such intermediate could proceed via O-demethylation of the 3-

http://dx.doi.org/10.5772/58359

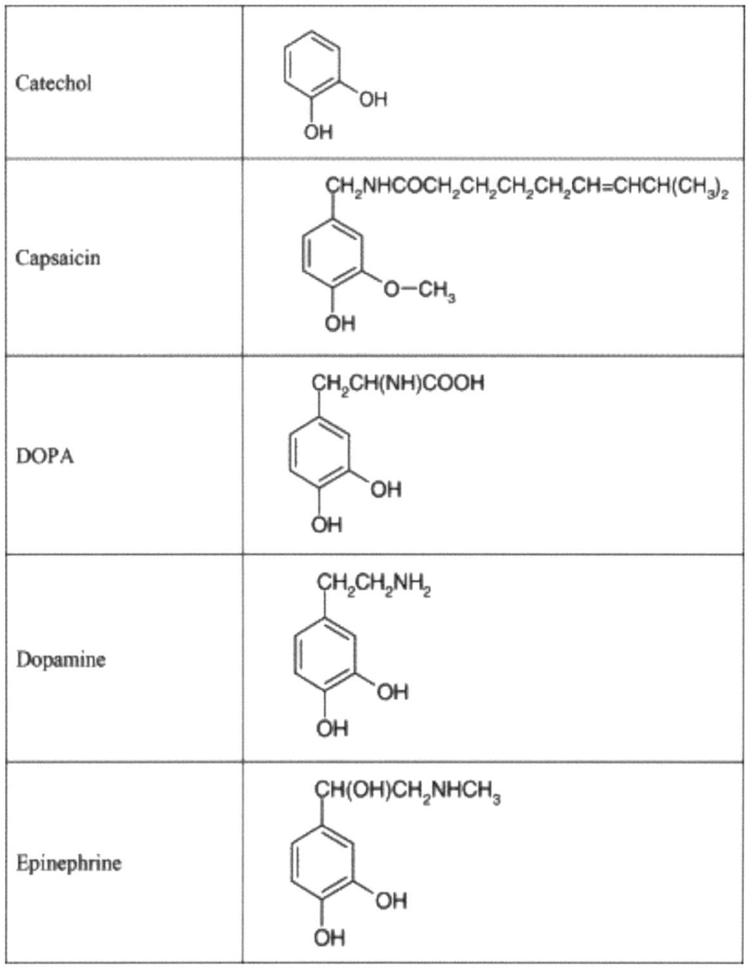

Figure 15. Structures of selected compounds containing cathecol moieties, including capsaicin. (Chanda et al., 2004)

methoxy group on the vanillyl moiety with concomittant oxidation to the semiquinone and *ortho*-quinone derivates. The same of *ortho*-quinone metabolite could be generally through O-demethylation of the aforementioned phenoxy radical intermediate of capsaicin (Table 1). This process will also lead to the formation of an extremely reactive CH_3 radical, which is wel known to alkylate cellular nucleic acids and proteins. The above mentioned reactions are likely to occur in presence of microsomal O-demethylase activity and relatively high reactivity of the catechols. The antineoplastic agent, etoposide, for instance, has been known to exert its cytotoxic effect by enzymic O-demethylation of one of its methoxy groups to the *ortho*-quinone derivative capable for binding covalently to cellular macromolecules (Haim et al., 1987a; 1987b; Mans et al., 1991; Relling et al., 1992; 1994). Similarly, initial ring epoxidation of capsaicin and subsequent NIH shift resulting benzoepoxide derivate would generate a catechol intermediate without O-demethylation

4.3.6.3. Effects of capsaicin on xenobiotic metabolism and chemically induced mutagenesis and carcinogenesis

Capsaicin has been suggested to exert such chemopreventive effects through modulation of metabolism of carcinogens and their interactions with tareget cell DNA. It has been reported that capsaicin displays a dose-related inhibition of the activity of rat epithelial aryl hydrocarbon hydroxylase (Modly et al., 1986), a marker enzyme for metabolism of polycyclic aromatic hydrocarbons such as benzo(α)pyrene. Furthermore, capsaicin suppressed the metabolism and covalent DNA binding of benzo(α)pyrene and human as well as murine keratocytes (Modly et al., 1986). The results of different studies suggested the interaction of capsaicinoids with microsomal mixed-function oxidases.Thus, the pretreatment of rats with subcutaneous dosages of capsaicin resulted in pronounced prolongation of fenobarbital or hexobarbital sleeping time (Miller et al., 1983; Surh et al., 1995; Rauf et al., 1985). Capsaicin also competitively inhibited the ethylmorphine demethylase activity in rat liver microsomes and produced a type I spectral change (Miller et al., 1980). Oral administration of capsaicin (50 mg/kg) together with 10% ethanol in drinking materials resulted much greater xenobitic metabolizing enzyme activity, than that induced by ethanol alone (Iwama et al., 1989). Capsaicin pretreatment also induced 4-hydroxylation of biphenyl in the rat liver (Rauf et al., 1985).

Yagi has reported that capsaicin and dihydrocapsaicin repress the energy-transducing NADH-quinone oxidoreductase activity (Yagi, 1990). This finding confirms an earlier observation by investigations of inhibitory effects of capsaicin on rat hepatic mitochondial energy metabolism through supression of energy flow from NADH to coenzyme Q (Chudapongse and Jathanasoot, 1881). Capsaicin was shown to inhibit calmodulin-mediated oxidative burst in rat macrophages as determined by attenuetion of Ca^{2+}ionophore-triggered production of superoxide anion and hydrogen peroxide (Savitha et al., 1990). Joe and Lokesh (1994) have also shown that capsaicin can strongly block the generation of reactive oxygen species in rat peritoneal macrophages *in vitro*. Capsaicin fed to animals was also inhibitory onto these macrophages (Joe and Lokesh, 1994). Pretreatment of rats with capsaicin (1.68 mg/kg, intraperitoeally) for three consequeutive days resulted in enhancement of activities of pulmonary antioxidant enzymes such as superoxide dismutase, catalase and peroxidase while long-term treatment caused an opposite effect on the latter two enzymes (De and Ghosh, 1989). Since reactive oxygen species are known to play an important role in phorbol-12-myristate-13-acetate (PMA)-mediated tumor promotion as well as in inflammation (Kensler and Trush, 1989), it would be worth determining whether capsaicin with potential anti-inflammatory activity (Joe and Lokesh, 1994; Flynn and Rafferty, 1986) could act as an anti-tumor promoter. It is noteworthy that the inhibition of prostaglandin synthesis by curcumin, the product of tumeric, correlates well with its protective activity against curcumin by inactivate xanthine dehydrogenase/oxigenase, which may account for its anti-promotional activity.

Capsaicinoids have also been found to retain inhibitory effects on liver microsomal CYP2E1 activity (Gannett el al., 1990; Lee et al., 1994; Shlyankevich et al., 1995). Capsaicin inhibits the metabolism and mutagenicity (Guengerich et al., 19991; Koop, 1992; Espinosa-Aguirre et al., 1993), which is known to be activated by CYP2E1. The vinyl carbamate-induced CYP2E1-mediated mutagenicity and tumorigenicity has been showns to be reduced by capsaicin (Lee et al., 1995). The initiation of papillomas in mouse skin by benzo(α)pyrene was also significantly reduced by topical application of capsaicin prior to the carcinogen (Lee et al., 1995). This finding is in agreement with *in vitro* inhibition of rodent epidermal arylhydrocarbon hydroxylase activity by capsaicin as previously reported by Moody et al. (1986). Chilli extracts have been found to modulate the mutagenic activity of particulate organic matter in urban air samples (Espinosa-Aquuirre et al., 1993).

In a series of observations, it has been observed that capsaicin has a protective effect on the metabolism, DNA binding, and/or mutagenicity of some carcinogens [aflatoxin Bl, tobacco-specific nitrosoamine and 4-(methylnitroso)-1-(3-pyridyl)-1-butanone)]. These findings suggest that capsaicin might act as a chemoprotective agent by modulating the activities of microsomal mixed-function oxidases which play key roles in metabolic activation as well as detoxication of a wide array of chemical carcinogens and mutagens (Surh and Lee, 1995).

4.3.6.4. Hepatoprotection of capsaicin in rats

Recently Abdel Salam et al. observed in details the dose dependent hepatoprotective effect of orally given capsacin (2 mL/kg followed by 1 mL/kg after one week) in rats treated with carbon tetrachloride (CCl_4) (2006). Capsaicin at three dose levels (10,100 and 1000 μg/kg) or silymarin (22 mg/kg) was administered orally for 10 days, starting at the time of administration of CCl_4. The daily administration of capsaicin conferred significant protection against the hepatotoxic effect of CCl_4 in rats. It decreased the increases of of serum alanine aminotransferase (ALT) and aspartate aminotransferase (AST) and also prevented the development of histological hepatic necrosis caused by CCl_4 as determined 10 days after drug administration. Thus, compared with CCl_4 control group, serum ALT decreased by 39.3, 59.3 and 71.1 %, while AST decreased by 14.3, 21.5 and 23.3%, after the capsaicin administration (given it in doses mentioned above), respectively. Serum bilirubin was decreased by 10 and 100 μg/kg (46.4 and 66.5% reduction, respectively), but an increased bilirubin and ALP was observed after the highest dose of capsaicin. Meanwhile, silymarin reduced serum ALT by 65.3%, AST by 18.9%, ALP by 22% and bilirubin by 13.4%, compared to controls. Serum proteins were significantly increased by 16.9 to 22.9% after treatment with capsaicin compared, whilst marked increased in serum glucose by 66.9% was observed after highest dose of capsaicin compared with vehicle-treated group.

Quantitative analysis of the area of damage by image analysis technique showed a reduced area of damage from 13.6% to 7.5, 4.3 and 2.8% by application of capsaicin (used in the above mentioned doses) respectively (Abdel-Salam et al., 2006). Haematoxylin-eosin staining indicated markedly less hepatic necrosis in rats treated with capsaicin or silymarin. Histochemical alterations such as decreased nuclear DNA, cell glycogen and proteins contents caused by CCl_4 in hepatocytes were prevented by capsaicin as well as by silymarin.

It has been concluded from these results that orally applied capsaicin exerts beneficial effects on liver histopathologic changes and enzymatic release caused by CCl_4 in rats, but high doses are likely to result cholestasis (Abdel Salam et al., 2006).

4.3.7. Genotoxicity studies of capsaicin or trans-capsaicin

Published information on the potential genotoxicty of capsaicin is inconsistent, both positive and negative effects have been found in classic genetic toxicology assays (Surh and Lee, 1995; Azazan and Blevins, 1995).

Eight bacterial point mutation tests (including Ames assays) were performed from 1981 to 1995 on capsaicin of carying origins, using variuos strains of S.typhimurium. Variopus forms of S9 activation were provided seven of the eight assays. Four of these tests resulted in a positive responses and four resulted in a negative response. Point mutation tests in Chinese hamster V79 cells were conducted twice, resulting in positive and one negative response. The *in vivo* micronucleus test was conducted once in mice and it was positive (Nagabhushan and Bhide, 1985). Data from one micronucleus and sister chromatid exchange study in human lymphocytes was interpreted to show that capsaicin is genotoxic (Marques et al., 2002). Capsaicin was also reported to induce DNA strand breaks in human neuroblastoma cells (Richeus et al., 1999).

The most of these studies were carried out with natural extracts, and these may not exhibit the same toxicological profile with pure capsaicin.

Recently different studies were carried out to evaluate the genotoxic potential of *trans*-capsaicin using different genotoxic assays used by international regulatory agencies to evaluate drug product safety (Chanda et al., 2004). These included the Ames assay, mouse lymphoma cell mutations assay, mouse *in vivo* bone marrow micronucleus assay and chromosomal aberration assay in human peripheral blood lymphocytes (HPBL). All studies were conducted accoring to the Organization of Economic Cooperation and Development (OECD) principles Good Laboratory Practice (GLP)

4.3.7.1. Ames assay

Ames assay described in the paper of Chanda et al. (2004) was based on the method described by Ames et al. (1975). The thimidi kinase (TK) heterozygote system was described by Clive et al. (1972), in which tk+tk-is mutated to tk-tk-. It's measured on the L5178Y mouse lymphoma cell line established by Fischer (1958).

In this assay, cell deficient tk+/ tk-to tk-tk-are resistant to cytotoxic effects of pyrimidine analoque triflurothymidine (TFT). Thymidin kinase proficient cells are sensitive to TFT, which causes the inhibtion of cellular metabolism and stops further cell division. Thus, the mutant cells are able to proliferate in the presence of TFT, whereas normal cells containing thymidine kinase are not (Moore et al., 2002).

Salmonella typhimurium TA 1535, TA 1537, TA 98 and TA 100 were used. The assays were performed in presence and absence of S9, using the direct method and preincubation method. Capsaicin did not induce mutagenic activity in any of bacterial strains.

4.3.7.2 Mouse lymphoma cell mutation assay

The tk+/tk-3.7.2C heterozygote of L5178Y mouse lymphoma cells were used in these studies (details of the methods used, see in paper of Chanda et al., 2004).

Both assays in presence of S9 mix gave weak mutagenic responses. Both assays contained at least two treatment groups of capsaicin that tested sinificant (for log mutant fraction) at the level of 5%. Both assays showed linear trend (of mutant fraction with concentration) that was significant at *P< 0.001*. The increases in the mutant fraction obtained were small, the largest was 190 mutants per million above the control value obtained at near the maximum acceptable level of toxicity (12% relative total growth).

In the absence of S9 mix, the 4 hour exposure assay gave a very weak mutagenic response, while the 24 hour assay gave no significant responses at dose levels resulting acceptable level of genotoxicity, throughout the test linear trend was significant (*P=0.022*).

Colony size distribution patterns were difficult to assess due to the very small sample sizes. The same situation occurs for vehicle control groups, which show a high level of variation between the experiments, and within experiments. The numbers of mutant colonies assessed in the capsaicin treatments resulting significant increases were found very low.

4.3.7.3. *Mouse in vivo micronucleus assay*

For details of this methodology, see the paper of Chanda et al. (2004). At least 2000 polychromatic erythrocytes were scored for frequency of micronucleated cells. The numbers of mironucleated normochromic erythrocytes (NCE), which were observed within the same microscope fields, were similarly recorded. The PCE/NCE ratio was assessed by scoring a total of at least 500 PCE+NCE. All assessment was performed on coded slides.

In preliminary toxicity tests the maximum tolerated dose of capsaicin was determined to be around 800 mg/kg per day in males and around 200 mg/kg per day in females. Three groups of male mice were dosed with 200, 400 and 800 mg/kg per day and one group of females was dosed with 200 mg/kg per day of capsaicin at 0 and 24 hours. Five mice per sex from each test material dose groups were selected to provide the normal assessment base. Current vehicle and positive groups were included.

Treatment-related animal deaths and clinical signs were observed in the middle and high dose level groups. One death occurred in the male vehicle control group, immediately after dosing and was considered to be as a result of a dosing error.

The frequencies of micronucleated polychromatic erythrocytes (MN-PCE) in the capsaicin-treated groups were 0.04, 0.10, 0.09 % (males) and 0.05% (females). All of these frequencies were within the historical control range for negative responses (0.01-0.23 % for a group of five mice). The frequencies of MN-PCE in the concurrent vehicle control groups were 0.07% (males) and 0.11% (females), whereas the MN-PCE frequency in the positive control group was 1.57%, demonstrating the sensitivity of the test system.

4.3.7.4. *Chromosomal aberration in human peripheral blood lymphocytes (HPBL)*

Human venous blood from healthy, adult donors (nonsmokers without any history of radiotherapy, chemotherapy or drug usage and lacking current viral infections) was used. The whole blood cultures were initiated in 15 ml centrifuge tubes by adding 0.6 mL of fresh heparinized blood and the final volume of culture medium and test arcticle was 10 mL.

Cultures were incubated with loose caps at 37±2 ºC in a humidified atmosphere of 5± 1.5 ºC in air. The medium was RPMI 1640 supplemented with HEPES buffer (25 mM), about 20% heat-activated fetal bovine serum (FBS), penicillin (100 U/mL), streptomycin 100 μg/mL, L-glutamine (2 mM) and 2% phytohemagglutinin-M (PGA-M). Negative (untreated controls) and vehicle controls (cultures treated with 10 μL of DMS0/mL) were used. The positive control agents used in the assays were mitomycin-C (MMMC) for the nonactivation series and CP (cyclophosphamide) in the metabolic activation series.

The *in vitro* metabolic activation system (Maron and Ames, 1983) consisted of liver post-mitochondrial fraction (S9) and an energy-producing system (NADP at 1.5 mg/mL (1.8 mM) and isocitric acid at 2.7 mg/mL (10.5 mM). S9 was prepared 5 days after a single dose of 500 mg/kg of Aroclor® 1254.

Two trials were conducted. In the initial trial, cultures were treated for about 3 hours with and without S9 and harvested about 22 hours after initiation of treatment. In the second trial, cultures were treated for about 22 hours without S9 and about 3 hours with S9 and harvested about 22 hours after initiation of treatment. This harvested time corresponds to 1.5 times a cell cycle time (Galloway et al., 2004). The time of cell cycle is approximatively 15 h after the lymphocytes was included to divide by the addition of PHA-M. At harvest, cells were swollen by 75 mM KCl hypotonic solution and fixed with absolute methanol-glacial acetic acid (3:1 v/v). Cells were selected from each duplicate culture were analyzed for the different types of chromosomal aberrations (Evans, 1962; Evans, 1976). Mitotic index was evaluated from the negative control, vehicle control and a range of test article concentrations and this was used for measurement of toxicity and selection of doses for analysis. Percent of polyploidy and endoreduplication were also analyzed. For control of bias, all slides were coded prior to analysis and read blind.

In the first trial, 6.78, 9.69, 13.8, 19.8, 28. 2, 40.4, 57.6, 82.4, 118, 168, 240, 343, 490, 700 and 1000 μg/mL of capsaicin were evaluated with and without metabolic activation by S9. The highest concentration was limited due to the presence of a precipitate dosing. In the first trial, a precipitate was observed at > 240 μg/mL, and hemolysis was observed prior to washing and harvesting of these cultures. Only dead cells were present on slides prepared from cultures treated with > 343 μg/mL due to excessive toxicity (Chanda et al., 2004). Chromosomal aberrations were analyzed from the cultures treated with 82.4, 118, 168 and 240 μg/mL. The high concentration had > 50% reduction in mitotic index. No increase in structural or numerical chromosomal aberrations was observed (Chanda et al., 2004).

Based on the results from the initial assay, the second trial was conducted at concentrations of 6.15, 12.3, 24.6, 49.2, 98.4, 154, 192, 240 and 320 μg/mL without metabolic activation and 49.2, 98.4, 123, 154, 192, 240 and 320 μg/mL with metabolic activation. Treatment periods were for about 22 and about 3 h without and with metabolic activation, respectively, and the cultures were harvested at 22 h from the initiation of treatment. In the assay without metabolic activation, a precipitate was observed in cultures treated with > 92 μg/mL and hemolysis was found prior to harvest of the cultures treated with > 240 g/mL. Only dead cells were present on slides prepared from cultures treated with > 192 μg/mL, due to excessive toxicity. Severe toxicity was observed also in case of 98.4 μg/mL dose (92% reduction in mitotic index). Chromosomal aberrations were analyzed from the cultures treated with 24.6, 49.2 and 123 μg/mL. Due to toxicity, < 100 metaphases were available for analysis in the duplicate cultures treated with 123 μg/mL dose. The highest tested concentration (240 μg/mL) had > 50% reduction on mitotix index. No increase in structural or numerical chromosomal aberrations was observed.

In the assay with metabolic activation, a precipitate was observed after dosing at > 192 μg/mL and hemolysis was observed prior to harvest of the cultures treated with 320 μg/mL. Since the cultures treated with 240 μg/mL had excessive toxicity (100% reduction in mitotic index) and the slides prepared from cultures treated with 192 μg/mL were selected as the highest concentration for analysis. Chromosomal aberrations were analyzed from the cultures treated with 98.4, 123, 154 and 192 μg/mL. No increase in structural or numerical chromosomal aberrations was observed (Chanda et al., 2004).

Although there are a number of publications focussing on genotoxic potential of capsaicin or spicy pepper extracts, the test substances used in these studies were various according to source,purity and impurity profile. Consequently, there has not been any systemic observation of the genotoxic potential of *trans*-capsaicin.

The majority of the studies found in the literature (Marques et al., 2002; Richeux et al., 1999; Ames et al., 1975; Fischer, 1972) used the Ames assay. There was one study using either micronucleus assay, the sister chromatoid exchange assay or the assay investigating DNA strand breaks in human neuroblastoma cells (Surh and Lee, 1995; Azizan and Blevins,1995; Nagabhushan and Bhide, 1985; Marques et al., 2002; Ames et al., 1999). None of the studies were conducted using systematically pure capsaicin preparations, and it is very important to be able to attribute the results of capsaicin alone, not the impurities.Chanda et al. (2004) applied synthetic capsaicin alone (the purity > 99%) to perform to genotoxicity studies.

In the Ames assay with pure synthetic capsaicin, no increase in mutation frequency was observed in any assays, with and without S9. It was concluded from these studies that the capsaicin is not genotoxic in the bacterial assay, with and without metabolic activation (at the highest concentrations that could be tested).

Capsaicin was found to be weakly mutagenic in mouse lymphoma L5178Y cells, in presence of S9, when it was dissolved in DMSO at concentrations that extended into the toxic range. The lowest positive concentration in the presence of S9 in any individual test was 12 μg/mL. Limited evidence of very weak activity was also noted in the absence of S9.The lowest positive concentration in absence of S9 was 65 μg/mL. Although criteria for the determinations a positive response in the lymphoma assay remained controversial according to the criteria used by the laboratory that conducted in these studies (Clive et al., 1979; Moore et al., 2003). These results can be interpreted as week toxicity. With longer exposures (about 24 hours), higher capsaicin concentrations were too toxic for analysis and the mutant fractions were not significantly different from the controls at the usable concentrations.Thus, it can be concluded that capsaicin is non-mutagenic at concentrations up 28 μg/mL after 24 h exposure in the absence of S9.

In the *in vivo* micronucleus study in mice, the frequency of MN-PCEs was 0.04-0.10 % in the treated group compared to 0.07-0.11% in the vehicle treated control mice. Both were within the historical control range, which was started to be 0.07 ± 0.08%. The frequency of MN-PCE for the positive control (50 mg/kg of cyclophosphamide) was 1.5%. However, in this study a difference was observed between the maximum tolerated doses estimated for males (800 mg/kg) and females (200 mg/kg). These values are higher than previous reports in the literature (Glinsukon et al., 198O; Saito and Yamamoto, 1996), which probably may reflect the quality of the current drug substance, and do not reflect to sex difference.

Capsaicin was evaluated for its ability to induce clastogenicity in cultured human lymphocytes with and without an exogenous metabolic activation system. Clastogenecity was evaluated at concentrations that induced severe toxicity to no toxicity. Cultures were harvested within 22 hours from the initiation of treatment. Capsaicin did not induce structural and numerical chromosomal aberrations.

It can be concuded from the rsults of genotocity observations with pure *trans*-capsaicin that its genotocity potential is very limited and differs when the impured capsaicin or chilli extracts were used in assays.

These data have important implications for analysis of risks associated with dietary or environmental capsaicin exposures. Although the majority of epidemiological data suggests that dietary capsaicin consumption is not associated with enhanced risk of cancer (Surh and Lee, 1995). It is true that a positive matematical correlation can be observed between the intake of Chilli pepper and the gastric cancer in Mexico (Lopez-Carrilo et al., 2003), other factors than capsaicin should be investigated as the causal link in such epidemiological evaluation (Table 9).

Test compound	Animal/Cells tested	Hepatic S9 for metabolic activation	Endpoint	Response
CAP, Chilli	S. typhimurium	Aroclor 1254-induced rat	His+ reversion	+
CAP, Chilli	Chinese hamster V79	Aroclor 1254-induced rat	Azaguanine resistance	-
CAP, Chilli	Swiss mice	In vivo	Micronuclei formation	+ CAP(only)
CAP	S. typhimurium TA98	Aroclor 1254-induced rat	His+ reversion	+
CAP, DHC,	typhimurium TA98,	Aroclor 1254-induced rat	His+ reversion	-
ChilliS	TA1535			
CAP, DHC, Chilli	Chinese hamster V79		Azaguanine resistence	+
CAP, Chilli	S. typhimurium	Phenobarbital-induced rat	His+ reversion	-
CAP, Chilli	S. typhimurium		Streptomycin-resistance	+ (Chilli); -(CAP)
CAP, DHC,	S. typhimurium TA98,	+ (source unclear)	His+ reversion	- or + (CAP)
Chilli	TA100			
Chilli	Mouse bone marrow	In vivo	Micronuclei formation	+
CAP	Albino mice	In vivo	Pregnancy frequency	-
CAP	Mouse epididymis	In vivo	Sperm abnormality	-
CAP	Human lymphocytes		Chromosome aberrations	+

CAP, capsaicin; DHC, dihydrocapsaicin; Chilli, planet extract (after Surh J., Lee S.S. Life Science 56: 1845-1855, 1995) (with modification)

Table 9. Genotoxicity of chilli extracts and its major pungent constituents capsaicin and dihydrocapsaicin up to 1995

4.3.8. Chronic toxicity studies in animals

The chronic toxicological studies are absolutely required to drug candidate in species (one from the rodents and dog) for 6 months time period. None of these types of observations could be found in the literature, consequently these studies should be done in the fourthcoming time with our preparation.

4.3.9. Brief summary of the main results of observations with capsaicin in animals

Capsaicin is a very active compound acting at the levels of capsaicin sensitive afferent nerves. Capsaicin has dual action, namely given in small doses it produces a biological significant gastrointestinal mucosal protective effect, meanwhile it enhances the gastrointestinal mucosal damages to different chemical, osmotic and pressure stimuli.

It is important to note that the doses (10 to 100 μg/kg) produce gastrointestinal mucosal defensive actions are significantly lower than those (100-200 mg/kg) induce gastrointestinal mucosal damage.

The capsaicin is absorbed well from gastrointestinal tract in animals, and its metabolization is carried out by the liver (in pathways of enzymatic oxidation and non enzymatic oxidation). The production of epoxyns (arene) is suggested; however, it was not clearly proven.

There is specific and important observation that the capsaicin dose-dependently prevents the CCl_4-induced hepatic injury during one week treatment.

The genotoxicity studies indicated a very limited positivity, which dominantly depends on the extents of capsaicin purity from plants.

No chronic toxicological studies have been published in two species (rodent, dog) and applied for 6 months.

4.4. Human observations with capsaicin

4.4.1. Observations with capsaicin in healthy human subjects

The capsaicin studies were carried out from 1997, by the permission of Regional Ethical Committee of Pécs University, Hungary. These studies were carried out in randomized, prospective manner, respecting the Helsinki Declaration. The observations were carried out according to the Good Clinical Practice (GCP), at the same methods as those are required to classical drug (or drug candidate) studies.

The First Department of Medicine, Medical and Health Centre, University of Pécs, Hungary, is one of the Hungarian Accreditated Centres for the studies of the human phase I-II. examinations. This institute has been participating in the drug developments since 1968.

4.4.1.1. Dose-response curves of capsaicin in the human stomach acute observations

The dose-response curves were identified on the gastric basal acid secretion (BAO) in healthy human subjects, and on the measurements in gastric transmucosal potential difference (GTPD) without and with topically (intragastrically) applied ethanol (Mózsik et al., 2005). We tested 100, 200, 400 and 800 μg capsaicin dissolved in 100 saline solution given intragastrically via nasogastric tube on the gastric BAO values and on GTPD.

In other series of observations, the gastric microbleeding was produced by orally given indomethacin (3x25, plus 25 mg at the starting of examinations) in healthy human subjects. Indomethacin was given alone, or in combination of capsaicin (200, 400 and 800 μg). The results were compared with the results obtained without application of indomethacin (baseline).

The effect of capsaicin given in smaller dose than 100 μg, no effect was observed. The ED_{50} value was obtained in experiments using 400 μg dose on the gastric BAO, GTPD (without and with topically applied ethanol), and Indomethacin-induced gastric microbledings (Mózsik et al., 2005; Mózsik et al., 2007).

It was also observed that gastric microbleeding produced by both inhibition of COX-1 and COX-2 was completely prevented by the application of 400 μg capsaicin (Mózsik et al., 2007; Sarlos et al., 2003).

When capsaicin was given in dose of ED_{50} intragastrically, the "parietal component" decreased ($P < 0.001$), meanwhile the "non-parietal component" (buffering secretion) and gastric emptying increased significantly ($P < 0.001$) in human healthy subjects (Mózsik et al., 2004; 2005; 2007; Debreceni et al., 2001). Recently, it was observed that capsaicin (given in dose of 400 μg orally) enhanced the glucose absorption and glucagon release during standard glucose loading test in human healthy subjects (Dömötör et al., 2006).

4.4.1.2 Changes in laboratory parameters and complaints of human healthy subjects during the study with capsaicin

No systemic laboratory changes were noted in the biochemical parameters except the observations with gastric juice (Mózsik et al., 2004; 2005), glucose loading test (Dömötör et al., 2006). No subjective complains were observed in patients (pain, diarrhoea, vomit).

4.4.2. Subchronic observations with capsaicin in human healthy subjects

4.4.2.1. Two weeks treatment with capsaicin

The group of healthy human subjects received capsaicin treatment for two weeks (3 x 400 μg given orally) in prospective, randomized study. The gastric microbleeding was produced by indomethacin application before and after the two week capsaicin treatment. At baseline indomethacin-induced gastric microbleedings applied without and with different doses of capsaicin were measured before and after two-week capsaicin treatment.

No changes were obtained at baseline, indomethacin-induced gastric microbleding, and on the other hand, the gastric mucosal protective effects of capsaicin remained the same after the two-week capsaicin treatment as those were found at baseline (Mózsik et al., 2005; Mózsik et al., 2007a).

4.4.2.2. Biochemical meaurements and complaints in human healthy subjects during two weeks capsaicin treatment

No changes were noted in the biochemical parameters and no complaints registered in the human healthy subjects.

4.4.3. Human chronic observations with capsaicinoids

In a case-control study in Mexico City included 220 cases of gastric cancer and 752 controls randomly selected from the general population. Chilli pepper consumers were found to be having a 5.5 fold greater risk for gastric cancer than non-consumers. Persons who stated themselves as heavy consumers of chilli peppers were at a 17 fold greater risk. However, when chilli consumption was measured as frequency per day, a significant dose-response relationship was not observed (Lopez-Carrillo et al., 1994).

In another case-control study in India, red chilli powder was found to be a risk factor for cancer of the oral cavity, pharynx, esophageus and laryngx compared with population controls, but not with hospital controls (Notani and Jayant, 1987).

In an Italian case-control study, chilli was briefly mentioned as being protective against stomach cancer (Buiiatti et al., 1989). Chilli pepper, however, are not heavily consumed in Northern Italy, where this study was conducted, and it is possible that chilli consumption rather correlated with other used protecting spices such as onions and garlic, which are heavily consumed in Italy.

The Committee of Experts on Flavouring Substances of the Council of Europe concluded that the available data do not allow to establish a safe exposure level of capsaicinoids for foods (Opinion of the Scientific Committee on Food on Capsaicin, adopted on 26 February, 2002).

It was also observed that the non-selective COX-1 and COX-2 inhibiting nonsteroidal anti-inflammatory drug-induced gastric microbleeding can completely be prevented by 400 μg capsaicin administrations in human healthy subjects (Mózsik et al., 2007).

4.4.4. Preventive effects of capsaicin against the selective and nonselective inhibitory actions produced by nonsteroidal anti-inflammatory drugs on COX-1 and COX-2 enzymes

The indomethacin (as non selective COX inhibitor) was used to provoke gastric microbleeding in healthy human subjects, and capsaicin itself, as a specific stimulator of capsaicin receptor (TRVP1) was applied in small doses to healthy human subjects. The capsaicin treatment was carried out for two weeks, it was given in 3 x 400μg dose orally daily (400 μg capsaicin dose was obtained to be equal to ED_{50} value in previous human observations) (Mózsik et al., 1999; 2004; 2005) (Table 10-11).

NSAID	Ratio COX-1 : COX-2
Aspirin	0.12
Diclofenac	38.00
Etodolac	179.00
Ibuprofen	0.86
Indomethacin	0.30
Loxoprofen-SRS	3.20
NS-398	1263.00
Oxaprozin	0.061
Zaltoprofen	3.80

*After Kawai, S. et al. Eur. J. Pharmacol 347: 87-94 (1998)

Table 10. Comparison of inhibitory effects (IC_{50}) by giving the COX-1 and the various NSAIDs using human platelet COX-1 and synovial cell COX-2*

- **IC_{50} VALUE OF INDOMETHACIN TO RATIO OF COX-1/COX-2 = 0,30 (1: 3.25)**
- **MICROBLEEDING IN THE STOMACH**

← 2 weeks capsaicin treatment →

	Before	After
Baseline	**2,1 ± 0,1 mL/day**	**2,0 ± 0,1 mL/day**
After IND	**8,25 ± 0,25 mL/day**	**7,8 ± 0,3 mL/day**
Δ IND-induced	**6,15 ± 0,2 mL/day**	**5,8 ± 0,3 mL/day**

(= inhibition on COX-1 + COX-2) (= 100%)

COX-1:	**1.447±0.1 mL/day**	**1.364±0.1 mL/day**
COX-2:	**4.70±0.2 mL/day**	**4.44±0.2 mL/day**

- **400 µg CAPSAICIN (IG GIVEN) INDUCED DECREASE OF IND-GASTRIC MICROBLEEDING**

6±0.2 mL/day	**5.9±0.2 mL/day**

* means±SEM in 14 human healthy subjects.

Table 11. Correlation between the capsaicin actions, COX-1 and COX-2 systems and gastric microbleedings produced by indomethacin in human healthy subjects before and after 2 weeks capsaicin (3x400µg orally) treatment.*

4.5. Summary of the observation with capsaicin alone or in combination with selectively and non-selectively inhibition of COX-1 and COX-2 enzymes by nonsteroidal anti-inflammatory compounds in animal experiments and in human observations

The capsaicin chemically representing a mixture of compounds of capsaicinoid (capsaicin, dihydrocapsaicin, norcapsacin, nordihydrocapsaicin) has been widely used in the population nutrition of different countries for the last 9000-9500 years.

It was a significant internationally accepted discovery that capsaicin (capsaicinoids) significantly stimulates (stimulate) a subgroup of the afferent nerves (named under as "capsaicin-sensitive afferent nerves") responding upon various chemical agents, heat, pH gradients in animal experiments and human observations.

The doses of capsaicin (capsaicinoids) are significant in the biological actions, because when it (those) is (are) given in small doses then it (those) prevents (prevent) tissue protection (including the gastrointestinal tract), however, capsaicin (capsaicinoids) enhances (enhance) the organ's damage (including the gastrointestinal tract). The capsaicin (capsaicinoids) produces (produce) organ damaging effects as a consequence of capsacin-induced desensitation proceeded by the application of capsaicin (capsaicinoids) in higher doses. The existence of these principle observations was scientifically proven in animal experiments and human observation.

The application of capsaicin has been carried out as a tool to approach the different physiological and pharmacological regulation of different diseases and their prevention.

The study of the afferent nerves has been carried out from the years of 1970. The results of this research clearly proved the principle and important role of the afferent nerves in the physiological regulation of various organs and as well as in the development of damage and prevention of these different organs.

The human observations with capsaicin were carried out randomized, prospective studies by the permission of Regional Ethical Committee of our Univesity of Pecs, Hungary. These studies were carried out in accordance of the Good Clinical Practice (GCP) together with respect of the Helsinki Declaration.

The results of the animal experiments and human observations clearly proved the gastrointestinal protection by application of small doses of capsaicin (capsaicinoids) (including the application of nonsteroidal anti-inflammatory drugs).

The anti-inflammatory drugs (acting by the properties of drugs of selective and non-selective inhibitions of COX-1 and COX-2 enzymes) are widely used in the prevention of thromboembolic episodes, in the prevention of reinfarction in patients who underwent myocardial infaction, in the treatment of patients with acute and chronic pains with degerative chronic joint diseases, malignant diseases and healthy persons for preventing gastrointestinal cancers, etc.

Capsaicinoids absorbs well from the gastrointestinal tract. They are metabolized in the pathways of enzymatic oxidation of liver and as well as non enzymatic oxidation. It is very important that capsaicin alone dose-dependently prevents the hepatic damage produced by carbon tetrachloride (in a significantly higher level that it was found for silymarin). The studies with genotoxicity clearly indicated that the pure capsaicin has a very limited toxicity (this value is higher if the capsaicin preparation is not chemically clear and contaminated with different toxicological agents of plants, e.g. aflatoxin, pesticides).

The human observations also clearly indicated that capsaicin actions can be reproduced well in human healthy subjects. The capsaicin application produces an dose-dependent increase in GTPD (without and with combined ethanol), decreases BAO, and totally prevents the indomethacin-induced gastric mucosal microbleedings (in range of 100 to 800 μg given intragastrically). Furthermore two weeks treatment with capsaicin (3x 400 μg given intragastrically) did not modify the sensitivity of the gastric mucosa to capsaicin-sensitive afferent nerves and the gastric mucosal protective effects against indomethacin remained at the same dose-dependent level after 2-week capsaicin treatment.

The conclusions of these animal and human observations clearly proved that the application of capsaicin in small doses is completely able to prevent the nonsteroidal anti-inflammatory drug-induced gastrointestinal side effects. By the other ways capsaicin is able to inhibit the functions of COX-1 and COX-2 enzymes in animal experiments and in human observations.

The further scientific research may offer an absolutely new pathway(s) for the development of drug (s) by the stimulation of capsaicin-sensitive afferent nerves by the usage of small doses of capsaicinoids to patients, who have to be treated with nonsteroidal anti-inflammatory drugs and for other diseases requiring cyclooxygenase inhibition (inflammations, tumors).

4.6. Summary of expters' opinion

The plant origin capsaicinoids (capsaicin, dihydrocapsaicin, norcapsaicin, dihydrocapsaicin, homocapsaicin, homodihydrocapsaicin) are well known and used as nutritional additive agents in the every day nutronal practice from the last 7000 years, however, we have a very little scientifically based knowledge of their chemistry, physiology, pharmacology in animal observations, and in humans up till the end of 20th century. Our knowledge from their chemistry, physiology and pharmacology entered to be scientifically based evidence from the years of 1980s, dominantly upon animal observations. The human observations with capsaicin (capsaicinoids), in terms of good clinical practice, have been started only in the last ten years in randomized, prospective, multiclinical studies. The name of "capsaicin" used only in the physiological and pharmacological research both in animal experiments and in human observations. The "capsaicin" (as a"chemically" used natural compound) modifies the "so-called" capsaicin-sensitive afferent nerves, depending on their doses of application.

Aims: The specific action of capsaicin (capsaicinoids) on sensory afferent nerves modifying gastrointestinal (GI) function offers a possibility for the production of an orally applicable drug or drug combinations, which can to be used for human medical therapy. The production of a new drug needs to be based on the critical interdisciplinary review of the results obtained with capsaicinoids.

Materials and methods: This paper gives an interdisciplinary and critical overview on the chemical, physiological, pharmacological and toxicological actions of the natural origin capsaicinoids (from the point of drug production) under conditions of acute, subacute and chronic administration in animal experiments and human observations for toxicology and pharmacokinetics.

This interdisciplinary review covers the following main chapters: 1. Physiological and pharmacological research tool by capsaicin in the animals and human beings; 2. capsaicin research in animals (including the acute, subacute and chronic toxicology, metabolism as well as genotoxicology); 3. Pharmacological observation with capsaicin in human beings.

Conclusion: 1. The capsaicin used in the physiological and pharmacological observations (in animals and human beings) chemically represents heterogenous chemical compounds, which can be obtained from the plants (paprika, chilli, etc). 2. Capsaicinoids are able to modify the capsaicin-sensitive afferent nerves, which play principle roles in the defence of various organs (including the gastrointestinal tract (against heat, stress, chemical-induced damage). 3. The beneficial effects of capsaicin (capsaicinoids) application on gastrointestinal tract obtained in animal experiments can be converted for humans observations. After this interdisciplinary and critical review, this paper demonstrates well-planned research pathways of discoveries on capsaicinoid chemistry, physiology, pharmacology and toxicology in animal experiments and human observations.

5. Some general scientific problems in the application of the plant origin compounds in the every used foods and drugs

The evaluation of effectiveness and safety of chemically produced compound(s) is very strickly regulated testing program both in animals and in humans.

After very careful and critical overview of plant origin compounds, it was very surprising to see that health and scientific requirements differ so much in regards of their application as dietary (Response to EMEA Consultation Document CPMP/QWP/2819/00 REV 1 AKA EMEA/CVMP/814/00 REV 1: Guideline on Quality of Herbal Medicinal Products/Traditional Herbal Medicinal Products (Released 21 July 2001/Consultation Date 30th September 2005) and as a drug terapy (this Notice to Applicants (NTA) prepared by the European Commission in consultation with the competent authorities of the Member States, the European Medicines Agency and interested parties in order to fulfil the Commission's obligations with respect to article 6 of Regulation (EC) No. 726/2004, and with respect to the Annex I to Directive 2001/83/EC as amended (Directive 2003/63/EC, OJ L 159 27.6.2003 p.46 NTA, Vol. 2B-CTD, foreword & introduction, edition June 2006).

We, the authors of this review could not understand the extremely high number of application of plant origin compounds needed to be applied for foods, food additive agents, health modification compounds and classical drugs (especially orally applicable preparations).

A lot of chemical compounds are used during the culturation of different plants, which are be used as sources of various compounds of food or drug preparations. Furthermore, during the preparation of the cultivated plant are treated with different chemicals to result aimed chemical compounds (we can use only "Drugs Master File", surprisingly up to now no "Food Master File"). These aspects are remained out off the scientific area up till present time.

The medical sciences emphasize the prevention of different diseases. Our main question is why these aspects remained out of the scope of science?

In case of capsaicin, we have the following main problems:

1. The research of physiology and pharmacology only "capsaicin" is mentioned all the time, while the capsaicin as a plant source compound chemically does not represent one chemical entity;
2. The content of capsaicin (Sigma-Aldrich, USA) is also not standard, because its content of capsaicin, dihydrocapsaicin, nordihydrocapsaicin and other capsaicinoids can vary;
3. No correct Drug Master File (DMF) for capsaicin (capsaicinoids) has been prepared;
4. No classical animal toxicological (including the germinative function) examinations have been carried out for capsaicin (capsaicinoids);
5. No classical preclinical dossier exists for capsaicin;
6. No classical human clinical pharmacological study (human phase I-II) exists in the international literature.

Our research team works in capsaicin research from 1980 using mostly animal experiments, but starting form 1997 we are studiing capsaicin physiology in human investigations (under permission of the the Regional Ethical Committee of Pécs University, Hungary).

We actively participated in innovative research of capsaicin (capsaicinoids) to produce a new drug or new drug combinations affecting capsaicin sensitive afferent nerve function offering an absolutely new gate for gastrointestinal pharmacology (Mózsik et al., 2009a,b; 2010)

6. Chemical composition of capsaicinoids originated from plants and their botanical backgrounds

In physiological and pharmacological research capsaicin is generally used as "one chemical compound". Capsaicin (capsaicinoids) is (are) active chemical substance(s) extracted from paprika, chilli, chillies, which is (are) able to modify the capsaicin-sensitive afferent nerves. This (these) compound(s) stimulates (stimulate) in smaller doses and inhibits (inhibit) in higher doses of capsaicin-sensitive afferent nerves.

Szolcsányi and Barthó demonstrated first that capsaicin given in doses of 5-50 μg/mL inhibits the development of gastrointestinal mucosal damage (Szolcsányi and Barthó, 1981). Similar

http://dx.doi.org/10.5772/58359

results were obtained in systematic research on gastrointestinal tract in animals (Mózsik et al., 1997) and human healthy subjects treated with indomethacin (Mózsik et al. 2005; Mózsik et al., 2009a,b).

The action of capsaicin expresses itself as an initial short-lasting stimulation that can be followed by desensitation to capsaicin itself and to other stimuli of afferent sensory neurons. Capsaicin applied in ng to μg/ kg doses to the peripheral or central endings or cell bodies of sensory neurons induces transient excitation. In response to stimulation peptide mediators are released from the central and peripheral nerve endings (Szolcsányi, 1984; Maggi, 1995). These four response stages could be separated: 1. excitation, 2. sensory-blocking, 3. long-term selective neurotoxic impairment and 4. irreversible cell destruction. From the point of gastro-intestinal mucosal protection only the small doses of capsaicin have clinical relevancy (these doses 200-1200 μg/person) (Mózsik et al., 2005; Mózsik et al., 1997; Mózsik et al., 2009a,b; 2010, Szabó et al., 2013).

Seven capsaicinoids and their chemical structures have been identified from different *Capsicum* species: *C. annuum; C. frutescens; C. chinese; C. baccatum; C. pubescens*) (Table 9) (Basu and De, 2003; Anu and Peter, 2000; Jurenitsch et al., 1979): *capsaicin, dihydrocapsicin, nordihydrocapsaicin, homodihydrocapsicin; homocapsaicin; nonanoic acid vanillylamide and decanoid acid vanillylamide* (Basu and De, 2003, Anu and Peter, 2000; Jurenitsch et al., 1979). The first five compounds represent capsaicin homologues, meanwhile the last two represent capsaicin analogues (Fig. 16).

The fine chemical trading firms (including Sigma Aldrich and others) obtain the capsaicin from plants (*Capsicum*). According to the chemotaxonomic key, the different species of *Capsicums* contain different amounts of capsaicin homologues and analogues (Jurenitsch et al., 1979) (Table 13).

Species	Flower colour	Number flw/node	Seed colour	Calyx constriction
C. annuum	white	1	tan	absent
C. frutescens	greenish	2–5	tan	absent
C. chinese	white/greenish	2-5	tan	present
C. baccatum	white with yellow spot	1–2	tan	absent
C. pubescens	purple	1–2	black	absent

* For further informations, see Ref. Mózsik et al.(2009b)

Table 12. The morphological identification of the five major species*

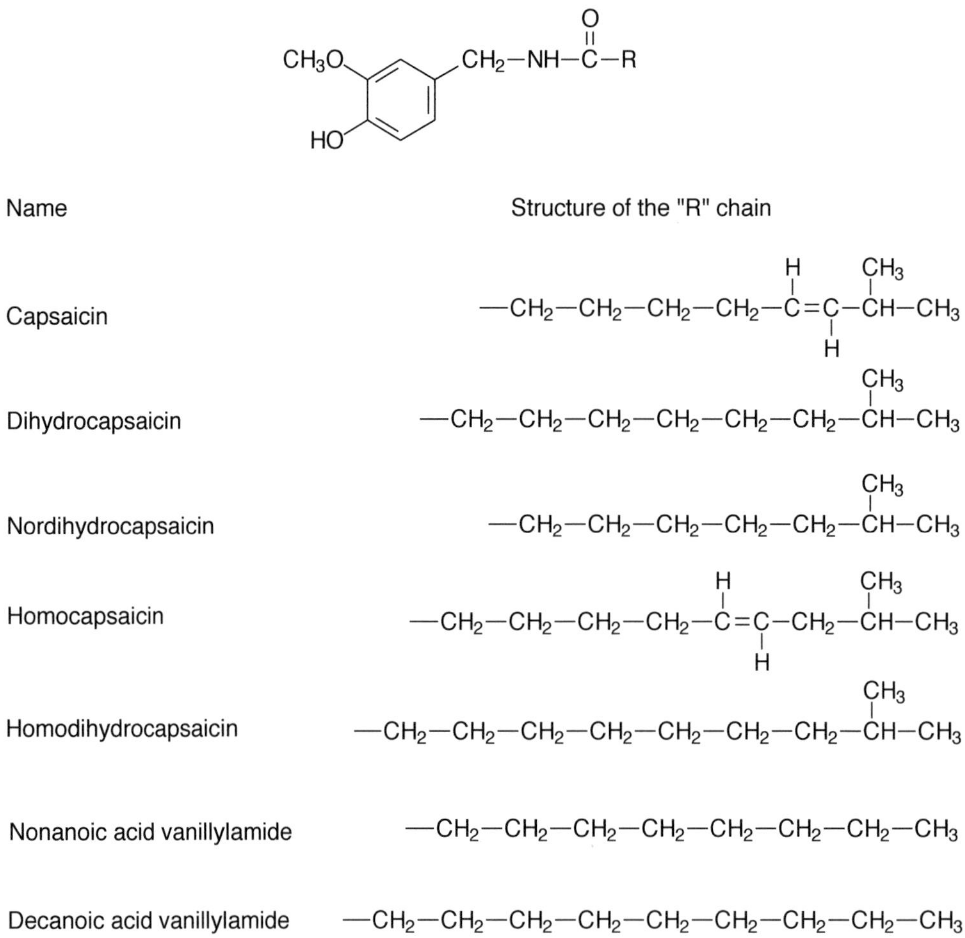

Figure 16. Structure of capsaicin and natural capsaicinoids (Mózsik et al, 2009b).

Accordingly, the commercially available natural capsaicin preparations are mixtures of capsaicin and natural capsaicinoids (Fig. 17).

The capsaicin preparation can be used as an active pharmaceutical ingredient (Capsaicin Natural) is described by the United States Pharmacopeia (USP). The 2006 edition of USP30-NF25 described its definition, identification, melting range and the content of capsaicin, dihydrocapsicin and other capsaicinoids. According to the USP requirements Capsaicin Natural should contain not less than 90 percent of total capsaicinoids. The content of capsaicin and dihydrocapsaicin should not be less than 75 percent, and the content of other capsaicinoids should not be more than 15 percent calculated on dried basis [USP30-NF25 Page 1609].

The principal requirements of the European Authorities for capsaicinoid content of natural capsaicin preparations usable in medical therapy are the same as those of USP30-NF25.

http://dx.doi.org/10.5772/58359

1.	NDHC fraction over 9.5 %		
	1.1	Cfraction over 56 %	*Capsicum baccatum var. pendulum*
	1.2	C fraction under 56%	*Capsicum annum var. annum*
2.	NDHC C Fraction 9,5 %		*Capsicum annum var. annum*
	2.1	C fraction, 42 to 57 %	
	2.2	C fraction under 42 %	*Capsicum baccatum var. pendulum*
	2.3	C fraction, 57 to 73 %	
		DHC fraction 26 to 34 %	
		Total capsaicinoids, under 0,35 %	*Capsicum baccatum var. pendulum*
	2.4	C fraction over 63%	
		DHC Fraction under32 %	
		Total capsaicinoids, over 0,35 %	*Capsicum fritescens – Capsicum chinense complex*

Abbreviations: C, capsaicin; NDHC, nordihydrocapsaicin; DHC, dihydrocapsaicin

* For further I nfromations, see Ref. Mózsik et al.(2009b).

Table 13. A chemotaxonomic key to the identification of cultivated *Capsicums**

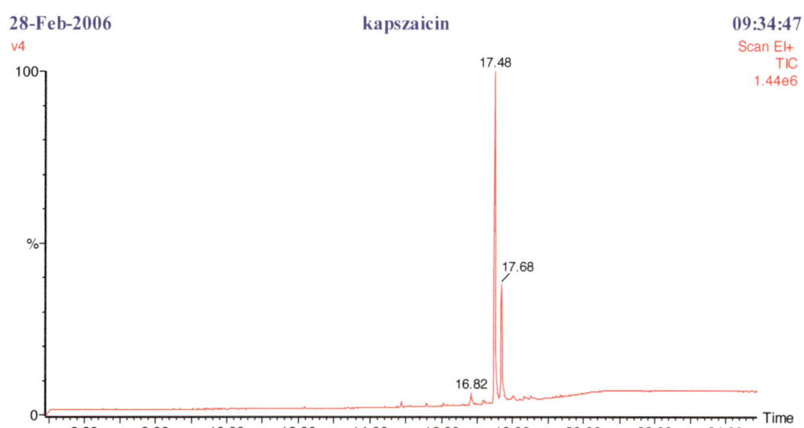

Figure 17. Gas-chromatographic (GC-MS) analysis of a commercially available natural capsaicin preparation. Retention times: 16.8 min: nordihydrocapsaicin, 17.5 min: capsaicin, 17.7 min: dihydrocapsaicin [36].

For pharmaceutical industry and human clinical pharmacology the presence of several components of natural capsaicin preparations represent special technological and clinical pharmacological difficulties. Namely, we have to quantify these components of capsicum extract in the pharmaceutical preparations as well as in the human biological blood samples, consequently we have to use specific and sensitive analytical methods.

7. Drug Master File (DMF)

To receive permission for human use of capsaicin preparations from the National and International Regulatory Authorities we have to present the following details: 1. specification of the *Capsicum* species; 2. climatic regulations of places of *Capsicum* cultivation; 3. chemical treatments of *Capsicum* plants during their cultivation; 4. details of treatment of *Capsicum* plants (their collections, drying, extractions storages, etc.), analytical results supporting the chemical composition of the plant origin capsaicinoids extract; 6. chemical stability of the natural capsaicin (capsaicinoids); 7. analytical results showing the (possible) contamination of the natural capsaicin product with organic phosphates, pesticides, fusariums, aflatoxin; 8. international certification (including Food and Drug Administration, FDA) on capsaicin (capsaicinoids) content of the natural preparation. Data of above mentioned facts need to be given by internationally accredited laboratories. These data are collected in the Drug Master File (DMF).

The leading chemical trading firms-concerning capsaicin supply-had no DMF for their capsaicin preparations. Independently, several trading firms keep the natural capsaicin (capsaicinoids) preparation on the market without the exact knowledge on the circumstances of cultivation, details of extraction and stability of the product. They have no exact information on the quantities of residues of organic phosphates, pesticides, fusariums, aflatoxin in their preparation of capsaicin (proved by certifications of various internationally accredited laboratories).

According to the observations of Foodnews Enviromental Working Group (food-news.org;http://www.drgreene.org/body.cfm?xyzpdqabc=21&action=detail& ref=1920), the most sweet peppers are contaminated with more than one pesticide. Pesticides were not detected only in 32 % of the samples, and 7 pesticides were observed in 1 % of tested samples. The samples of Sweet Bell Peppers contain *acephate, dicophol, dimethoate, diphenylamine, fenvalerate, metalaxyl, methamidophos, methomyl, fermethrin; malathion, endosulfanes, azinphos-methyl, o-phenylphenol,* which may produce animal carcinogens, birth defects, brain and nervous system damage as well as the damage of immune system and endocrine system (Report Card www.ewg.org).

In our case we found only one natural capsaicin preparation with Drug Master File (DMF) from India, which signed by the Food and Drug Administration, USA. Along with this preparation, we could not exact information from the manufacturer on above mentioned data to be incorporated into the DMF.

8. Preparation of human clinical pharmacological studies

We wanted to use capsaicinoid preparation as an orally applicable drug or part of a drug combination in human beings.

We compiled the below listed documentations for the National Institute of Pharmacy to apply permission for human clinical pharmacological studies with capsaicin preparation

1. experts' opinion; 2. results of all toxicological studies; 3. chemical stability of the natural capsaicin preparation; 4. results of pharmaceutical industrial formulation from the natural capsaicin; 5. various permissions from our University; 6. documentation of health insurance of volunteers; 7. preclinical dossiers; 8. documented valid permission on the accreditation of Clinical Pharmacological Unit for human phase I and II examinations (accreditation controlled by the National Institute of Pharmacy in Hungary); 9. exact protocols for human clinical pharmacological studies; 10. written information on the planned examinations for the volunteers; 11. request for authorization of a clinical trial on medical product for human use to the competent authorities and ethical committees in the community; 12. lists of investigators (together with their CV), data of involved institutes (departments participating in the study).

9. The National Instute of Pharmacy in Hungary requested additional exmainations with natural capsaicin (capsaicum natural usp 27) obtained from India on geno-and other toxicological examinations

The National Institute of Pharmacy in Hungary requested additional examinations with natural capsaicin (Capsaicin Natural USP 27) obtained form India on geno-and other toxicological studies due to having limited knowledge of circumstances of cultivation, collection, storage, stability and preparation. In the literature some data were available supporting genotoxic property of some natural capsaicin preparations by different researchers. Some positivities were indicated with natural capsaicin on its genotoxicity and the different researchers suggested that these mostly depend on various enviromental factors of natural capsaicin, since these tests were negative with synthetic capsaicin.

These requisted studies with the natural capsaicin obtained from India were 1. testing of natural capsaicin with bacterial reverse mutation assay; 2. testing of mutagenic effect of natural capsaicin by mouse micronucleus test; 3. 14-day oral average dose range finding study with natural capsaicin in rats (30–60 and 120 mg/ kg. b. w. orally for 14 days); 4. oral dose range finding toxicity study of natural capsaicin in Beagle dogs (0.3 – 0.6 – 0.9 mg /kg. b. w. /day orally for 14 days); 5. 28-day oral toxicity study of natural capsaicin in rats (placebo, 5, 15 and 30 mg/kg b. w orally for 28 days); 6. 28-day oral toxicity study of test item natural capsaicin in Beagle dogs (placebo, 0.1 – 0.3 – 0.9 mg/kg b. w/day orally for 28 days) (together with capsaicin kinetics).

Determination of LOD and LOQ (Reilly et al.,2002).: Limit of detection (LOD) was determined experimentally, and taken as the concentration producing a detector signal that could be clearly distinguished from the baseline noise (3 times baseline noise). The limit of quantification (LOQ) taken as the concentration that produced a detector signal ten times greater than the baseline noise. The LOD and LOQ values of capsaicin and dihydrocapsaicin in dog's plasma were found to be 2 ng/mL and 10 ng/mL, respectively.

The sensitivity of the present method exceeds that of the HPLC-MS methods previously reported for determination of the two main capsaicinoids in rat plasma and tissues (Reilly et al., 2002). Furthermore, the method is practical and less expensive than current methodology.

In our experience, after *per os* administration of Capsaicin natural (USP 29) in dogs neither capsaicin nor dihydrocapsaicin could be detected in the plasma samples. Our HPLC-FLD results were confirmed by investigation of the samples by HPLC-MS. Ex vivo animal investigation of pharmacokinetics of per os administered capsaicinoids are under way by means of the present method for better understanding of the gastrointestinal fate of capsaicinoids.

In the 2005-2008 time period our innovative drug research produced the following main subjects: 1. developed and validated methods for testing of drug active agents, and for testing of biological samples: 7 methods; 2. developed of a validated liquid chromatography-mass spectrometry (LC-MS) method for testing of drug(s) (and their metabolites) in biological samples; 3. developed other validated analytical protocols: 7 protocols; 4. validated genotoxicity examinations were carried out with natural capsaicin; 5. internationally validated 14-day oral gavage range finding studies were carried out with natural capsaicin in rats and dogs; 6 internationally validated complete 28-day oral toxicity studies were carried out with natural capsaicin in rats and Beagle dogs (Mózsik et al., 2008 a,b,c,d,e,f,g,h).

After compilation of the results of these observations we received permissions from the National Institute of Pharmacy in Hungary for human phase I. clinical pharmacological studies for natural capsaicin (Capsaicin Natural USP27) used alone and natural capsaicin plus NSAID combinations. Our industrial partner was PannonPharma Ltd., Pécsvárad Hungary, who did the pharmaceutical industrial research in the field.

10. Human phase I. single-blind study comparing the pharmacokinetic properties of asa and its platelet aggregation after single administration alone and co-administration with two different doses of capsaicin (400 and 800 μG) and evaluating their safety in healty male jubjects

(protocol number: 1.4.1; EudraCT number: 2008-007048-32)

10.1. Main aims of these studies

We planned to produce various drugs combinations, in which ASA, diclofenac, Naproxen (as NSAIDs) were combined with capsaicin(oids) in tablet [suggesting that the NSAIDs induced GI mucosa damage can be prevented by the capsaicin(oids)].

1. To plan the chemical compositions of these drug combinations for their pharmaceutical industrial productions (dosages, bioadhesive compounds of tablets) and to produce them. We wanted to start with a human clinical pharmacological phase I. examinations (respective all the national and international experts' requirements and necessary permissions form different (18) Authorities) (Mózsik et al., 2010).

2. We wanted to study whether the capsaicin(oids) (orally given in different doses, which only stimulate the capsaicin-sensitive afferent nerves) is(are) able to modify the absorption, metabolism, excretion of NSAIDs and their specific pharmacological actions (e.g. the platelet aggregation in case of ASA) in human healthy subjects.

This book chapter deals with the problems and results of ASA+capsaicin(oids) combination in healthy male subjects during "classical human pharmacological phase I. examinations".

Inclusion and exclusion of so-called healthy persons for the human phase I. examination (according the principals of clinical pharmacology) and characterizations of different somatic parameters of included healthy subjects into the phase I. study,

3. Schedule of the protocol for whole study (including the clinical phase, detections of capsaicin(oids), measurements of ASA – and salicylic acid (as one of the metabolites) of ASA and platelet aggregation produced by capsaicin(noids) (given in two doses) alone or in combination with ASA),
4. The registrate the tolerance and safety of these combinations in these clinical pharmacological studies,
5. Definitive results of measurements of plasma capsaicin and dihydrocapsaicin, and their evaluation,
6. Pharmacokinetic measurements of ASA, salicylic acid after application of ASA alone and in combinations with capsaicin(oids) (given orally in two doses),
7. Platelet aggregation studies with capsaicin(oids) alone and capsaicin(oids) in combination with ASA.

10.2. Clinical pharmacological aspects of the planned examinations: pharmaceutical preparation of tested preparations of tested drugs

1. ASA (acidum acetylsalicylicum 500, manufactured by PannonPharma Ltd, Pécsvárad, Hungary);
    - Active ingradient: acidum acetylsalicylicum,
    - Batch number: F005/2008-4,
    - Formulation: Tablet.
2. Capsaicin(oids) (capsaicin 400 μg manufactured by PannonPharma Ltd, Pécsvárad, Hungary);

Formulation: film-coated tablet,

Active ingradient: capsaicin (Capsaicin USP as manufactured in Andhra Pradesh, India, and Drug Master File was assigned by Drug and Food Aministration in USA: "17856 A II 26.10.2004 Asian Herbex Ltd" for as orally applicable drug substance in humans),

3. Placebos (indentical with capsaicin film-coated tablet and with acetylsalicylic acid tablet, manufactured by PannonPharma Ltd., Pécsvárad, Hungary).

The following doses of drugs were studied in this human phase I. examination:

- ASA : 500 mg,
- Capsaicin(oids) : 400 μg and 800 μg,
- ASA placebo,
- Capsaicin(oids) placebo.

"Human phase I. single-blind study comparing the pharmacokinetic properties of ASA after single administration alone and co-administration with two different doses of capsaicin (400 and 800 μg) and evaluating their safety in healthy male subjects"

Protocol number: 1.4.1

EudraCT number:2008-007048-32

The study for human clinical phase I. examination was permitted by

the Hungarian Institute of Pharmacy (Budapest, Hungary) (dated by June 4, 2009),

the National Ethics Commitee for Clinical Pharmacology, Medical Research Council (Budapest, Hungary) (dated by March 11, 2009).

The clinical pharmacological study was carried out at Clinical Pharmacological Unit of the First Department of Medicine, Medical and Health Centre, University of Pécs, Hungary.

The pharmacokinetic measurements were done at PannonPharma Pharmaceutical Ltd., Pécsvárad, Hungary.

The initiation date: March 10, 2011 and finished (including the clinical examinations, pharmacokinetic measurements, mathematical analysis, closing of written reports) by December 6, 2012.

[Selected references to the preparation of protocols:

1. Declaration of Helsinki (1964) as revised in Tokyo (1975), Venice (1983), Hong Kong (1989), Somerset West, RSA (1996) and Edinburg, Scotland (2000) with the Note of Clarification on Paragraph 29,Washington (2002),

2. ICH Topics E3. Structure and Content of Clinical Study Reports. Step 4, Consensus Guidelines from 30,11, 1995.Note for Guidance on Structure and Content of Clinical Study Reports (CPMP/ICH/137/95). July 1996.

3. ICH Topics E6. Guidelione for Good Clinical Practice. Step 5. Consolidated Guideline from 01.05.1996.Note for Guidance on Good Clinical Practice (CPMP/ICH/135/95). January 1997.

4. R.H.B. Meyboom, Y.A. Hekster, A.C.G. Egberts, F.W.J. Gribnau, R. Edwards: Causal or Causal? The Role of Causality Assessment in Pharmacovigilance – Drug Safety. 17.12.1997.

http://dx.doi.org/10.5772/58359

5. ICH Topic E2. A Clinical Safety data Management: Definitions and Standards for Expediting Reporting Step 5. 01.06.1995. Note for Guidance on Clinical Data Management: Definitions and Standards for Expecditing Reporting (CPMP/ICH/377/95),

6. ICH Topic E9. Statistical Principles for Clinical Trials Step 4. Consensus Guideline 05.02.1998. Note for Guidance on Statistical Principles for Clinical Trials (CPMP/ICH/363/96),

7. CPMP/PhVWP (III/3445/91): Causality classification in pharmacovigilance in the European Community.]

10.3. Requested permissions from the different authorities before the start of human phase I. examinations

We compiled the documentations for the National Institute of Pharmacy in Hungary to ask for human clinical pharmacological studies with this capsaicin preaparation (all the documents listed below were requested for receiving permissions):

1. Experts' opinion (Mózsik et al., 2007b; Mózsik et al.,2009b´),
2. Results of all toxicological studies,
3. Chemical stability of the natural capsaicin preparation,
4. Results of pharmaceutical industrial formulation from the natural capsaicin,
5. Different permissions from University (Regional Ethics of Committee),
6. Documentation of health insurance of volunteers,
7. Preclinical dossiers (protocols for the planned clinical pharmacological studies),
8. Documented valid permission on the accrediation of Clinical Pharmacological Unit for human phase I. and II. examinations – which accrediatation controlled by the National Institute of Pharmacy – was prepared for the National Institue of Pharmacy in Hungary,
9. Exacts protocols for the human clinical pharmacoligical studies,
10. Written information on the planned examinations, for the volunteers,
11. Request for authorization of a clinical trial on medical product use to the competent authoririties and for of opinion of the ethical committees in the community,
12. Lists of investigators (together with their CV), place institutes (departments) participating in the study and of course, the all written agreements and permissions.

10.4. Collection, screening of the healthy male volunteers Selection on volunteers:

- In this study fifteen healthy male subjects, age between 18-55, BMI 18-29.9 kg/m^2 were involved,

- A person is healthy if medical examination did not find any pathological signs and other screening test parameters stated in this protocol were within the normal range and the subject did not mention any significant disease when taking the case history,
- If, in the course of initial screening, some pathological values would be observed, these findings had to be regarded as an exclusion criterion. Having a laboratory parameter out of the normal range could generally not regarded as an exclusion criterion provided that:
- they were not accompanied by clinical symptoms,
- the context of related laboratory values gave no indication of pathological process and
- the Investigator regarded them as clinically irrelevant in a written form in the Case Report File (CRF) from the accepted protocoll.

Inclusion criteria:

The subject could be involved in the trial if the following criteria had been fulfilled:

- Voluntary participation after given information (Informed Consent signed and dated before the start of the screening period),
- Age between 18 and 55 years,
- Healthy male subjects,
- BMI: 18-29.9 $kg/m^{2,}$
- Negative physical status by physical examinations,
- Laboratory parameters within the normal range,
- Normal ECG findings – standard 12 leads.

Exclusion criteria:

- Unwillingness or incapacity to sign the written Informed Consent Form,
- Any clinically significant acute or chronic abnormalities during the physical examinations at screening,
- Clinically significant history or presence of any clinically significant gastrointestinal pathology (e.g. gastric or duodenal ulcer, gastro-oesophageal reflux, chronic diarrhoea, IBD), unresolved gastrointestinal symptoms (diarrhoea, vomiting),
- Clinically significant liver or kidney disease, or other condition which known to interfere with the absorption, metabolism and excretion of the study drug,
- Clinically significant cardiac and neurological disease in the medical history,
- Any clinically significant changes of laboratory tests from blood and/or urine,
- Donation of blood within 3 months prior to the study,

- Acute infection,
- Positive virological testing,
- Pathological findings on the standard 12 lead ECG,
- Hypertension (blood pressure higher than 140/90 mmHg (systolic/diastolic),
- Heart rate outside the range of 50-100 beats per minute,
- History of psychiatric diseases and treatment,
- Known hypersensitivity to any component of the study drugs,
- Use of any drugs known to induce or inhibit hepatic metabolism (inducers for example: barbiturates, carbamazepine, phenytoin, glucocorticoids omeprazole; examples for inhibitors: SSRIs, cimetidine, diltiazem, macrolides, imidazoles, neuroleptics, verapamil, flouroquinolones, and antihistamines) within 1 month prior to study drug administration,
- Use of any prescribed medication within 14 days or over-the-counter medication within 7 days prior to study drug administration,
- Any depo injection or medication implant within 3 months prior to administration of study medication,
- Any food allergy, intolerance, restriction or special diet i.e. vegetarian, which in the opinion of the investigator could contraindicate the subject to participate in the study,
- Participation in another clinical trial within 3 months prior to this study,
- Positive screen on drug abuse,
- Positive alcohol breath test (at time of hospitalisation),
- Known drug or chronic alcohol abuse, drug addiction,
- Malignant disease,
- Smoking more than 10 cigarettes/day (or comparable),
- Excessive caffeine drinking (more than 3 cups a day),
- Legal incapacity and/or other circumstances rendering the volunteer unable to understand the nature, scope and possible consequences of the study,
- Evidence of an uncooperative attitude,
- Vulnerable subject.

10.6. Clinical parameters of included healthy male volunteers (Table 14)

Age of subjects from 20 to 44 years (average is 34.5± 6.7 years),
Body heights form 170 to 196 cm) (average is 180.8± 6.9 cm),
Body weights from 69.5 to 101 kg) (average is 84.8± 9.6 kg),
Body Mass Index (BMI) from 20.77 to 29.68 kg/m^2 (average is 25.97 ± 2.87 kg/m^2).

Table 14. Clinical parameters of included healthy male subjects in our human phase I. studies. (Number of volunteers=15) (average ± SD):

10.7. Study design (Figure 18)

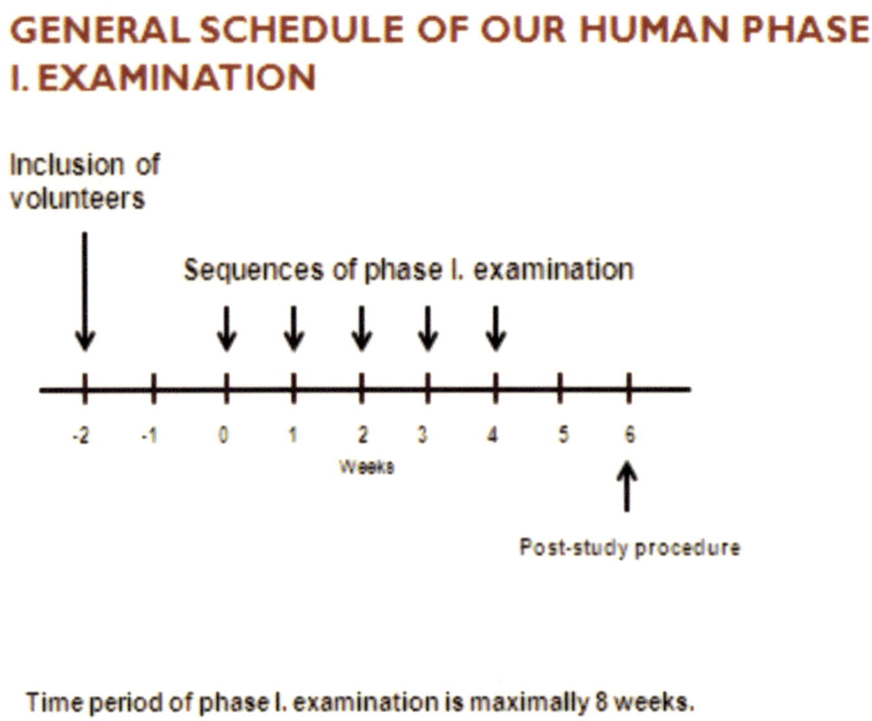

Figure 18. Study design of human phase I.examination of capsaicin alone or co-adminsiration with Aspirin (ASA)

10.8. Study procedures and treatment periodes – Study procedure in both treatment periods

Hospitalisation of subjects:

Subjects were required to attend the Unit on the evening preceding dose administration not later than 8:00 p.m. Subjects should fast for 10 hours (9:00 p.m. – 7:00 a.m.) prior to dosing. Only water may be drunk after the evening meal until 6:00 a.m. and then no fluids will be taken prior dosing. Subjects had to remain in upright position (i.e. sitting, standing) for 30 minutes after dosing. Meals were provided within the Unit. Subjects were allowed to leave the clinic after the last blood sampling post dose or after blood drawing for safety laboratory tests.

Daily activities during the trial:

Period 1:

Day 0: This day was the day before administration of the study medication and had to be not later than 2 weeks after screening. Subjects had to report to the clinic at 8 p.m. on the day before dosing. The subjects received an evening snack which had to be consumed until 9 p.m.,

- Short interview for possible presence of exclusion criteria,
- Physical examination, temperature, blood pressure, pulse rate ECG,
- Alcohol breath test,
- Urine drug test was performed.

Day 1-2: The following procedures were carried out or checked prior to the drug administration in all subjects:

- Insertion of the intravenous canule, if applicable,
- Blood sampling for pharmacokinetic analysis before dose (0:00 h),
- Study drug administration between 7 and 9 a.m. according to the randomization list. Compliance check had to be performed. Subjects took the medication with 150 ml water in upright position and remained upright for 30 minutes after dosing.
- Additional 150 ml water had to be drunken 2 hours after drug administration,
- Blood sampling (4 ml) for pharmacokinetic analysis up to 24:00 h after administration (pre-dose and 0:10, 0:20, 0:40, 1:00, 1:30, 2, 4, 6, 10, 12, 16, and 24 hours post dose) with separation of plasma,
- 12-lead ECG examination after the 4 hour blood sample, and before the meal,
- Standard meal 4 hours post dose,
- Questioning for and registration of adverse events.
- **Wash-out period**: A wash-out period of at least 3 days followed the all but one each treatment period; registration of adverse events.
- **Following study periods**: Procedures over 3 days (please see day 0 to 1 in period 1) identical with period 1. After the last study period completed final examinations were carried out.
- **Water intake**: During the period from two hours prior to dose administration until after the 4 hour blood sample was taken, each subject took 150 ml of water with the dose and 150 ml of water after the 2 hour blood sample. No other fluid was permitted during this time. Subjects were allowed to drink water ad libitum.

- **Diet**: Four hours after the drug treatment, subjects consumed a standard meal, well-balanced in carbohydrates, lipids and proteins and resume their normal rate of fluid intake.

Concomitant medication:

- Concomitant medication was generally not allowed for the duration of the study. If this was considered to be necessary for the volunteer's welfare it could be given at the discretion of the Investigator. The volunteers had to inform the Investigator about any intake of other medicine in the course of the trial. Any intake of concomitant medication had to be documented in the Case Report Form (CRF).
- Additional intake of acetylsalicylic acid was considered as exclusion criteria.

Post-study procedure:

- Within one week after the last blood sampling time point of the last treatment period follow-up examinations was performed:
- Physical examination (incl.: blood pressure, heart rate, body weight, temperature), ECG,
- Laboratory test: haematology, blood chemistry and urine (after 10 hours fasting condition),
- Clinically relevant deviations of laboratory parameters (with the exception of those measured during the screening period) were regarded as adverse events.

10.9. Drug administration schedule and randomization of healthy male volunteers included into the study

			Treatments		
Sequence 1	400	400+ASA	800	800+ASA	ASA
Sequence 2	400	400+ASA	800	ASA	800+ASA
Sequence 3	400	400+ASA	ASA	800	800+ASA
Sequence 4	400	ASA	400+ASA	800	800+ASA
Sequence 5	ASA	400	400+ASA	800	800+ASA

The table above indicates only the active drugs. The remaining drugs are placebos.

It means the following:

400:1 tablet of 400 μg capsaicin+1 ASA placebo+1 capsaicin placebo

800:2 tablets of 400 μg capsaicin+1 ASA placebo

ASA:1 tablet of ASA+2 capsaicin placebo

ASA+400:1 tablet of ASA+1 tablet of capsaicin 400 μg+1 capsaicin placebo

ASA+800:1 tablet of ASA+2 tablets of capsaicin 400 μg

Table 15. Drugs administration schedule for healthy male voluneteers

10.10. Randomization of volunteers for this pharmacokinetic study (Table 16).

	Sequence 1	Sequence 2	Sequence 3	Sequence 4	Sequence 5
Subject number	6	4	3	2	1
	10	8	11	9	5
	13	14	12	15	7

The numbers in the table indicates the order of volunteers in time of inclusion. The time of the study was five weeks (3 days for the kinetic measurements, 3 days for wash-out) (see later)

Table 16. Random allocation of healthy male volunteers in this study

10.11. Chemical composition of "capsaicin" (capsaicinoids)

The United States Pharamcopeia defines capsaicin as product with contains >55% capsaicin, and combination of capsaicin and dihydrocapsaicin >75%; total capsaicinoids may be as little as 90% (United States Pharmacopoeia, 2005; USP 37).

This capsaicin definition is used as capsaicin in the animal researches and as well as in human observations.

The measurements of capsaicin and dihydrocapsaicin are accepted in the animal and human pharmakokinetic observations.

10.12. Measurements of Capsaicin and Dihydrocapsaicin from the plasma of volunteers

Measurements were performed:

- by High Pressure Chromatography (HPLC)-limit of detection by HPLC is 20 nanogram /mL plasma,
- by Liquid Chromatography – Mass Spectromery (LC-MS)-limit of detection is 26 fentogram/ mL for capsaicin and 20 fentogram/mL for dihydrocapsaicin.

Results:

No capsaicin and no dihydrocapsaicin could be detected in any samples of plasma of volunteers, after oral application of capsaicin (given orally in doses of 400 μg and 800 μg) in time period of 0 to 24 hours. If we applied the capsaicinoids externally to the equipments, then we were able to detect both capsaicin and dihydrocapsaicin.

(Similar negativ results were obtained in Beagle dogs treated different doses (0.1, 0.3 and 0.9 mg/kg/body weight orally in every day for one month period) *(Mózsik et al. 2008; Boros et al., 2008*).

10.13. Pharmacokinetic measurements of ASA alone and in combination with capsaicin(oids)

• ASA*
• ASA* + capsaicin(oids)** (400µg)
• ASA* + capsaicin(oids)** (800µg)
**500 mg orally given, ** orally given*
ASA metabolism in humans
by ASA esterase
ASA → salicylic acid + acetic acid
Measurements: ASA and Salicylic acid

Table 17. Combinations of pharmacokinetic measurements of human phase I. examinations

Blood sampling:

- Blood samples of 4 ml were taken from the forearm vein at the following times: pre-dose and 0:10, 0:20, 0:30, 0:40, 1:00, 1:30, 2, 4, 6, 10, 12, 16, and 24 hours post dose,
- Blood samples (14 in each period) were taken by vein puncture. Samples (4 ml) were collected into tubes using anticoagulation agent (potassium fluorid). The total amount of blood taken from each volunteer was not exceed 500 ml,
- After taking the blood sample for pharmacokinetic analysis, it was immediately transferred to a bath of melting ice and remained there for not more than 20 minutes. After centrifugation (1600 g, 4°C, 10 min), the separated plasma from each sample was divided into two aliquots (not less than 1 ml in each tube) using transparent, polypropylene tubes and they were immediately frozen and stored at a temperature below –20°C until analysis,
- Tubes were labelled. Each label contained the following information: study number, period and sample number, blood sampling time point, subject's randomisation number.
- After the end of clinical part, samples were transferred frozen directly to the analytical facility. Samples were packed with dry ice for transport, no interruption of the freeze cycle is allowed.

Pharmacokinetic and statistical evaluation:

The following pharmacokinetic parameters for the salicylic acid were calculated (by Prof. Mihály Klincsik, Department of Mathematics, Pollack Mihály Faculty of Engineering University of Pécs, Hungary) for each subject using model – independent approaches as follows:

- C_{max}observed maximal concentration,
- T_{max}time corresponding to the observed maximal concentration,
- $AUC_{0\text{-}tlast}$area under the plasma concentration time-curve, calculated by means of log-linear trapezoidal rule from time zero to the last data point above quantitation limit,

- $AUC_{0-\infty}$ area under the plasma concentration time-curve extrapolated from zero to infinity: $AUC_{0-\infty}=AUC_{0\text{-last}}+C_{\text{last, calc}}/\lambda_z$, where $C_{last,\ calc}$ represents the estimated plasma concentration by the regression line at the last sampling time point with measured concentration above the limit of quantitation, and
- λ_z represents the rate constant calculated from the regression line,
- $t_{1/2}$ terminal half-life calculated from the terminal elimination constant λ_z : $t_{1/2}=\ln 2/\lambda_z$,
- MRT(mean residence time): $MRT=AUMC_{0-\infty}/AUC_{0-\infty}$, where AUMC is the area under the first moment curve, calculated by the trapezoidal rule and extrapolated to infinit

Changes in pharmacokinetics of ASA metabolism:

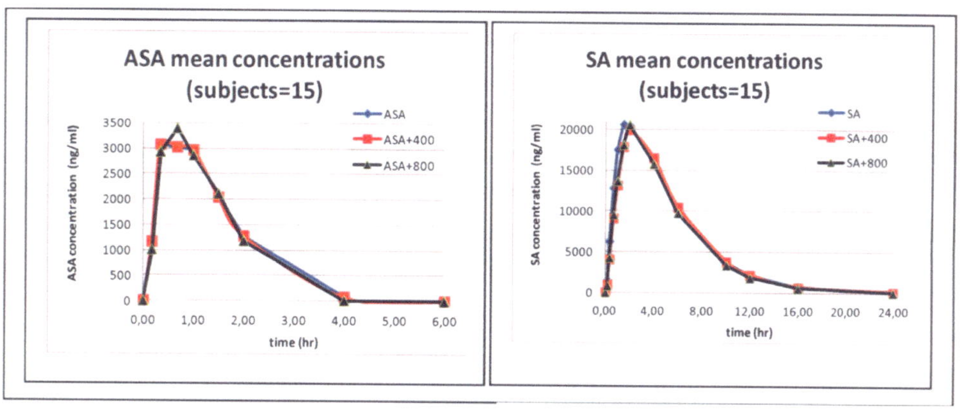

Figure 19. Mean concentration curves of aspirin (ASA)(left figure) and salicylic acid (SA)(right figure) plasma concentrations after oral administration of 500 mg ASA and co-administration of 400 and 800 µg capsaicin tablets in 15 healthy male volunteers

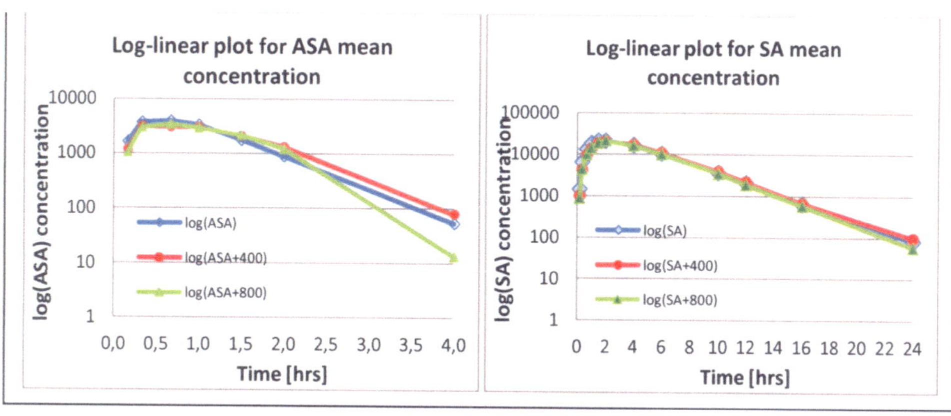

Figure 20. Log-linear plot curves of aspirin (ASA)(left figure) and salicylic acid (SA)(right figure) plasma concentrations after oral administration of 500 mg ASA and co-administration of 400 and 800 µg capsaicin tablets in 15 healthy male volunteers

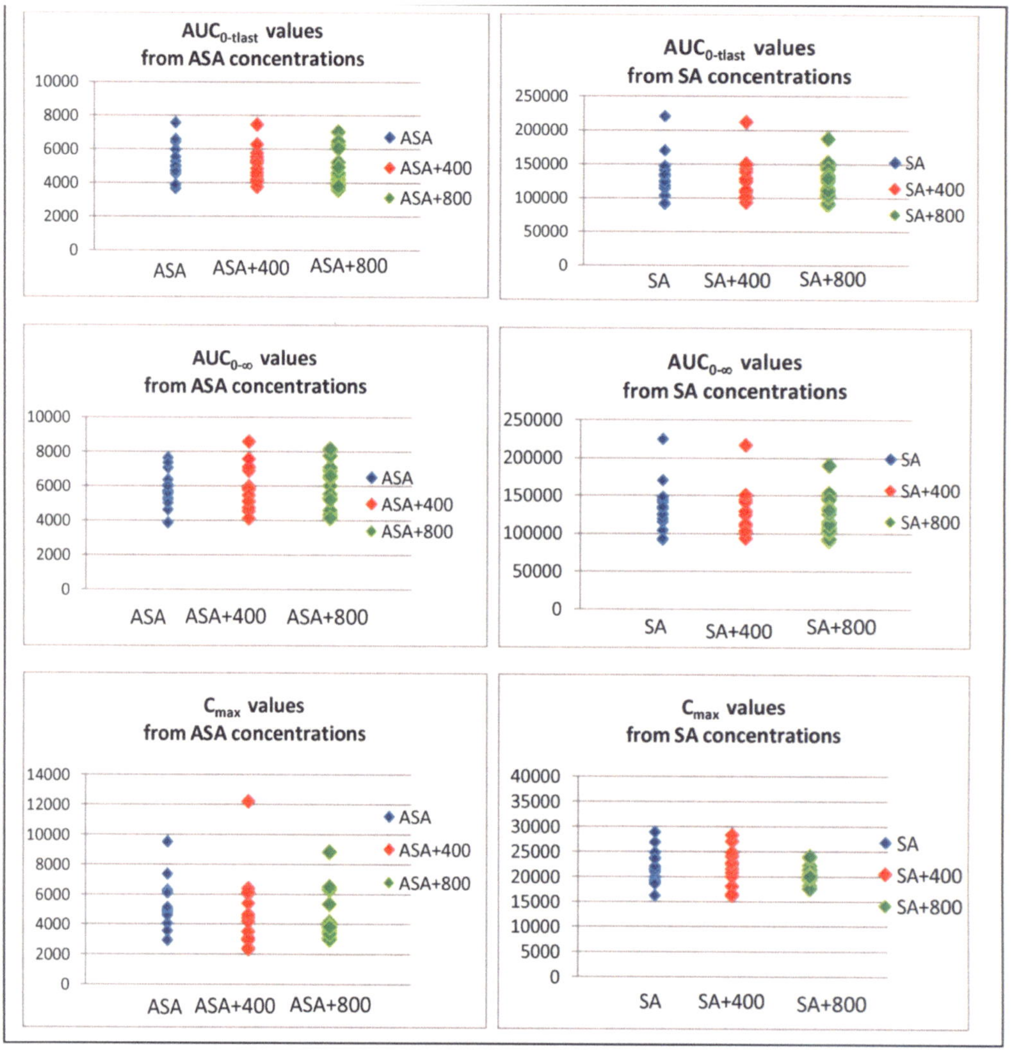

Figure 21. Changes of $AUC_{0\text{-tlast}}$, $AUC_{0\text{-}\infty}$ and C_{max} values for aspirin (ASA)(left figure) and salicylic acid (SA)(right figure) detected in plasma of 15 healthy male volunteers after oral administration of 500 mg ASA and co-administration of 400 and 800 μg capsaicin tablets

P-values from ANOVA tables* (No. of subjects=15)		from ASA concentration			from SA concentration		
		ASA (Reference)	ASA+400 (Test1)	ASA+800 (Test2)	SA (Reference)	SA+400 (Test1)	SA+800 (Test2)
Parameters	C_{max} [ng/ml]	p=0,42020			p=0,69971		
	T_{max} [hours]	p=0,19119			p=0,60419		
	$AUC_{0\text{-tlast}}$ [ng·hr/ml]	p=0,48281			p=0,76832		
	$AUC_{0\text{-}\infty}$ [ng·hr/ml]	p=0,96279			p=0,76929		
	$t_{1/2}$ [hr]	p=0,86917			p=0,78408		
	K_{el} [hr^{-1}]	p=0,86917			p=0,78408		

*All parameters were logarithmically transformed prior to data analysis (ie, assuming multiplicative model) except for T_{max} which was analyzed using untransformed data (ie, assuming additive model).

Table 18. P values from NOVA table comparing the mean values of the PK parameters

10.14. Platelet aggregation studies with ASA alone and in combination with capsaicin(oids)

10.14.1. Acetylsalicylic acid (ASA, Aspirin)

- high doses (500 mg) decreases pain, fever and inflammation,
- continuously taken low doses (75-325 mg) cause effective inhibition of platelet aggregation prevention of cardiovascular and cerebrovascular diseases,
- the incidence of coronary heart disease among ASA nonuser high cardiovascular risk patients is more than 15 cases per 1000 person-years,
- among low risk patients without ASA medication the incidence is less than 5 cases per 1000 person-years,
- high or low risk patients take low dose ASA everyday, the incidence of ACS became in the high risk group 4, in the low risk group only 1 event per 1000 patient-years.

10.14.2. Upper gastrointestinal tract complications (UGIC) (peptic ulcer, bleeding, perforation)

- among the general population 1 case / 1000 person-years,
- endpoints are 5-10%,
- UGIC among patients on ASA is 2-3 cases / 1000 person-years,
- endpoints are 10-20%,
- daily-users of low doses ASA have a 3-5 fold increased RR for UGIC as non-users.

10.14.3. Study design

- 15 healthy male volunteers,

- prescreening procedure demographic data BMI, medical history, physical examination laboratory blood tests, urine test, urine drug test and viral serology (HBsAg, Anti HCV, HIV),
- subjects were 18-55 years old and had a BMI of 18-29.9 kg/m^2.

Treatments	Tablets			
	400 µg capsaicin	**500 mg ASA**	**capsaicin placebo**	**ASA placebo**
400 µg capsaicin	1		1	1
800 µg capsaicin	2			1
500 mg ASA		1	2	
400 µg capsaicin + 500 mg ASA	1	1	1	
800 µg capsaicin + 500 mg ASA	2	1		

Table 19. Treatment protocol for ASA induced platelet aggregation on the epinephrine-induced platelet aggreagtion

10.14.4. Study of capsaicinoids alone, ASA and their combinations ont he epinephrine-induced platelet aggregation int he healthy male volunteers.

Materials: following the drug administration (according to the randomized schedule of the permitted human phase I. protocol) 8.1 ml blood was collected for platelet aggregation measurements before drug administration (0.0) (as control) and in 1.0, 2.0, 6.0 and 24.0 hours after drug administration.

Aggregation measurements: the epinephrine-induced platelet aggregation was studied by CARAT TX4 optical aggregometer (Carat Diagnostics Ltd, Budapest, Hungary at 37 ºC based on Born' method (Born, 1962; Koltai et al.,2008).

Method of evaluation of the obtained results: aggregation index below 40% was considered as clinically significant and effective inhibition of platelet aggregation.

Mathematical analysis of the obtained results was done by parired Student's t test (after using Kolmogonov-Smirnov' test to check the normality of the data distribution), one-way ANOVA test, Dunnett's post-hoc test.

http://dx.doi.org/10.5772/58359

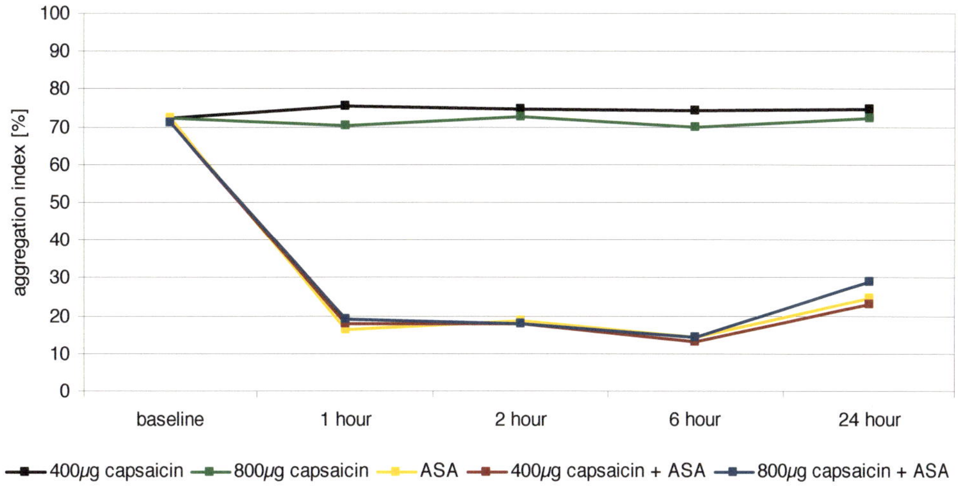

Figure 22. The platelet aggregation after oral capsaicin alone in two doses (400, 800 µg) and after co-administration of ASA (500 mg) in 15 male healthy subjects

10.15. Summaries and conclusions

- The human clinical pharmacological phase I. study (protocol number: 1.4.1; EudraCT number: 2008-007048-32) was successfully carried out in human healthy male volunteers.
- The capsaicin (oids) with using biodhesive compound was successfully pharmaceutically produced by PannonPharma Pharmaceutical Ltd. (Pécsvárad, Hungary
- The presence of capsaicin and dihydrocapsaicin (from the orally given capsaicinoids) was not able to detect in the plasma of healthy male volunteers, who were treated with capsaicin (oids) (in doses of 400 and 800 µg orally given).
- The capsaicin (oids) (given in doses of 400 and 800 µg orally does (do) not modify the absorption, metabolism and excretion of orally given ASA.
- The capsaicin (oids) does (do) not modify the epinephrine-induced aggregation by ASA, meanwhile the different doses of capsaicin(oids) alone have no direct action on the epinephrine-induced platelet aggregation.
- The capsaicin(oids) acts (act) locally in the gastrointestinal tract (indicating a good selection of bioadhesive compounds during the pharmaceutical technological preparation of our ASA +capsaicin(oids) combination.
- The results of these phase I. examinations offer us further possibility to carried out the forthcoming phase II. and phase III. examinations in patients.

Acknowledgements

The study was supported by the grant of **National Office for Research and Technology, "Pázmány Péter program" (RET-II 08/2005).**

Authors express their thanks to physicians, medical nurses, assistants, technicians at First Department of Medicine and Institute of Cardiology, Medical and Health Centre, University of Pécs and chemists, techniciants at PannonPharma Pharmaceutical Ltd, Pécsvárad, Hungay for their excellent assistance.

This study was supported by the National Office for Research and Technology, "Pázmány Péter programme, RET-II 08/2005, by BAROS GÁBOR Programme, Hungary (REG_DKI_O, CAPSATAB) and by SROP-4.2.2.B-10/1/KONV-2010-029 (TAMOP 4.2.2./B).

Author details

Gyula Mózsik[1], Tibor Past[1], Tamás Habon[1], Zsuzsanna Keszthelyi[1], Pál Perjési[2], Mónika Kuzma[2], Barbara Sándor[1], János Szolcsányi[3], M.E. Abdel-Salam Omar[4] and Mária Szalai[5]

*Address all correspondence to: gyula.mozsik@aok.pte.hu; gyula.mozsik@gmail.com

1 First Department of Medicine, Medical and Health Centre, University of Pécs, Hungary

2 Institute of Pharmaceutical Chemistry, Medical and Health Centre, University of Pécs, Hungary

3 Department ofPharmacology and Pharmacotherapy, Medical and Health Centre, University of Pécs, Hungary

4 Department of Pharmacology, National Research Centre, Dokki, Cairo, Egypt

5 PannonPharma Pharmaceutical Ltd., Pécsvárad, Hungary

The authors confirm that this overview content has no conflicts of interest.

References

[1] Abdel-Salam, O.M.E., Szolcsányi, J., Barthó, L., Mózsik, Gy. (1994): Sensory nerve-mediated mechanisms, gastric mucosal damage and its protection: A critical overview. Gastroprotection 2: 4-12

[2] Abdel-Salam, O.M.E., Mózsik, Gy., Szolcsányi, J. (1995a): The effect of intragastrically administered capsaicin analogue in HCl and non-HCl dependent models of gastric mucosal injury. Z. Gastroenterol. 33; 80

[3] Abdel-Salam, O.M.E., Mózsik, Gy., Szolcsányi, J. (1995b): Capsaicin and its analogue Resiniferatoxin inhibit gastric acid secretion in pylorus-ligated rats. Pharmacol. Res. 31: 341-345

[4] Abdel-Salam, O.M.E., Mózsik, Gy., Szolcsányi, J. (1995c): Effect of Resiniferatoxin on stimulated gastric acid secretory responses in the rat. J. Physiology (Paris) 88: 353-358

[5] Abdel-Salam, O.M.E., Mózsik, Gy., Szolcsányi, J. (1995d): Studies on the effect of intragastric capsaicin on gastric ulcer and on the prostacyclin-induced cytoprotection in rats. Pharmacol. Res. 32: 209-215

[6] Abdel-Salam, O.M.E., Bódis, B., Karádi, O., Szolcsányi, J., Mózsik, Gy. (1995e): Modification of aspirin and ethanol-induced mucosal damage in rats by intragastric application of Resiniferatoxin. Inflammopharmacology 3: 135-147

[7] Abdel-Salam, OME, Bódis, B., Karádi, O., Szolcsányi, J., Mózsik, Gy. (1995f): Nature of gastric H+ back-diffusion approached by cimetidine, vagotomy, RTX and sucralfate. Ceska Slovenská Gastroenterologie. 49: 175-185

[8] Abdel-Salam, O.M.E., Bódis, B., Karádi, O., Nagy, L., Szolcsányi, J., Mózsik, Gy. (1995g): Stimulation of capsaicin-sensitive sensory peripheral nerves with topically applied Resiniferatoxin decreases salicylate-induced gastric H+ back-diffusion in the rat. Inflammopharmacology 3: 121-133

[9] Abdel-Salam, O.M.E., Szolcsányi, J., Mózsik, Gy. (1996a): Differences in action of topical and system cystamine on gastric blood flow, gastric acid secretion and gastric ulceration in the rat. J. Physiology (Paris) 90:63-73

[10] Abdel-Salam, O.M.E., Szolcsányi, J., Porszász, R., Mózsik, Gy. (1996b): Effect of capsaicin and resiniferatoxin on gastrointestinal blood flow in rats. Eur. J. Pharmacol. 305: 127-136

[11] Abdel-Salam, O.M.E., Mózsik, Gy., Szolcsányi, J. (1997a): The effect of capsaicin and Resiniferatoxin on the indomethacin-induced gastric mucosal damage in rats. In: Mózsik, Gy., Nagy, L., Király, Á. (eds.) (1997): Cell Injury and Protection in Gastrointestinal Tract. From Basic Science to Clinical Perspectives. Kluwer Academic Publisher, Dordrecht. pp.: 95-105

[12] Abdel-Salam, O.M.E., Mózsik, Gy., Szolcsányi, J. (1997b): The role of afferent sensory nerve in gastric mucosal protection. In: Mózsik, Gy., Nagy, L., Király, Á. (eds.): Twenty Five Years of Peptic Ulcer Research in Hungary. From Basic Science to Clinical Practice 1971-1995. Akadémiai Kiadó, Budapest, pp: 295-308

[13] Abdel-Salam, O.M.E., Szolcsányi, J., Mózsik, Gy., (1997c): The effect of Resiniferatoxin on experimental gastric ulcer in rats. In: Gaginella, T., Mózsik, Gy., Rainsford K.D.

(eds): Biochemical Pharmacology as Approach to Gastrointestinal Disease. From Basic Science to Clinical Perspectives. Kluwer Academic Publisher, Dordrecht. pp.: 269-285

[14] Abdel-Salam, O.M.E., Szolcsányi, J., Mózsik, Gy., (1997d): The indomethacin-induced gastric mucosal damage in rats. Effect of gastric acid, acid inhibition, capsaicin-type agents and prostacyclin. J. Physiology (Paris) 97: 7-19

[15] Abdel Salam O.M.E., Sleem A.A., Hassan N.B., Sharaf H.A., Mózsik Gy. (2006): Capsaicin ameliorates hepatic injury caused by carbon tetrachloride in the rat. J. Pharmacol. Toxicol. 1:147-156.

[16] Abdel Salam, O. M. E., Czimmer, J., Debreceni, A., et al. (2001): Gastric mucosal integrity: Gastric mucosal blood flow and microcirculation. An overview, J. Physiol. 95, 105-127.

[17] Abdel Salam, O. M. E. Debreceni, A. and Mózsik, Gy. (1999). Capsaicin-sensitive afferent sensory nerves in modulating gastric mucosal defense against noxious agents, J. Physiol. 93, 443-454.

[18] Aijoka, H., Matsuura, N., Miyake, H. (2002): High quality of ulcer healing in rats by lafutidine and new-tipe histamine H2-receptor antagonist: involvement of capsaicin of sensitive sensory neurons. Inflammopharmacology 10, 483-493.

[19] Aijoka, H., Miyake, H., Matsuura, N. (2000): Effect of FRG-8813, a new-tipe histamine H2-receptor antagomist, on the recurrence of gastric ulcer healing by drug treatment. Pharmacology 61, 83-90.

[20] Alföldi, P., Obál, F. Jr., Tóth, E., Hideg, J. (1986): Capsaicin pretreatment reduces the gastric acid secretion elicited by histamine but does not affect the responses to carbachol and pentagastrin. Eur. J. Pharmacol. 123: 321-632

[21] Alföldi, P., Tóth, E., Obál, F., Hideg, J. (1987): Capsaicin treatment reduces histamine-induced gastric acid secretion in the rat. Acta Physiol. Hung. 69: 509-512

[22] Ames, B.N., McCann J., Yamasaki E. (1975): Methods for detecting carcinogens and mutagens with the Salmonella/microsoma test assay of 300 chemicals. Mutat Res. 31:347-364.

[23] Anonymus (1986): Metabolism and toxicity of capsaicin. Nutr. Rev. 44:20-22.

[24] Anu, A., Peter, K.V. (2000): The Chemistry of Paprika. Indian Species 37:15-18

[25] Ato, A., Yamamoto, M. (1996): Acute oral toxicity of capsaicin in mice and rats. J. Toxicol. Sci. 21:195-200.

[26] Azizan, A., Blevins, R.D. (1995): Mutagenecity and antimutagenecity testings of six chemicals associated with the purgent properties of specific spices as revelated by the Ames salmonella microsomal assay. Arch. Environ. Contam. Toxicol. 28:248-258.

[27] Basu, S.K., De, A.K. (2003): Capsicum: Historical and Botanical Perspectives. Taylor and Francis Ltd., London. pp 1-15

[28] Berkesy, L. (1934): Effect of paprika on gastric secretion (in Hungarian). Orv. Hetil. Hung. Weekly Med. J. 78: 397-399

[29] Bevan, S., Szolcsányi, J. (1990): Sensory neuron-specific actions of capsaicin: mechanisms and application. Trends. Pharmacol. Sci. 11: 330-333

[30] Bevan, S., Yeats, J. (1990): Protons activate a cation conductance in a subpopulation of rat dorsal root ganglion neurons. J. Physiology (London) 433: 145-161

[31] Bley, K.R. (2004): Recent developments in transient receptor potential vanilloid 1 agonist-based therapies. Expert Opin Investig Drugs. 13:1445-1456.

[32] Boersch A., Calligham B.A., Lembeck F., Sharman D.F. (1991): Enzymatic oxidation of capsaicin. Biochem Pharmacol 41: 1863-1969.

[33] Born, CV. (1962): Aggregation of blood platelets by adenosine diphosphate and its reversal. Nature 194: 927-929.

[34] Boros, B., Dörnyei, Á., Felinger, A. (2008): Determination of capsaicin and dihydrocapsaicin in dog plasma by Liquid Chromatography –Mass Spectrometry (Analytical method report). PTE TTK Analitikai Kémiai Tanszék, Pécs, Hungary.

[35] Brash, AR., Baertschi, SW., Ingram, C.D., Harris, TM. (1988): Isolation and characterization of natural allene oxides: unstable intermediates in the metabolism of lipid hydroperoxides. Proc. Natl. Acad. Sci. USA 85: 3382-3386.

[36] Bruggeman, T.M., Wood, J.G., Davenport, H.W. (1979): Local control of blood flow in the dog's stomach: vasodilatation caused by acid back-diffusion following topical application of salicylic acid. Gastroenterology 77: 736-744.

[37] Buck, S.H., Miller, M.S., Burks, T.F. (1982): Depletion of primary afferent substance P by capsaicin and dihydrocapsaicin without altered thermal sensitivity. Brain Res. 233:216-220.

[38] Buck, S.H., Burks, T.F. (1986): The Neuropharmacology of capsaicin: review of some recent observation. Pharmacol. Rev. 38:179-226.

[39] Buiatti, E., Palli, D., Dacarli, A., Amaddori, D., Avelini, C., Biachi S., Biserni, S., Cipriani, E., Cocco, P., Giacoso, A., Marubini, E., Puntoni J., Blot, Jr. W. (1989): A case-control study of gastric cancer and diet in Italy. Int. J. Cancer 44:611-616.

[40] Cabanac, M., Cormareche-Leyder, M., Poirior, L.J. (1976): The effect of capsaicin on the temperature regulation of the rat. Flügers Arch. Ges. Physiol. 366: 217-221.

[41] Castle, N.A. (1992): Differential inhibition of potassium currents in rat ventricular myocytes by capsaicin. Cardivasc. Res. 26:1137-1144.

[42] Caterina, M.J., Schumacker, M.A., Tomigana, M., Rosen, T.A., Levine, J.D., Julius, D. (1997): Capsaicin receptor: a heat activated ion channel in the pain pathyway. Nature 389:816-624.

[43] Chanda, S., Erexson, G., Riach, C., Innnes, D., Stevenson, F., Murli, H., Bley, K. (2004): Genotoxicity studies with pure trans-capsaicin. Mutat Res. 557:85-97.

[44] Chanda, S., Mould, A., Esmail, A., Bley, K. (2005): Toxicity studies with pure trans-capsaicin delivered to dogs via intravenous administration. Reg. Toxicol. Pharmacol. 43:66-75.

[45] Chard, P.S., Bleakman, D., Saridge J.R. (1995): Capsaicin-induced neurotoxicity in cultured dorsal root ganglion neurons: involvement of calcium-activated proteases. Neuroscience 65: 1099-1108.

[46] Cheng, Y.P., Wang, Y.H. Cheng, L.P., He, R.R. (2003): Electrophysiologic effects of capsaicin on pacemaker cells in sinoatrial nodes of rabbits. Acta Pharmacol. Sin. 24:826-830.

[47] Chudapongse, P., Janthasoot, W. (1981): Mechanism of the inhibitory action on capsaicin on energy metabolism by rat liver mitochondria. Biochem. Pharmacol. 30: 735-740.

[48] Clive, D., Flamm, W.G., Machesko, M.R., Bernheim, N.J. (1972): A mutational assay system using the thymidine kinase locus in mouse lymphoma cells. Mutat Res. 16:77-87.

[49] Clive, D., Johnson, K.O., Spector, J.F., Batson, A.G., Brown, M.M. (1979): Validation and characterization of the L5178Y/TK+/- mouse lymphoma and mutagens assay system. Mutat Res. 59:61-108.

[50] Cordell, G.A., Araujo, O.D. (1993): Capsaicin: identification, nomenclature, and pharmacology. Ann. Pharmacother. 27:330-336.

[51] Couzin, J. (2004a): Withdrawal of Vioxx casts shadow over COX-1 inhibitors. Science 306: 3844-3850.

[52] Couzin, J. (2004b): Nail-biting time for trials of COX-2 drug. Science 306:1673-1675

[53] Csáky, T.Z. (1969): Introduction to general pharmacology. Appleton Century-Craft Educational Division, Meredith Corporation, New York, 17-34

[54] De, A.K., Ghosh, J. J. (1990): Inflammatory responses induced by substance P in rat paw. Indian J. Exp. Biol. 28: 946-948.

[55] De Lille, J., Ramirez, E. (1935): Pharmacodynamic action of the active principle of chilli (Capsicum annum). Chem. 4836 (abstract).

[56] Debreceni, A., Juricskay, I., Figler, M., Abdel-Salam O.M.E., Szolcsányi, J., Mózsik Gy. (1999): A direct stimulatory effect of small dose of capsaicin on gastric emptying

rate in healthy human subjects measured by ^{13}C labeled octanoid acid breath test. J. Physiol. 93: 455-460.

[57] Desai, H.G., Venugopalam, K., Anita, F.P. (1973): Effect of red chili powder on NDA content of gastric aspirates. Gut 14: 974-976

[58] Donnerer, J., Lembeck, F. (1983): Capsaicin-induced reflex fall in rat blood pressure is mediated by afferent substances P-containing neurones via a reflex centre in the brain stem. Naunyn-Schmiedeber's Arch. Pharmacol. 324:293-295.

[59] Donnerer, J., Amann, R., Schuligoi, R, Lembeck, F. (1990): Absorption and metabolism of capsaicinoids following intragastric administration in rats. Naunin-Schmiedeberg's Arch Pharmacol. 342:357-361.

[60] Dugani, A.M., Galvin, G.B. (1986): Capsaicin effects on stress pathology and gastric acid secretion in rats. Life Sci. 39: 1531-1538.

[61] Dömötör. A., Szolcsányi, J., Mózsik, Gy. (2006): Capsaicin and glucose absorption and utilization in healthy human subjects. Eur. J. Pharmacol. 534: 208-283.

[62] Endoh, K., Leung, F.W. (1990): Topical capsaicin protects the distal but not the proximal colon against acetic acid injury. Gastroenterology 98: A 446.

[63] Espinosa-Aquire, JJ., Reyes, RE., Rubio, J., Ostrosky-Wegman, P., Martinez, G. (1993): Mutagenic activity of urban air samples and its modulation by chilli extracts. Mutat. Res. 303:55-61.

[64] Esplugues, J.V., Whittle, B.J.R., Moncanda, S. (1989): Local opioid-sensitive afferent sensory neurons in the modulation of gastric damage induced by PAF. Br. J. Pharmacol. 97: 579-585.

[65] Esplugues, J.V., Ramos, E.G, Gil, L., Esplugues, J. (1990): Influence of capsaicin-sensitive afferent neurons on the acid secretory responses of the rat stomach in vivo. Br. J. Pharmacol. 100: 491-496.

[66] Esplugues, J.V., Whittle, B.J.R. (1990): Morphine potentiation of ethanol-induced gastric mucosal damage in the rat. Role of local sensory afferent neurons. Gastroenterology 98: 82-89.

[67] Esplugues, J.V., Whittle, B.J.R., Moncanda, S. (1992): Modulation by opioids and by afferent sensory neurons of prostanoids protection of the rat gastric mucosa. Br. J. Pharmacol. 106: 846-852.

[68] Evangelista, S., Meli, A. (1989): Influence of capsaicin-sensory fibres on experimentally-induced colitis in rats. J. Pharm. Pharmacol. 41: 574-576.

[69] Evangelista, S., Santicioli, P., Maggi, C.A., Meli, A. (1989): Increase in gastric acid secretion induced by 2-deoxy-D-glucose is impaired in capsaicin pretreated rats. Br. J. Pharmacol. 98: 35-37.

[70] Evans, H.J. (1962): Chromosomal aberrations produced by ionizing radiation. Int Rev Cytol 13:221-231.

[71] Evans, H.J. (1962): Cytological methods for detecting chemical mutagens. In: Hollander, A. (ed.) Chemical Mutagens, Principles and Methods for their Detection.Vol. 4. Plenum Press., New York and London, 1976. pp. 1-29.

[72] Expert Consensus Document on the Use of Antiplatelete Agents. ESC Eur. J. 2004.

[73] Fischer, G.A. (1958): Studies of the culture of leukemic cells in vitro. Ann. N. Y. Acad. Sci. 76:673-680.

[74] Flynn, D.L., Rafferty, M.F. (1986): Inhibition of human neutrophil 5-lipoxygenase activity by ginerdione, shogaol, capsaicin and related pungent compounds. Prostagland. Leucotrien. Med. 24:195-198.

[75] Freudenberg, K. (1962): Research on lignin. Fortschr. Chem. Org. Naturst. 20:41-72.

[76] Galloway, S.M., Aardema, M.J., Ischidate, M., et al. (1994): Report from working group on in vitro tests for chromosomal aberrations. Mutat Res. 312:241-261.

[77] Gislason, H., Guttu, K., Sorbye, H., Schifter, S., Waldum, L.H., Svanes, K. (1995): Role of histamine and calcitonin gene-related peptide in the hyperemic response to hypertonic saline and H^+ back-diffusion in the gastric mucosa of cats. Scand. J. Gastroenterol. 30: 300-310.

[78] Goso, C., Evangelista, S., Tramontana, N., Manzini, S., Blumberg, P.M., Szallasi, A. (1993): Topical capsaicin protects against trinitrobenzene sulfonic acid-induced colitis in the rat. Eur. J. Pharmacol. 249: 185-190.

[79] Govindarajan, V.S., Sathyanarayana, M.N. (1991): Capsicum-production, technology, chemistry, and quality. Part V. Impact on physiology, pharmacology, nutrition, and metabolism: structure pungency, pain, and desensitization sequences. Crit. Rev. Food Sci. Nutr. 29: 435-474.

[80] Glinsukon, T., Stitmunnaitnum, Y., Toskulkao, C., Buranawuth, T., Tandkrisanavinont, V. (1980): Acute toixicity of capsaicin in several animal species.Toxicon. 18:215-220.

[81] Gray, J.L., Bunnet, N.W., Orloff, S.L., Mulvihill, S.J., Debas, H.T. (1994): Role for calcitonin gene-related peptide in protection against gastric ulceration. Ann. Surg. 219: 58-64

[82] Green MD (2005). Causation, Vioxx and legal issues. Science 310: 973.

[83] Guengerich, FP., Kim, D.H., Iwasaki, M. (1991): Role of human cytochrome P-450 IIE1 in the oxidation of many low molecular weight cancer suspects. Chem. Res. Toxicol. 4: 168-179.

[84] Gulbekian, S., Merighi, A., Wharton, J., Varndell, I.M., Polak, J.M, (1986): Ultrastructural evidence for the coexistence of calcitonin gene-related peptide and substance P in secretory vesicles of peripheral nerves in the guinea-pig. J. Neurocytol. 15: 535-542.

[85] Gunnett, P.M., Shi X., Lawson T., Kolar C., Toth B. (1997): Aryl radical formation during the metabolism of arylhydrazines by microsomes. Chem. Res. Toxicol. 10:1372-1377.

[86] Haim, N., Nemec, J., Roman, J., Sinha, BK. (1987a): In vitro metabolism of etoposide (VP-16-213) by liver microsomes and irreversible binding of reactive intermediates to microsomal proteins. Biochem. Pharmacol. 36: 527-536.

[87] Haim, N., Nemec, J., Roman, J., Sinha, BK. (1987b): Peroxidase-catalyzed metabolism of etoposide (VP-15-213) and covalent binding of reactive intermediates to cellular macromolecules. Cancer Res. 47: 5835-5840.

[88] Holzer, P., Sametz, W. (1986): Gastric mucosal protection against ulcerogenic factors in the rat mediated by capsaicin-sensitive afferent neurons. Gastroenterology 91: 975-981

[89] Holzer, P., Lippe, I.T. (1988): Stimulation of afferent nerve endings by intragastric capsaicin protects against ethanol-induced damage of gastric mucosa. Neuroscience 27: 981-987

[90] Holzer, P., Pabst, M.A., Lippe, I.T. (1989): Intragastric capsaicin protects against aspirin-induced lesion formation and bleeding in the rat gastric mucosa. Gastroenterology 96: 1425-1433.

[91] Holzer, P., (1990): Capsaicin-sensitive nerves in the control of vascular effector mechanisms. In: Green, B.G., Mason, J.R., Kare, M.R. (eds.): Chemical Senses. Irritation. MarcelDekker, New York. 2: 191-210.

[92] Holzer, P., (1991a): Capsaicin: cellular targets, mechanisms of action, and selectivity for thin sensory neurons. Pharmacol. Rev. 43: 144-202

[93] Holzer, P., (1991b): Afferent nerve-mediated control of gastric mucosal blood flow and protection In: Costa, M., Surrenti, C., Gorini, S., Maggi, C.A., Meli, A. (eds.): Sensory Nerve and Neuropeptides in Gastroenterology. From Basic Science to Clinical Perspective. Plenum Press, New York, pp.: 97-108.

[94] Holzer, P., (1992a): Capsaicin: selective toxicity for thin primary sensory neurons. Selective neurotoxicity. In: Herken, H., Hucho, F. (eds.): Handbook of Experimental Pharamacology. Springer Verlag, Berlin, pp.: 419-481.

[95] Holzer, P., (1992b): Peptidergic sensory neurons in the control of vascular functions: mechanisms and significance in the cutaneous and splanchnic vascular beds. Rev. Physiol. Biochem. Pharmacol. 121: 50-146.

[96] Holzer, P., (1998): Neural emergency system in the stomach. Gastroenterology 114: 823-839

[97] Holzer, P. (1999). Capsaicin cellular targets, Mehanisms of action, as selectivity for thin sensory neurons, Phamacol. Res. 43. 143-201.

[98] Iwama, M., Tojima, T., Itol, Y., Takahashi N., Kanke, Y. (1990): Effects of capsaicin and ethanol on hepatic drug-metabolizing enzymes in rat. Int. J. Vit. Nutr. Res. 60:100-103.

[99] Jancsó, N., Jancsó-Gábor, A., (1959): Dauerausschaltung der Chemischen Schmerzempfindlichkeit durch capsaicin. Naunyn-Schmiedebergs Arch. Exp. Path. Pharmacol. 236: 142-145.

[100] Jancsó, N., Jancsó-Gábor, A., Szolcsányi, J. (1967): Direct evidence for neurogenic inflammation and its prevention by denervation and by pretreatment with capsaicin. Brit. J. Pharmacol. 31, 138-151.

[101] Jancsó, N., Jancsó- Gábor, A., Szolcsányi, J. (1968): The role of sensory nerves endings in the neurogen inflammation induced in human skin and in the eye and paw of the rat. Brit. J. Pharmacol. 33, 32-41.

[102] Jancsó-Gábor, A., Szolcsányi, J., Jancsó, N. (1970): Irrevesible impairement of the irregulation induced by capsaicin and similar pungent substances in rat and guinea-pigs. J. Physiol. (London) 206, 495-507.

[103] Jaiarj, P., Kitphati, C., Sinchaipanid, N., Lertsin, N., Siripanyachan, P. (2000): Stability testing of capsaicinoid cream, Mahidol University Annual Research Abstracts 371

[104] Joe, B., Lokesh, B R. (1994): Role of capsaicin, curcumin and dietary n-3 fatty acids in lowering the generation of reactive oxygen species in rat peritoneal macrophages. Biochim. Biophys. Acta 1224:255-263.

[105] Jurenitsch, J., Kubelka, W., Jentzsch, K. (1979): Identification of cultivated taxa of Capsicum. Taxonomy, anatomy and composition of purgent principles. Plant. Med. 35: 175-183.

[106] Karádi, O., Mózsik, Gy. (2000). Surgical and chemical vagotomy on the gastrointestinal mucosal defense. Akadémiai Kiadó, Budapest.

[107] Kawada, T., Suzuki, T., Takahashi, M., Iwai K. (1984): Gastrointestinal absorption and metabolism of capsaicin and dihydrocapsaicin in rats. Toxicol. Appl. Pharmacol. 72:449-456.

[108] Kawada, T., Iwai, K. (1985): In vivo and in vitro metabolism of dihydrocapsaicin, a pungent principle of hot pepper, in rat. Agric. Biol. Chem. 49:441-448.

[109] Kawai, S., Nishida, S., Kato, M., Furumaya, Y., Okomoto, T., Mizushima Y. (1998): Comparison of cyclooxigenase-1 and-2 inhibitory activities of nonsteroidal anti-in-

flammatory drugs using humaín platelets and synovial cells. Eur. J. Pharmacol. 347:87-94.

[110] Kensler, T.W., Egner, PA, Davidson, NE., Roebuck, BD, Pikul, A, Groopman, JD. (1986): Modulation of aflatoxin metabolism, aflatoxin-N7-guanine formation, and hepatic tumorigenesis in rats fed ethoxyquin: role of induction of glutathione S-transferases. Cancer Res. 46: 3924-3931.

[111] Ketusinh, O., Dhorranintra, B., Juengjareon, K. (1966): Influence of capsaicin solution on gastric acidities. Am. J. Protocol. 17: 511-515.

[112] Koop, DR. (1992): Oxidative and reductive metabolism by cytochrome P450 2E1. FASEB J. 6: 724-730.

[113] Koltai, K., Fehér G., Kenyeres, P., Lenard, I., Alexy, T., Horváth, B., Márton, Z., Késmárky, G., Tóth K. (2008): Relation of platelet aggregation and fibrinogen levels to advancing age in aspirin- and thioenopyrimide-treated patients. Clin. Hemorheol. Microcirc. 40: 295-302.

[114] Kopec, S.E., DeBellis, R.J., Irwin, R.S. (2002): Chemical Analysis of Freshly Prepared and Stored Capsaicin Solutions: Implications for Tussigenic Challenges. Pulm. Ther. 15: 529-534.

[115] Lawler, A. (2005): The law.Vioxx verdict: too little or too much science? Science 309:1481.

[116] Lawson, T., Gannett, P. (1989): The mutagenicity of capsaicin and dihydrocapsaicin in V79 cells. Cancer Lett. 49:109-113.

[117] Lee, S.S., Kumar, S. (1980): Microsomes, Drug Oxidations, and Chemical Calcinogenesis. Vol.2. In: Coon, M.J., Conney, A.H., Estabrook, R.W., Gelboin, H.V., Gillette, J.R., O' Brien, P.J. (eds.): Academic Press, New York, pp. 1009-1012.

[118] Lenzer, J, (2004): FDA is incapable of protecting of US "against another Vioxx". Brit. Med. J. 329:1253.

[119] Li, D.S., Raybould, H.E., Quintero, E., Guth, P.H. (1992): Calcitonin gene-related peptide mediates the gastric hyperemic response to acid back-diffusion. Gastroenterology 102: 1124-1128.

[120] Lippe, I.T., Pabst, M.A., Holzer, P. (1989): Intragastric capsaicin enhances rat gastric acid elimination and mucosal blood flow by afferent nerve stimulation. Br. J. Pharmacol. 96: 91-100.

[121] Lippe, I.T., Holzer, P. (1992): Participation of endothelium-derived nitric oxide but not prostacyclin in the gastric mucosal hypeaemic response due to acid back-diffusion. Br. J. Pharmacol. 105: 708-714.

[122] Maga, J.A., (1975): Capsicum. Crit. Rev. Food. Sci. Nutr. 177-199.

[123] Maggi, C.A., Meli, A. (1988): The sensory-efferent function of capsaicin-sensitive sensory neurons. Gen. Pharmacol. 19: 1-43.

[124] Maggi, C.A., Santicioli, P., Geppetti, P., Parlani, M., Astolfi, M., DelBianco, E., Patacchini, R., Giuliani, S., Meli, A., (1989): The effect of calcium free medium and nefidipine on the release of substance P-like immunoreactivity and contractions induced by capsaicin in the isolated guinea-pig bladder. Gen. Pharmacol. 40: 445-456.

[125] Maggi, C.A., (1995): Tachykinins and calcitonin gene-related peptide (CGRP) as co-transmitters released from peripheral endings of sensory nerves. Progress in Neurobiology 45: 1-98.

[126] Makara, G.B., Frenkl, C.R., Somfai, Z., Szepesházi, K. (1965): Effect of capsaicin on the experimental ulcer in the rat. Acta. Med. Sci. Hung. 21: 213-216.

[127] Mans, D.R., Lafleur, M.V., Westmijze E.J., van Maanen, J.M., van Schaik, M.A., Lankelma, J., Retel, J. (1991): Formation of different reaction products with single-and double-stranded DNA by the ortho-quinone and the semi-quinone free radical of etoposide (VP-16-213). Biochem. Pharmacol. 42: 2131-2139.

[128] Maron, D.M., Ames, B.N. (1983): Revized methods for the Salmonella mutagenecity test. Mutat Res. 113:173-215.

[129] Marques, S., Oliveira, N.G., Chaveca, T., Rueff, J. (2002): Micronuclei and sister chromatid exchanges induced by capsaicin in human lymphocytes. Mutat Res. 517:39-46.

[130] Martin, R.L., McDermott, S.J., Salmen, H.J., Palmatier, J., Cox, B.F., Gintant, G.A. (2004): The utility of hERG and repolarization assays in evaluating delayed cardiac reporalization: influence of multi-channel block. J. Cardiovasc. Pharmacol. 43:369-379.

[131] Mcgettigan, P., Henry, D (2006): Cardiovascular Risk and Inhibition of Cyclooxygenase. A System Review of the Observational Studies of Selective and Nonselective Inhibitors of Cyclooxygenase 2 JAMA 2006; 296.

[132] Merighi, A., Polak, J.M., Gibson, S.J., Gulbekian, S., Valentino, K.L., Peirone S.M., (1988): Ultrastructural studies on calcitonin gene-related peptide-, tachykinin- and somatostatin-immunoreactive neurons in rat dorsal root ganglia: Evidence for colocalization of different peptides in single secretory granules. Cell Tiss. Res. 254: 101-109.

[133] Miller, M.S., Brendel, K., Burks, T.F., Sipes, I.G. (1983): Interaction of capsaicinoids with drug-metabolizing systems. Relationship to toxicity. Biochem. Pharmacol. 32:547-551.

[134] Modly, C.E., Das, M., Don, P.S., Marcelo C.L., Mukhtar, H., Bickers, D.R. (1986): Capsaicin as an in vitro inhibitor of benzo(a)pyrene metabolism and its DNA binding in human and murine keratinocytes. Drug. Metab. Dispos. 14: 413-416.

[135] Molnar, J.(1965): Die pharmakologischen wirkungen des capsaicin, des schaf schmeckenden wirkstoffers im paprika. Arzeilmittel-Forsh. L5: 718.

[136] Molnar, J., György, L. (1967): Pulmonary hypertensive and other haemodynamic effect of capsaicin in the cat. Eur. J. Pharmacol.1: 86-92.

[137] Monsereenusorn, Y. (2001): Subchronic toxicity studies of capsaicin and capsinum in rats. Res. Commmun. Chem. Path. Pharmacol. 41:95.110.

[138] Moore. M.M., Honna, M., Clements, J., et al. (2003): Mouse thymidine kinase gene mutation assay: International workshop on genotocicity test. Workgroup Report. Plymouth, UK. 2002. Mutat Res. 540:127-140.

[139] Mózsik, Gy., Moron, F., Jávor, T. (1982): Cellular mechanisms of the development of gastric mucosal damage and of gastroprotection induced by prostacyclin in rats. A pharmacological study, Prostagland. Leukot. Med. 9, 71-84.

[140] Mózsik, Gy., Király, Á., Sütö, G., Vincze, Á. (1993): ATP breakdown and resynthesis in the development of gastrointestinal mucosal damage and its prevention in animals and human (an overview of 25 years ulcer research studies). In: Mózsik, Gy., Pár, A., Kitajima, M., Kondo, M., Pfeiffer, CJ., Rainsford, KD., Sikiric, P., Szabó, S. (eds.): Cell Injury and Protection in the Gastrointestinal Tract: From Basic Science to Clinical Perspectives. Akadémiai Kiadó, Budapest, pp.: 39-80.

[141] Mózsik, Gy., Abdel-Salam, O.M.E., Bódis, B., Karádi, O., Nagy, L., Szolcsányi, J. (1996a): Role of vagal nerve in defense mechanisms against NSAIDs-induced gastrointestinal mucosal damage. Inflammopharmacology 4: 151-172.

[142] Mózsik, Gy., Abdel-Salam, O.M.E., Bódis, B., Karádi, O., Király, Á., Sütö, G., Rumi, Gy., Szabó, I., Vincze, Á. (1996b): Gastric mucosal protective effects of prostacyclin and β-carotene, and their biochemical backgrounds in rats treated with ethanol and HCl in dependence of their doses and of their time after administration of necritizing agents. Inflammopharmacology 4: 361-378.

[143] Mózsik, Gy., Nagy, L., Király, Á. (eds.) (1997a): Twenty Five Years of Peptic Ulcer Research in Hungary. From Basic Science to Clinical Practice 1971-1995. Akadémiai Kiadó, Budapest, pp.: 1-448.

[144] Mózsik, Gy., Nagy, L., Pár, A., Rainsford, K.D. (eds.) (1997b): Cell Injury and Protection in the Gastrointestinal Tract: From Basic Science to Clinical Perspectives. Kluwer Academic Publisher, Boston, Dordrecht.

[145] Mózsik, Gy., Abdel-Salam, O.M.E., Szolcsányi, J. (1997c): Capsaicin-Sensitive Afferent Nerves in Gastric Mucosal Damage and Protection. Akadémiai Kiadó, Budapest.

[146] Mózsik, Gy., Debreceni, A., Abdel-Salam, OME., Szabó, I., Figler, M., Ludány, A., Juricskay, I., Szolcsányi, J. (1999): Small doses capsaicin given intragastrically inhibit gastric secretion in healthy human subjects. J. Physiol. Paris 93: 433-436

[147] Mózsik, Gy., Vincze, Á., Szolcsányi, J. (2001): Four responses of capsaicin sensitive primary afferent neurons to capsaicin and its analog. Gastric acid secretion, gastric mucosal damage and protection. J. Gastroenterol. Hepatol. 16, 193-197.

[148] Mózsik, Gy., Belágyi, J., Szolcsányi, J. (2004a): Capsaicin-sensitive afferent nerves and gastric mucosal protection in the human healthy subjects. A critical overview. in: Takeuchi K., Mózsik Gy. (eds.) Research Signpost Kerala, India pp. 43-62.

[149] Mózsik, Gy., Pár, A., Pár, G. et al. (2004b). Insight into the molecular pharmacology to drugs acting on the afferent and efferent fibres of vagal nerve in the gastric mucosal protection in: Ulcer Research, Proceedings of the 11th International Conference, Sikirič P., Seiwerth P., Mózsik Gy., Arakawa T., Takeuchi K. (eds.): pp. 163-168. Monduzzi, Bologna.

[150] Mózsik, Gy., Rácz, I., Szolcsányi, J. (2005): Gastroprotection induced by capsaicin in healthy human subjects. World J. Gastroenterol. 11:5180-5184.

[151] Mózsik Gy.(2006a).Molecular pharmacology and biochemistry of gastroduodenal mucosal damage and protection. In: Mózsik, Gy. (ed.) Discoveries in Gastroenterology: from Basic Research to the Clinical Perspectives.Akadémiai Kiadó, Budapest, pp 139-224.

[152] Mózsik Gy., Dömötör, A., Abdel-Salam O.M.E. (2006b): Molecular pharmacological approach to drug actions on the afferent and efferent fibres of the vagal nerve in the gastric mucosal protection in rats. Inflammopharmacology 14: 243-249.

[153] Mózsik, Gy., Szolcsányi, J., Dömötör, A. (2007a): Capsaicin research as a new tool to approach of the human gastrointestinal physiology, pathology and pharmacology. Inflammopharmacology 15: 232–245.

[154] Mózsik Gy., Past T.,Perjési P. (2007b): Capsaicinoids,nonsteroidal antiinflammatory drugs and gastrointestinal protection. An expert' opinion. Pécs, Hungary.

[155] Mózsik, Gy., Past, T., Perjési, P., Szolcsányi, J. (2008a): Original Reports on Toxicology of Capsaicin I. The Testing of Capsaicin Natural USP 27 with Bacterial Reverse Mutation Tests. The date of final report 13 September 2007. Study code: 07/496-007M. Veszprém, LAB International Research Centre Hungary Ltd. 2008; 1-33 (7 appendix).

[156] Mózsik, Gy., Past, T., Perjési, P., Szolcsányi J. (2008b): Original Reports on Toxicology of Capsaicin II. Testing of Mutagenic Effect of Test Item Capsaicin Natural USP 27 by Mouse Micronucleus Test. The date of final report 12 October 2007. Study Code: 07/019-008E. Budapest, Toxic-Coop Ltd. 2008; 1-18 (5 appendix).

[157] Mózsik, Gy., Past, T., Perjési, P., Szolcsányi, J. (2008c): Original Reports on Toxicology of Capsaicin III. 14-Day Oral Gavage Dose Range Finding Study with Capsaicin Natural USP 27 in the Rats. The date of final report 15 October 2007. Study Code: 07/018-100PE. Dunakeszi, Toxic-Coop Ltd. 2008; This report consists of 27 pages of text, 51 pages of appendices.

[158] Mózsik, Gy., Past, T., Perjési, P., Szolcsányi, J. (2008d): Original Reports on Toxicology of Capsaicin IV. Oral Dose Range Finding Toxicity Study in Beagle Dogs with Capsaicin Natural USP 27. The date of final report 08 October 2007. Study Code: 07/496-100KE. Veszprém, LAB International Research Centre Hungary Ltd. 2008; 1-26 (17 appendix)

[159] Mózsik, Gy., Past T., Perjési, P., Szolcsányi, J. (2008d): Original Reports on Toxicology of Capsaicin V. Oral Dose Range Finding Toxicity Study of Capsaicin Natural USP 27 in Beagle Dogs (Supplementary Final Report). The date of final report 08 October 2007. Study Code: 07/496-100KE. Veszprém, LAB International Research Centre Hungary Ltd. 2008; 1-20 (10 appendix)

[160] Mózsik Gy, Past T, Perjési P, Szolcsányi J. (2008e): Original Reports on Toxicology of Capsaicin VI. 28-Day Oral Toxicity Study of Capsaicin Natural USP 27 in Rats (Final Report). The date of final report 21 May 2008. Study Code: 07/018-100P. Dunakeszi Toxic-Coop Ltd. 2008; This report consists of 31 pages text and 166 pages of appendix.

[161] Mózsik, Gy., Past, T., Perjési, P., Szolcsányi J. (2008f): Original Reports on Toxicology of Capsaicin VII. 8-Day Oral Toxicity Study of Test Item Capsaicin Natural USP 27 in Beagle Dogs (Final Report). The date of final report 13 June 2008. Study Code: 07/496-100K. Veszprém, LAB International Research Centre Hungary Ltd. 2008; 1-35 (90 appendix).

[162] Mózsik, Gy., Past, T., Perjési, P., Szolcsányi, J. (2008g): Original Reports on Toxicology of Capsaicin VIII. Amendment 2 to Study Plan. 28-Day Oral Toxicity Study of Test Item Capsaicin Natural USP 27 in Beagle Dogs. The date of final report 03 June 2008. Study Code: 07/496-100K. Veszprém, LAB International Research Centre Hungary Ltd. 2008; 1-4.

[163] Mózsik, Gy., Past, T., Perjési, P., Szolcsányi, J. (2008h): Determination of capsaicin and dihydrocapsaicin content of dog's plasma by HPLC-FLD method. In.: Mózsik Gy., Past T., Perjési P., Szolcsányi J.: Original Reports on Toxicology of Capsaicin VII. 8-Day Oral Toxicity Study of Test Item Capsaicin Natural USP 27 in Beagle Dogs (Final Report). The date of final report 13 June 2008. Study Code: 07/496-100K LAB. Veszprém, International Research Centre Hungary Ltd. 2008; 1-35 (190 appendix).

[164] Mózsik, Gy., Past, T., Abdel Salam, O.M.E, Kuzma, M., Perjési, P. (2009a): Interdisciplinary review for the correlation between the plant origin capsaicinoids, non-steroidal antiinflammatory drugs, gastrointestinal mucosal damage and prevention in animals and human beings. Inflammopharmacology 17: 113-150.

[165] Mózsik, Gy., Dömötör, A., Past, T., Vas, V., Perjési, P., Kuzma, M., Blazics, Gy., Szolcsányi, J. (2009b): Capsaicinoids: From the plant cultivation to the production of the human medical drug. Akadémiai Kiadó, Budapest.

[166] Mózsik, Gy., Past, T., Dömötör, A., Kuzma, M., Perjési P. (2010): Production of orally applicable new drug or drug combinations from natural origin capsaicinoids for human medical therapy. Curr. Pharm. Des. 16: 1197-1208.

[167] Nagabhuslan, M., Blide, S.V (1985): Mutagenecity of chili extract and capsaicin in short term tests. Environ. Mutagen 7: 881-888.

[168] Nopanitaya, W. (1974): Effects of capsaicin in combination with diets of varying protein content on the duodenal absorptive cells of the rat. Am. J. Dig. Dis. 19: 439-449.

[169] Notani, P.N., Jayant, K. (1987): Role of diet in upper aerodigestive tract cancers. Nutr. Cancer. 10:203-113.

[170] Newmark H.L. (1984): A hypothesis for dietary componets as blocking agents of chemical carcinogenesis: plant phenolics and pyrole pigments. Nutr.Cancer 6:58-70.

[171] Newmark H.L. (1987): Plant phenolics as inhibitors of mutational and precarcinogenic events. Can J Physiol Pharmacol 65:461-466.

[172] Oi, Y., Kawada ,T., Watanabe, T., Iwai, K. (1992): Induction of capsaicin- hydrolyzing enzyme activity in rat liver by continuous oral administration of capsaicin. J. Agric. Food Chem. 40:467-470.

[173] Onodera, S., Shibata, M., Tanaka. H, et al. (1999): Gastroprotective mechanisms of lafutidine, a novel anti-ulcer drug with histamine H_2-receptor antagonist activity, Artneim. Forsch., Drug. Res. 49, 519-526.

[174] Onodera, S., Shibata, M., Tanaka, H., et al. (2002). Gastroprotective activity of FRG-8813, a novel histamine H_2-receptor antagonist, in rats, Jpn. J. Pharmacol. 68, 161-173.

[175] Opez-Carrillo, L., Lopez-Cervantes, M., Bobles-Diaz, G., Ramilez-Espitia, A., Mohar-Betancourt, A., Menses-Gratia, A., Lopez-Vidal, Y., Blair A. (2003): Capsaicin consumption Helicobacter pylori positivity and gastric cancer in Mexico. Int. J. Cancer 106:277-282.

[176] Patrono, C., Bachmann, F., Baigent, C., Bode, C., De Caterina, R, Charbonnier, B., et al. (2004): Expert consensus document on the use of antiplatelet agents. The task force on the use of antiplatelet agents in patients with atherosclerotic cardiovascular disease of the Europen Society of Cardiology. Eur. Heart J. 25: 166-181.

[177] Pabst, M.A., Schöninkle, E., Holzer, P. (1993): Ablation of capsaicin-sensitive afferent neurons impairs defense but not rapid repair of rat gastric mucosa. Gut 34: 897-903.

[178] Park, Y.H., Lee, S.S. (1994): Identification and characterization of capsaicin-hydrolyzing enzymes purified from rat liver microsomes. Biochem. Mol. International 34:351-360.

[179] Pique, J.M., Esplugues, J.V., Whittle, B.J.R. (1990): Influence of morphine or capsaicin pretreatment on rat gastric microcirculatory response to PAF. Am. J. Physiol. 258: G352-357.

[180] Rauf, M., Bachmann, E., Metwally, S.A. (1985): J. Drug. Res. Egypt 16:29-36.

[181] Raybould, H.E., Taché, Y. (1989): Capsaicin-sensitive vagal afferent fibres and stimulation of gastric acid secretion in anesthetized rats. Eur. J. Pharmacol. 167: 237-243.

[182] Reilly, C.A., Crouch, D.J., Yost, G.S., Fatah, A.A. (2002): Determination of capsaicin, noivamide and dihydrocapsaicin in blood and tissue by liquid chromatography-tandem mass spectrometry. J. Anal. Toxicol. 26: 313-319.

[183] Reinshage, M., Pate, A., Sottili, M., Nast, C., Davis, W., Muellr, K., Eysselein, V.E. (1994): Protective functions of extrinsic sensory neurons in acute rabbit experimental colitis. Gastroenterology 106: 1208-1214.

[184] Richeux, F., Cascante, M., Ennamary, F., Sabourcau, D., Creppy, E.E. (1999): Cytotoxicity and genotoxicity of capsaicin in human neuroblastoma cells SHSY-5Y. Arch. Toxicol. 73:403-409.

[185] Ritchie, W.P. Jr. (1991): Mediators of bile acid induced alterations in gastric mucosal blood flow. Am. J. Surg. 161: 126-129.

[186] Robert, A., Olafsson, A.S., Lancaster, C., Zhang, W. (1991): Effects of capsaicin and of capsaicin denervation on gastric secretion and gastric lesions produced by ulcerogenic agents. Exp. Clin. Gastroenterol. 1: 5 (abst.).

[187] Rozin, P. (1990): Getting to like the burn of chili pepper. Biological, physiological, and cultural perspective. In: Green, B.G., Manson, J.R., Kare, M.R. (eds.): Chemical Senses. Irritation. Vol 2. Marcel Dekker, New York, pp.: 231-269.

[188] Saito, A., Yamamoto, M. (1996): Acute oral toxicity of capsaicin in mice and rats. J. Toxicol. Sci. 21: 195-200.

[189] Sarlós, P., Rumi, Gy., Szolcsányi, J., Mózsik, Gy., Vincze, Á. (2003): Capsaicin prevents the indomethacin-induced gastric mucosal damage n human healthy subject. Gastroenterology 124, Suppl. 1, A-511.

[190] Savitha, G., Panchanathan, S, Salimath, B.P. (1990): Capsaicin inhibits calmodulin-mediated oxidative burst in rat macrophages. Cell Signal. 2: 577-585.

[191] Schneider, M.A., de Luca, V., Gray, S.J. (1956): The effect of spice ingestion upon the stomach. Am. J. Gastroenterlol. 26: 722-732.

[192] Schweiggert, U., Schieber A., Carle R. (2006): Effects of blanching and storage on capsaicinoid stability and peroxidase activity of hot chili peppers. Innovative Food Science and Emerging Technologies.

[193] Solanke, T.F. (1973): The effect of red pepper (Capsicum frutescens) on gastric acid secretion. J. Surg. Res. 15: 385-390.

[194] Starlinger, M., Schiessel, R., Hung, C.R. (1981a): H+ back-diffusion stimulating mucosal blood flow in the rabbit fundus. Surgery 89: 232-236.

[195] Surh, Y.J., Ahn, S.H., Kim, K.C., Park, J.B., Sohn, Y.W., Lee, S.S. (1995): Metabolism of capsaicinoids: evidence for aliphatic hydroxylation and its pharmacological implications. Life Sci. 56, pp 305-311.

[196] Surh, Y.J., Lee, S.S (1995): Capsaicin a double-edged swort: toxicity, metabolism, and chemopreventive potential. Life Sci. 56:1845-1855.

[197] Szállasi, A., Blumberg, M. (1999): Vanilloid (capsaicin) receptors and mechanisms. Pharmacol. Rev. 51, 159-211.

[198] Szabo, IL., Czimmer, J., Szolcsányi, J., Mozsik, Gy. (2013): Molecular pharmacological approaches to effects of capsaicinoids and of classical antisecretory drugs on gastric basal acid secretion and on indomethecin-induced gastric mucosal damage in human healthy subjects (Mini review) Curr. Pharm. Des. 19: 84-89.

[199] Szolcsányi, J., (1977): A pharmacological approach to elucidation of the role of different nerve fibres and receptor endings in mediation of pain. J. Physiology (Paris) 73: 251-259.

[200] Szolcsányi, J., Barthó, L. (1981): Impaired defense mechanisms to peptic ulcer in the capsaicin-desensitized rat. In: Mózsik, Gy., Hänninen, O., Jávor, T. (eds.): Advances in Physiological Sciences. Vol. 29. Gastrointestinal Defense Mechanisms. Pergamon Press and Akadémiai Kiadó, Oxford and Budapest, pp.: 39-51.

[201] Szolcsányi, J., (1982): Capsaicin type pungent agents producing pyrexia. In: Milton, A.S. (ed.): Handbook of Experimental Pharmacology. Vol. 60. Pyretics and Antipyretics. Springer-Verlag, Berlin pp.: 437-478.

[202] Szolcsányi, J., (1984): Capsaicin-sensitive chemoceptive neural system with dual sensory-efferent function. In: Chahl, L.A., Szolcsányi, J., Lembech F. (eds.): Antidromic Vasodilatation and Neurogenic Inflammation. Akadémiai Kiadó, Budapest, pp.: 27-56

[203] Szolcsányi, J., (1985): Sensory receptors and the antinociceptive effect of capsaicin. In: Hakanson, R., Sundler, F. (eds.): Tachykinin Antagonists. Elsevier, Amsterdam, 45-54

[204] Szolcsányi, J. (1990a): Capsaicin, irritation, and desenzitation: Neurophysiological and future perspectives. In: Vo. 2. Green, B.G., Mason, J.R., Kare, M.R. (eds.): Chemical Senses. Irritation. Marcel Dekker, New York, pp.: 141-169.

[205] Szolcsányi, J. (1990b): Effect of capsaicin, rediniferatoxin and piperine on ethanol-induced gastric ulcer of the rat. Acta Physiol. Hung. 75: 267-268

[206] Szolcsányi, J. (1993): Actions of capsaicin on sensory receptors. In: Wood, J.N. (ed.): Capsaicin in the Study of Pain. Academic Press, London, pp.: 1-33.

[207] Szolcsányi, J., Pórszász, R., Pethő, G., (1994): Capsaicin and pharmacology of nociceptors. In: Besson, J.M., Besson, G., Ollat, H. (eds.): Peripheral Neurons in Nociception. Physicopharmacological Aspects, Paris, John Libby Eurotext. pp.: 109-124.

[208] Szolcsányi, J., (1996): Capsaicin-sensitive sensory nerve terminals with local and systemic efferent functions: facts and scopes of unorthodox neuroregulatory mechanisms. In: Kumazawa, T., Kumazawa, L., Mizumura, K. (eds.): The Polymodal Receptor – A Gateway to Pathological Pain. Progress in Brain Research. Vo.113. Elsevier, Amsterdam, pp.: 343-359.

[209] Szolcsányi, J. (1997): A pharmacological approach to elucidation of the role of different nerve fibres and receptor endings inmediation of pain. J. Phisiol. Paris 73, 251-259.

[210] Szolcsányi, J. (2004): Forty years in capsaicin research for sensory pharmacology and physiology. Neuropeptide 38, 377-384.

[211] Tominata, M., Caterina, M.J., Malmberg, A.B., Rosen, T.A., Gilbet, H., Skinner, K., Raumann, B.E., Basbaum, A.I., Julius, D. (1998): The cloned capsaicin receptor integrates multiple pain-producing stimuli. Neuron 21:531-543.

[212] Taurog, A., Dorris, M., Doerge, D.R. (1994): Evidence for a radical mechanism in peroxidase-catalyzed coupling. I. Steady-state experiments with various peroxidases. Arch Biochem Biophys 315:82-87.

[213] Takeuchi, K. (2006): Unique profile of lafutidine: a novel histamine H2-receptor antagonist: mucosal protection thronghout GI mucosal mediated by capsaicin-sensitive afferent nerves, Acta Pharmacol. Sinica Suppl. 27-35

[214] Takeuchi, K., Ohuchi, T., Okabe, S. (1994): Capsaicin-sensitive sensory neurons in healing of gastric lesions induced by HCl in rats. Dig. Dis. Sci. 39: 2543-2546

[215] Tanne, H.J. (2006a): NEJM stands by its criticism of Vioxx. Brit. Med. J. 332:505.

[216] Tanne, H.J. (2006b): NEJM editor gives pretrial evidence in Vioxx case. Brit. Med. J. 332: 255.

[217] Tanne, H.J. (2006c): Court awards claim 13.3 M dollars in rofecoxib lawsuit. Brit. Med. J. 332:927.

[218] Todd, P.A., Clissold, S.P. (1990): Naproxen. A reappraisal of its pharmacology, and therapeutic use in rheumatic disease and pain states. Drugs 40: 91-137.

[219] Tramontana, M., Renzi, D., Calabro, A., Panerai, C., Milani, S., Surrenti, C., Evangelista, S. (1994): Influence of capsaicin-sensitive afferent fibres on acetic acid-induced chronic gastric ulcers in rats. Scand. J. Gastroenterol. 29: 406-413

[220] Vaishnava, P., Wang, D.H. (2003): Capsaicin sensitive-sensory nerves and blood pressure regulation. Curr.Med. Chem. Cardiovasc. Hematol. Agents. 1: 177-188.

[221] Varga, L. (1936): Action of various stimulants on gastric chemistry (in Hungarian). Orv. Hetil. Hung. Med. Weekly J. 80: 702-704.

[222] Viranuvatti, V., Kalayasiri, C., Chearani, O. (1972): Effect of capsicum solution on human gastric mucosa as observed gastroscopically. Am. J. Gastroenterol. 58: 225-232.

[223] Walpole, C.S, Wrigglesworth, R., Bevan, S., et al. (1993b): Analogs of capsaicin with agonist activity as novel analgesic agents; structure-activity studies 1. The aromatic "A-region". J. Med. Chem. 36, 2362-2372.

[224] Walpole, C.S, Wrigglesworth, R., Bevan, S., et al. (1993a): Analogs of capsaicin with agonist activity as novel analgesic agents; structure-activity studies 2. The amide bond "B-region". J. Med. Chem. 36, 2373-2380.

[225] Walpole, CS, Wrigglesworth, R., Bevan, S., et al. (1993b): Analogs of capsaicin with agonist activity as novel analgesic agents; structure-activity studies 3. The hydrophobic side chain "C-region". J. Med. Chem. 36, 2381-2389)

[226] Winter, J., (1987): Characterization of capsaicin sensitive neurons in adult rat dorsal root ganglion culture. Neurosci. Lett. 80: 134-140

[227] Wehmeyer, Y., Kasting, G.B., Powell, J.H., Kuhlenbeck, D.L., Underwood, R.A., Bowman, L.A. (1990): Applications of liquid chromatography with on-line radiochemical detection to metabolism studies on a novel class of analgesic. J. Pharm. Biomed. Anal. 8:177-183.

[228] Whittle, B.J.R. (1977): Mechanisms underlying gastric mucosal damage induced by indomethacin and bile salts, and the action of prostaglandins. Br. J. Pharmacol. 60: 455-460.

[229] Whittle, B.J.R., Lopez-Belmonte, J. (1991): Interactions between the vascular peptide endothelin-1 and sensory neuropeptides on gastric mucosal injury. Br. J. Pharmacol. 102: 950-954.

[230] Wood, J.N, Winter, J., James, I.F., Rang, H. Ph., Yeats, J., Bevan, S. (1988): Capsaicin induced ion fluxes in dorsal root ganglion neurons in culture. J. Neurosci. 8: 3208-3220

[231] Yagi T (1990): Inhibition by capsaicin of NADH-quinone oxidoreductases is correlated with the presence of energy-coupling site 1 in various organisms. Arch. Biochem. Biophys. 281:305-311.